Childhood and Adolescent Diabetes

Other Titles in the Wiley Practical Diabetes Series

Diabetes in Old Age
Paul Finucane and Alan J. Sinclair (Editors)

Prediction, Prevention and Genetic Counseling in IDDM
Jerry P. Palmer (Editor)

Diabetes and Pregnancy: An International Approach to Diagnosis
and Management
Anne Dornhorst and David R. Hadden (Editors)

Diabetic Complications
Ken M. Shaw (Editor)

Forthcoming Titles

Towards Prediction and Prevention of NIDDM
Graham Hitman (Editor)

Diabetes and Hypoglycaemia
Brian M. Frier and B. Miles Fisher (Editors)

Childhood and Adolescent Diabetes

Edited by
SIMON COURT and BILL LAMB

JOHN WILEY & SONS
Chichester • New York • Weinheim • Brisbane • Singapore • Toronto

Other Wiley Editorial Offices

John Wiley & Sons, Inc., 605 Third Avenue,
New York, NY 10158-0012, USA

WILEY-VCH Verlag GmbH, Pappelallee 3,
D-69469 Weinheim, Germany

Jacaranda Wiley Ltd, 33 Park Road, Milton,
Queensland 4064, Australia

John Wiley & Son (Asia) Pte Ltd, 2 Clementi Loop #02-01,
Jin Xing Distripark, Singapore 129809

John Wiley & Sons (Canada) Ltd, 22 Worcester Road,
Rexdale, Ontario M9W 1L1, Canada

Library of Congress Cataloging-in-Publication Data

Childhood and adolescent diabetes / edited by Simon Court and Bill
  Lamb.
      p. cm. — (Practical diabetes series)
    Includes bibliographical references and index.
    ISBN 0–471–97003–4 (cased) : alk. paper)
    1. Diabetes in children. I. Court, Simon, Dr. II. Lamb, Bill,
  MD. III. Series: Practical diabetes (Chichester, England)
    [DNLM: 1. Diabetes Mellitus, Insulin-Dependent—in infancy &
  childhood. 2. Diabetes Mellitus, Insulin-Dependent—in adolescence.
  WK 810 C5351   1997]
  RJ420.D5C47   1997
  618.92´462,dc21
  DNLM/DLC
  for Library of Congress   97–3042
                                                             CIP

British Library Cataloguing in Publication Data

A catalogue record for this book is available from the British Library

ISBN 0–471–97003–4

Typeset in 10/12pt Palatino from the authors' disks by Dobbie Typesetting Ltd, Tavistock, Devon
Printed and bound in Great Britain by Biddles Ltd, Guildford and King's Lynn
This book is printed on acid-free paper responsibly manufactured from sustainable forestation, for which at least two trees are planted for each one used for paper production.

This book is dedicated to Professor Michael Parkin, whose humility and caring approach have influenced us all.

Contents

Contributors

J. Cane   *Paediatric Diabetes Specialist Nurse, Department of Child Health, Royal Victoria Infirmary, Newcastle upon Tyne NE1 4LP, UK*

Dr Simon Court   *Consultant Paediatrician, Community Division, Central Locality, Arthur's Hill Clinic, Douglas Terrace, Newcastle upon Tyne NE4 6BT, UK*

Dr Julie A. Edge   *Department of Paediatrics, John Radcliffe Hospital, Headington, Oxford OX3 9DU, UK*

A. English   *Consultant Clinical Psychologist, Child and Family Psychology Service, Huddersfield NHS Trust, Huddersfield Royal Infirmary, Acre Street, Lindley, Huddersfield, UK*

Dr Steve Greene   *Consultant Paediatrician, Department of Child Health, Ninewells Hospital & Medical School, Dundee DD1 9SY, UK*

Dr Ian Jefferson   *Consultant Paediatrician, Hull Royal Infirmary, Anlaby Road, Hull HU3 2JZ, UK*

Dr M. S. Kibirige   *Consultant Paediatrician, South Cleveland Hospital, Marton Road, Middlesborough TS4 3BW, UK*

Dr W. H. Lamb   *Consultant Paediatrician, Bishop Auckland General Hospital, County Durham DL14 6AD, UK*

Dr Geoff Lawson   *Consultant Paediatrician, Sunderland District General Hospital, Kayll Road, Sunderland SR4 7TP, UK*

Dr Debbie S. F. Matthews   *First Assistant in Child Health, Sir James Spence Institute of Child Health, Royal Victoria Infirmary, Newcastle upon Tyne NE1 4LP, UK*

Dr K. Matyka   *Research Fellow, Department of Paediatrics, John Radcliffe Hospital, Headington, Oxford OX3 9DU, UK*

Dr Caroline McCowen   *Consultant Paediatrician, North Tees General Hospital, Stockton, Cleveland TS19 8PE, UK*

Mrs Hilary Richardson   *Diabetes Specialist Nurse, Royal Victoria Infirmary, Newcastle upon Tyne NE1 4LP, UK*

Dr Ken Robertson *Consultant Paediatrician, Royal Hospital for Sick Children, Yorkhill, Glasgow G3 8SJ, UK*

Dr Mike Sills *Consultant Paediatrican, Huddersfield Royal Infirmary, Acre Street, Lindley, Huddersfield, UK*

Dr Peter J. Small *Consultant Paediatrician, Royal Aberdeen Children's Hospital, Cornhill Road, Aberdeen AB9 2ZG, UK*

C. J. Thompson *Adult Physician, Department of Child Health, Ninewells Hospital & Medical School, Dundee DD1 9SY, UK*

Dr J. Wales *Senior Lecturer in Paediatric Endocrinology, University Department of Paediatrics, Sheffield Children's Hospital, Western Bank, Sheffield S10 2TH, UK*

Mrs Shirley Watson *Senior Dietitian, Royal Victoria Infirmary, Newcastle upon Tyne NE1 4LP, UK*

Preface

Diabetes is presenting in childhood at a younger age and with increasing frequency. Although many of the principles of management apply across all ages, the problems and concerns identified by families of infants with diabetes, those with children in middle childhood and those with adolescents clearly differ. The child moves towards independence as parents relinquish the reins. This process has been likened to a game of chess where parents are actively but imperceptibly losing as their children win.

Health professionals are 'co-conspirators' and this book is aimed at providing practical guidance. Each chapter in large measure stands alone and has been written by individuals actively engaged in the care of diabetic children. They were specifically asked to present their own experience as well as the scientific literature in describing practical solutions. It seemed proper to provide an opportunity for children and parents to comment on their experiences — this proved amusing, salutory and at times sad.

The aim of the book is to share practical solutions to the everyday problems that confront children with diabetes and their carers. We would particularly like to thank those parents and children brave enough to share their feelings, but would extend this to all those who have contributed to this venture.

1

Aetiology, Epidemiology, Immunology, Environmental Factors, Genetics and Prevention

W. H. LAMB

AETIOLOGY

The majority of children with diabetes mellitus have Type I or insulin dependent diabetes mellitus (IDDM). However, there are other clinical conditions associated with an increased incidence of diabetes mellitus. Some of those associated with the onset of diabetes in childhood are listed in Table 1.1. Type I IDDM is probably neither a homogeneous condition nor due to a single disease process, but definite causes have still to be established. It is generally accepted that the majority of children develop IDDM as a result of genetic susceptibility combined with various environmental factors. This leads to the development of auto-immune disease directed at the insulin-producing β cells of the pancreatic islets of Langerhans. The cells are progressively destroyed, resulting in impaired glucose tolerance then increasing hyperglycaemia and ketosis. The process continues until all the β cells are destroyed, with total dependence on exogenous insulin. Figure 1.1 gives a schematic description of this process.

Childhood and Adolescent Diabetes. Edited by S. Court and B. Lamb.
© 1997 John Wiley & Sons, Ltd.

Table 1.1. Associations of other conditions with juvenile diabetes mellitus

Principal diagnosis	Type of diabetes
Cystic fybrosis	IDDM
Congenital absence or hypoplasia of pancreas	IDDM
Thalassaemia	NIDDM
MODY (maturity onset diabetes of the young)	NIDDM
Prader–Willi syndrome	NIDDM
DIDMOAD syndrome (diabetes mellitus–optic atrophy–diabetes insipidus–deafness)	IDDM
Congenital rubella syndrome	IDDM
Down's syndrome	IDDM
Turner's syndrome	IDDM
Kleinfelter's syndrome	IDDM

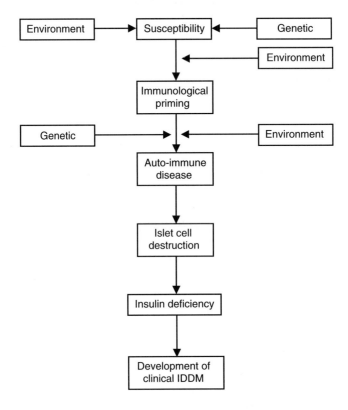

Figure 1.1. A mechanism for the aetiology of auto-immune IDDM

EPIDEMIOLOGY

INCIDENCE

Discovering the real incidence or prevalence of diabetes in a population is difficult. Few countries keep national registers, and it is important that the same methods and definitions are used to allow comparison of results. The WHO Multinational Project for Childhood Diabetes (WHO DIAMOND) with over 70 participating countries and the European based EURODIAB ACE reporting across 24 regions of Europe are two important international studies producing comparative information. Most of the more recent studies use an epidemiological method known as 'capture–recapture', i.e. the use of at least two independent data sources, thus allowing data validation and a better estimate of the true number of cases. The more sources of data used, the more accurate are the results.

The epidemiological information now available is fascinating even if the findings are not very consistent. The reported incidence of IDDM in children varies from 0.7/100 000 in China to 42.9 in Finland. In Europe there is a suggestion of a North–South gradient, with the highest incidence in Scandinavia and the lowest in Northern Greece, but this is not simply on geographical lines. There are surprises in that the Mediterranean island of Sardinia has the second highest incidence after Finland, and northern countries like Poland have low rates. Wide variations between genetically similar populations like Iceland and Norway or adjacent countries with differing lifestyles such as Estonia and Finland strongly support environmental factors including lifestyle as being important agents in the aetiology of IDDM. The variation within a nation can also be striking. A study of incidence in Great Britain for 1988 gave results ranging from a minimum rate of 6/100 000 in Southern England to 19.8 in Scotland. Another commonly reported finding is of a higher incidence in urban over rural populations, particularly where there is a low incidence generally. Table 1.2 gives information on incidence rates for a variety of countries and regions world-wide.

SECULAR TRENDS

There is evidence for a rising incidence of IDDM, particularly in the more developed nations where a doubling of incidence over 20 years has been described. Some countries have seen what amount to epidemics over one or more years followed by a subsequent return to lower incidence rates. This pattern is suggestive of an infective process, and geographical and spatial clustering of cases of IDDM has been reported.

Table 1.2. Some variations in the incidence of IDDM around the world (ranked by incidence rates)

Country	Region	Age range (years)	Rate/ 100 000	Year of study	Sex ratio	Rising incidence	Year published
Finland	All	0–14	42.9	1990	M>F	Yes	1992
Italy	Sardinia	0–14	34.4	1989–92	F>M	Yes	1995
USA	Pittsburgh	0–19	17.1	1985–9	M>F	Yes	1993
Kuwait	All	0–14	15.4	1992–3	M>F	Yes	1995
Australia	New South Wales	0–14	14.5	1985–9	F>M	No	1992
UK	All	0–14	13.5	1988	M>F	Yes	1991
New Zealand	Canterbury	0–19	12.7	1982–90		No	1992
Netherlands	All	0–14	12.4	1988–90		Yes	1995
France	Four regions	0–14	7.8	1990	M=F		1992
Greece	All	0–14	6.2	1992	F>M		1995
Argentina	Avellaneda	0–14	5.3–7.6	1985–90	M=F	No	1994
Barbados	All	0–14	5	1982–91	M>F	No	1994
Hong Kong	All	0–14	2	1990			1993
Japan	All	0–14	2	1985–9	M=F		1993
China	Shanghai	0–14	0.61	1980–91			1994

SEASONAL FACTORS

There is often a suggestion of seasonal variations in incidence, commonly during the winter months and at times of maximal viral respiratory tract infection. This again is more typical in countries with a high incidence. The variation is most marked in older children, particularly males.

AGE

Onset in infancy is unusual, but incidence steadily increases after the first year to a peak during early adolescence. Some countries have seen a rising incidence in the under-fives, giving a bi-modal distribution, and in the UK for example children diagnosed under the age of five will form over 40% of the childhood diabetes clinic population. It has been suggested that some of the apparent increase of incidence observed is because diabetes is developing earlier, although the total pool of susceptibles remains the same. This alone could not account for all the observed variations. Children diagnosed at a young age appear to have certain epidemiological features that suggest they may form a sub-group with a different aetiology. First, there is an absence of seasonal variation, with no mid-summer trough in the number of cases diagnosed. Secondly, there appears to be an increased incidence of positive family history of Type I diabetes in children developing the disease under two years of age (14.3% versus 4.8%), with fathers being the main contributors to this increase. This suggests that inherited susceptibility may play a more important role in this age group than environmental factors. Some studies have suggested a preponderance of boys diagnosed in this age group, compared with a slight preponderance of girls in the five- to 10-year group. A small group of young children have been identified where the diabetes is associated with other conditions, namely sensory neural deafness and dyserythropoeitic anaemia; this group is likely to be due to an autosomal recessively inherited condition (Barrett, unpublished results).

SEX DIFFERENCES

There seems to be a relationship between gender and the overall incidence of IDDM. Males in those countries with a higher incidence, such as Finland, USA, the Netherlands and the UK, tend to be at greater risk, whilst females seem to be at greater risk where the overall incidence is low. The risk also seems to be age-related, with higher rates reported in older males. There are several reports suggesting stable incidence rates for females but marked variations of seasonal or year-to-year incidence in males. There is no obvious reason why this should be, but some observers have speculated a role for male hormones, particularly as the fluctuations mainly occur in the older age groups.

RACIAL VARIATIONS

How much of the racial variation described is due to genetic difference and how much to different environments is difficult to clarify, and there is no consistency in reported findings. Caucasian populations in the USA have higher reported incidence rates than non-white groups, whereas in the UK some immigrant populations have acquired the same incidence rates as the indigents. In general, immigrant populations seem to acquire the incidence rates of the indigenous population over subsequent generations.

ENVIRONMENTAL FACTORS

The wide variation of incidence offers many possibilities for identifying environmental factors related to the development of IDDM. Viral infections and dietary factors are the two favourite candidates.

Viral Infections

There is both direct and indirect evidence of viral infections being a factor in the development of IDDM. Rubella, mumps, cytomegalovirus (CMV) and Coxsackie B viruses have been most often implicated. Epidemics of these viruses are often followed by an increased incidence of IDDM and many cases (15–40%) of congenital rubella develop IDDM. It is possible that in some instances a direct toxic effect of the infection is responsible, while in others the infections serve to either initiate or accelerate the auto-immune islet cell destruction, as in congenital rubella. The irony is, however, that the better the overall health of the childhood population the higher the incidence of IDDM seems to be. This could be due to improved diet, but the intriguing possibility exists that a high incidence of infectious disease could actually protect against IDDM possibly because of improved maternal immunity preventing congenital infections.

Dietary Factors

Birth weight could be considered to be an indirect dietary factor, and in contrast to the common finding that non-insulin dependent diabetes is associated with low birth weight, the risk of IDDM seems to be higher in the heavier babies. Breast feeding appears to provide protection in proportion to its duration. This may be due to a direct effect or simply to a delay in the introduction of cow's milk into the diet. A linear relationship between the per capita milk consumption and incidence of IDDM has been demonstrated. While Sardinia has a low cow's milk consumption compared with

Northern Europe, it is said to be much higher than in the rest of Italy. A mechanism for the relationship of IDDM to cow's milk has been suggested. One of the milk whey proteins, bovine serum albumin, shares antigenic similarities to a β islet cell antigen known as p69. The antigenic portions of this protein can pass unaltered across the infant gut and so stimulate an immune response. This may act as a trigger or adjunct to the auto-immune process. A direct relationship between per capita coffee consumption and IDDM incidence has also been suggested. This could be due to either a toxic effect of the coffee itself or of other foods taken with coffee, such as sucrose. Conversely the vitamin nicotinamide has been credited with having a protective effect. Other workers have linked total carbohydrate consumption, protein content of diet and other dietary components with risks of developing IDDM but there is still no proven link between diet and the development of IDDM.

Chemical Agents

Several chemicals can cause damage to the islet cells, including streptozotocin and a rat poison (RH-787, 'Vacor') which has been reported to cause IDDM in accidental ingestion. Nitrosamines are a group of chemicals found in water supplies and foodstuffs, particularly smoked foods. They have been shown to cause IDDM in animal models but no definite link between nitrosamine intake and IDDM in humans has been proven to date.

GENETICS

Most children with IDDM have no affected relatives at diagnosis, but information from the many population, family and twin studies reported from the 1930s onwards strongly points to genetic factors being important for the development of IDDM. For example, where one of monozygotic twins develops IDDM the lifetime risk to their twin also developing IDDM may eventually be more than 60%, although only 40% or less do so within 10 years. The overall risk for dizygotic twins who share the same environment is only 8%. More recently studies using multiplex families (two or more affected first-degree relatives within a family) offer the prospect of more accurate delineation of the genetic markers. While no proof exists, it seems most likely that susceptibility is linked to the major histocompatibility complex (MHC) on the short arm of chromosome 6 (Figure 1.2). This area codes for three classes of MHC molecules of which the Class I and Class II groups seem to be the most important in relation to risk of IDDM.

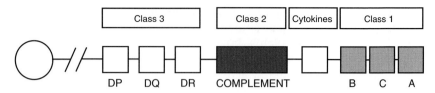

Figure 1.2. Cartoon of short arm of chromosome 6 showing MHC region

In particular the MHC molecules DR3 and DR4 have been the two most closely linked to IDDM susceptibility in Caucasian populations. While 50% of the Caucasian population have either DR3 or DR4 and very few develop IDDM, these two MHC types are found in 95% of Caucasian people with IDDM.

There are also MHC molecules that appear to offer protection against developing IDDM, in particular types DR2 and DR5. A more specific type DQB1.602 is so protective that no islet cell antibody (ICA)-positive first-degree relatives of patients with IDDM developed IDDM, whereas over a third of the individuals with similar MHC typing and antibodies but without the protective marker did.

Although inheritance of genes is usually predictable, some genes appear especially linked to others so that some gene combinations occur more or less frequently than expected. This is known as 'linkage disequilibrium'. DR3 and DR4 may not be specific markers for IDDM but linked instead to unidentified genes which may be more specific. Amongst the contenders is a gene in the DQ region of the MHC complex, coding for the β chain of the MHC DQ antigen. A mutation in this gene results in the substitution of aspartic acid at position 57 in the protein by another amino acid. In Caucasians, but not Asians, this seems strongly linked to Type I diabetes.

DIFFERENT FORMS OF IDDM

IDDM is probably not a homogeneous condition and it has been suggested that three main forms exist: an auto-immune form linked to DR3, an 'anti-insulin' form linked to DR4 and a mixed form combining DR3 and DR4. This would help to explain why some children with IDDM are at a greater risk of developing other auto-immune endocrine diseases. Those with MHC DR3 tend to have persistence of circulating ICA, low levels of insulin antibodies and a longer 'honeymoon' period of residual islet cell preservation and insulin secretion. DR3 status is also linked to auto-immune thyroiditis, Addison's disease, vitiligo and coeliac disease.

The MHC DR4 carriers seem to have a younger age of onset, high levels of insulin antibodies, transient ICA levels and a shorter honeymoon period. For those who carry both DR3 and DR4 the characteristics are combined.

RISK

Overall the risks of developing IDDM are low at 1/500. Having one affected parent or first-degree relative increases the risk to 1/14 but it is still low. It is possible to quantify the risk more precisely if MHC typing of the cases and their relatives is performed but as no easy, reliable and safe method of preventing IDDM exists, MHC typing is largely confined to research. Tables

Table 1.3. Risk of developing Type I IDDM in Caucasian populations

Identifiers	Risk
Overall population	1/500
Low-risk MHC	1/5000
One high-risk MHC (DR3 or DR4)	1/400
Two high-risk MHC	
DR3+DR3 or DR4+DR4	1/150
DR3+DR4	1/40

Table 1.4. Risk of developing IDDM in sibling of patient with IDDM

Identifier	Odds	Percentage risk
Overall risk	1/14	8
No MHC shared	1/100	1
DR3 or DR4 shared	1/20	5
DR3+DR3 or DR4+DR4	1/6	16
DR3+DR4	1/4 to 1/5	20–25
Monozygotic twin	1/3 to 2/3	30–60

Table 1.5. Risk of developing IDDM in children of a parent with IDDM

Identifier	Odds	Percentage risk
Overall risk	1/25	4
Risk if mother has IDDM	1/40 to 1/50	2–3
Risk if father has IDDM	1/20	5–6
Risk if both parents have IDDM	1/3–4	30

1.3, 1.4 and 1.5 give the risks for the general population, for siblings, and for children of parents with IDDM. The risk to children whose father has IDDM is double that if the mother has IDDM. There are several possible mechanisms for this. One is by linkage disequilibrium with increased transmission of the high-risk MHC genes from the father. Another is *in utero* protection granted by the altered immune status of the fetus. It has also been shown that stimulation of the β islet cells in animal models may be protective. With the likelihood of higher blood glucose levels in a pregnant mother with IDDM the fetal islet cells would be more stimulated than normal. The risk is even lower for children of older mothers.

The most important message to give to worried families is that the overall risk of another affected child is low.

IMMUNOLOGY AND PATHOGENESIS

All human cells express antigens on their surface but these are normally recognised as 'self' and not attacked by the immune system. Auto-immune disease results when the usual safeguards fail so that own tissues are mistaken as foreign and attacked by any of the cell-mediated or antibody-mediated immune responses. The MHC Class I and Class II molecules are needed for the recognition of foreign antigens by the immune system and this almost certainly explains their importance for genetic susceptibility.

Cytotoxic T cells are activated by being presented with antigen and a MHC class I molecule. Class I molecules are normally found on the β islet cell but it has been suggested that a trigger (viral, environmental, etc.) causes hyper-expression of the Class I molecule which leads to activation of the T cells and islet cell destruction. A more generalised immune process is initiated by T helper cells. These are activated by presentation of antigen with MHC Class II molecules and in turn activate antibody-producing B lymphocytes as well as other T cells and result in a cascade of immune activity. Normal islet cells do not express the Class II molecule but have been shown to do so in cases of IDDM. Again it is suggested that a combination of an environmental trigger together with genetic susceptibility results in Class II expression on the islet cell and initiation of auto-immune destruction.

Several antigens have been identified in association with IDDM. Islet cell cytoplasmic antibody was one of the earliest recognised and most studied, and is present in most newly diagnosed cases of IDDM. Islet cell surface antibody (ICSA) is also common at presentation. Insulin itself acts as an antigen and anti-insulin antibodies (AIA) are seen in a proportion of newly diagnosed cases. A more recently discovered antigen was known as the 64KD antigen but is now identified as glutamic acid decarboxylase (GAD).

Antibodies to GAD appear to persist for many years after diagnosis. It has been suggested that antibodies against GAD and insulin are more particularly found in individuals heterozygous for MHC DR4.

The various antibody markers have been used to try to identify family members at risk of developing IDDM. Their value and clinical use will obviously increase with the development of effective prophylaxis.

PREDICTION AND PREVENTION

Before the introduction of any programme to prevent disease certain conditions need to be met. First, there must be a reliable and specific means of identifying those at risk. Secondly, a safe and effective method is needed to prevent the disease developing in those subjects. Sadly neither of these conditions has been met for the prevention of IDDM, although much progress has been made in the past few years. A third condition is that the total cost of screening and prevention is less than that of supporting the disease itself in those who would otherwise succumb. The lifetime cost of treating childhood onset diabetes alone, even without the enormous costs of treating the major complications of visual impairment and renal failure, suggests that effective prevention of IDDM is worth trying for.

PREDICTION

Known risk factors have been discussed earlier. A genetic risk can be suggested at present through possession of specific MHC markers but is relatively non-specific as only a very small proportion of individuals with the high-risk MHC DR3/DR4 will develop IDDM. That proportion is increased in family members, particularly siblings of a child with IDDM, but is still not 100% predictive even with identical twins. Whilst full MHC typing of individuals would be prohibitively expensive as a screening method, the cost of using specific probes for the high-risk MHC molecules is much lower. Such probes are being used in research and may allow for effective whole population screening.

The several markers of auto-immune disease such as ICA, AIA and GAD alone have a low predictive value of IDDM and it has been suggested that only 2–3% of ICA-positive children would progress to IDDM within five years. The predictive power is improved if the antibody titre is measured, with greater risk at higher antibody titres. Other studies have looked at the development of islet cell antibodies in the children of parents with IDDM. Key findings are that the offspring of fathers have double the incidence of the various islet cell or insulin antibodies, and that antibodies appear very early and may be present in those at greatest risk before the age of six years.

Combining genetic markers and ICA is more predictive. Up to 70% of children with both high-risk genetic markers and positive ICA may develop IDDM. However, only 10% of children with IDDM have a positive family history, so any screening programme based on a positive family history, even if 100% predictive, would fail to identify 90% of the potential cases. Studies in Finland have used both MHC markers and islet cell antibodies to identify high-risk groups. Refinement of these techniques may allow for both high-risk and whole population screening.

Normally when glucose is given intravenously the β cell responds by secreting insulin in a bi-phasic manner. Insulin levels rise rapidly in the first 1–3 min followed by a return to baseline levels within 10 min. This is known as the first-phase insulin response. The second phase starts after 2 min with a gradual rise in insulin levels that persists for as long as glucose is infused. One of the first signs of islet cell damage is the abolition of the first-phase response, and this can be used to distinguish between healthy ICA-positive subjects and those who are pre-diabetic, long before significant islet cell damage has occurred.

In summary, a combination of genetic markers, auto-antibody markers and early clinical markers of islet cell destruction can be used confidently to predict those at highest risk of developing IDDM. It is not yet possible to contemplate whole population screening but screening of high-risk siblings is a practical option.

PREVENTION

The auto-immune attack against the islet cells is the likeliest cause of IDDM, and any measure to stop this happening could be considered primary prevention. Secondary prevention refers to the measures used to stop progression of the auto-immune process.

Primary Prevention

The inherited risk factors cannot be changed, so primary prevention would require elimination or modification of the trigger factors. As outlined earlier, these are most likely a combination of infectious agents, particularly viral, and other environmental factors such as diet.

Many viral agents have been associated with IDDM but none exclusively. Prevention strategy here means the identification of responsible viruses as well as the time when infection is most likely to lead to IDDM so that an appropriate vaccine and immunisation strategy can be developed. As antibodies against islet cells seem to appear very early in childhood, it may be that immunisation of the mother to prevent congenital infection may be needed. So far rubella is the only virus with a known association with IDDM where prenatal immunisation occurs. Immunisation of girls and young women against rubella prevents congenital infection and undoubtedly some cases of IDDM. Overall, however, better general immunisation coverage on its own does not seem to protect against IDDM.

Avoiding those factors with a known association with IDDM would seem to be the best currently available method of primary prevention. Of the suggested dietary factors, cow's milk is the one most associated with IDDM. Prolonged breast-feeding and the delayed introduction of cow's milk protein into the diet until at least nine months of age would seem sensible strategies, and could be applied to whole populations; indeed, prospective studies are currently under way. Other dietary measures could include the avoidance of smoked foods during pregnancy and possibly a reduction of coffee consumption.

Secondary Prevention

IDDM is an auto-immune disease and it seems logical to use immunosuppressives as a means to prevent further progression of the disease. The first attempts to do this used non-specific immunosuppressives such as corticosteroids and azathiaprine. These did seem to slow progression and extended the 'honeymoon' period after diagnosis. Unfortunately they did not prevent progression and the side-effects of general immunosuppresion were too great to consider this as acceptable therapy. More recently more specific immunotherapy using cyclosporin A has been attempted. It was found that if cyclosporin was given immediately after diagnosis then those children with a short duration of pre-diagnosis symptoms had extended honeymoon periods and some were able to stop insulin therapy completely. However, the protection lasted only as long as cyclosporin therapy continued and this drug is potentially very toxic. It is known to cause renal damage and is even toxic to islet cells but there are also concerns about the longer term risk of developing lymphoma. Well managed IDDM has the potential for a normal, complication-free life and there is currently no justification for using immunosuppressives to prevent progression of IDDM in childhood. Newer drugs are being developed and may prove more acceptable.

Two other therapies with much less potential for toxicity have been tried with some degree of success. Experiments with naturally diabetic strains of mice (NOD mice, non-obese diabetic) and rats (BB rats, Bio Breeding Laboratory) have shown that the water-soluble vitamin nicotinamide and insulin itself given either orally or parenterally have a protective effect on the development of IDDM.

Nicotinamide is thought to work through several mechanisms, including a direct immunosuppressive effect. The results of human trials have been variable but there is a suggestion that, given in large (but non-toxic) doses at a very early stage in the development of IDDM, it may delay or even prevent the progress to clinical diabetes. Larger trials are in progress and this may prove to be a useful therapy to prevent IDDM in high-risk children with detectable islet cell antibodies.

Oral insulin appears protective in the animal model but the most successful human trial involved high-risk antibody-positive siblings given daily low-dose subcutaneous insulin. None of the treated subjects and most of the controls had developed IDDM at the time the trial was reported. Whilst it may seem paradoxical to prevent IDDM and insulin therapy by giving injections of insulin, these children did benefit by not having to suffer the same dietary manipulations, regular testing and risk of complications that a child with IDDM might otherwise expect.

Practical Considerations

What advice can we offer to the family with a child newly diagnosed with IDDM and other siblings? First, the overall statistical risk is low, but statistics are not very comforting if your child happens to be one of the unlucky 8–16%. The siblings themselves may be very anxious about developing diabetes.

For most clinics caring for diabetes in the UK, specific MHC probes are not available and full MHC typing is too expensive to contemplate as a routine investigation. Likewise only simple ICA auto-antibody detection is available outside research laboratories, offering very limited facilities for identification of those most at risk.

Despite the limitations outlined above some families may be insistent on some further action being taken. As islet cell antibodies appear to be present at a very early age in those children who go on to develop IDDM the following is a suggested practical programme that could be offered to those families who demand further action.

All siblings could be screened for ICA. Children over six years old and antibody-negative are possibly at minimal risk. Children aged less than six years and antibody-negative may need annual screening for antibodies until the age of six. If ICA-positive, full MHC typing can be offered. Those children with high-risk MHC and positive ICA are most likely to develop IDDM, and this could be further refined by looking for an abnormal first-phase insulin response.

If all three factors are present then one of two options can be offered. The first is to give oral nicotinamide in pharmacological doses. Protection cannot be guaranteed and the vitamin may have to be taken for life in high doses. The second is to offer a single daily dose of subcutaneous long-acting insulin at, say, 2–4 units daily. Again this cannot guarantee protection and may have to be given for life.

Since no guarantees can be offered each family will need help to consider the risks, costs and potential benefits before making a decision.

SELECTED REFERENCES AND FURTHER READING

Bingley, P. J., Bonifacio, E., Gale, E. A. M. Can we really predict IDDM? *Diabetes*, 1993: **42;** 213–20.

Foulis, A. K. Pancreatic morphology/islet cellular morphology. In *Childhood and Adolescent Diabetes*, (Kelnar, C. J. H., ed.), Chapman and Hall, London, 1995: 169–82.

Foulis, A. K., Hitman, G. A., Marshall, B., Bottazzo, G. F., Bonifaco, E. Pathogenesis of Insulin Dependent Diabetes Mellitus. In *Textbook of Diabetes*, (Pickup, J., Williams, G., eds), Blackwell Scientific Publications, Oxford, 1991: 107–50.

Green, A., Gale, E. A. M., Patterson, C. C., for the EURODIAB ACE Study Group. Incidence of childhood-onset insulin-dependent diabetes mellitus: the EURO-DIAB ACE study. *Lancet*, 1992; **339:** 905–9.

Hamman, R. F., Klingensmith, G., Eisenbarth, G. S., Erlich, H. A. Newborn screening for HLA markers associated with IDDM: Diabetes autoimmunity study in the young (DAISY). *Diabetologia*, 1996; **39:** 807–12.

Keller, R. J., Eisenbarth, G. S., Jackson, R. A. Insulin prophylaxis in individuals at high risk of type 1 diabetes. *Lancet*, 1993; **341:** 927–8.

Kelnar, C. J. H. (ed.). *Childhood and Adolescent Diabetes*, Chapman and Hall, London, 1995.

LaPorte, R. E., Tuommilehto, J., King, H. WHO multinational project for childhood diabetes. *Diabetes Care*, 1990; **13:** 1062–8. [article]

Mandrup-Poulsen, T., Nerup, J. Pathogenesis of childhood diabetes. In *Childhood and Adolescent Diabetes*, (Kelnar, C. J. H., ed.), Chapman and Hall, London, 1995: 183–9.

Metcalfe, M. A., Baum, J. D. Incidence of insulin dependent diabetes mellitus in children aged under 15 years in the British Isles during 1988. *British Medical Journal*, 1991; **302:** 443–7.

Pickup, J., Williams, G. (eds). *Textbook of Diabetes*, Blackwell Scientific Publications, Oxford, 1991.

Pugliese, A., Gianani, R., Morimisato, R., Awdeh, Z. L., Alper, C. A., Ehrlich, H. A., Jackson, R. A., Eisenbarth, G. S. HLA-DQB1*602 is associated with dominant protection from diabetes even amongst islet cell antibody positive first-degree relatives of patients with IDDM. *Diabetes*, 1995; **44:** 608–13.

Rewers, M., Bugawan, T. L., Norris, J. M., Blair, A., Hoffman, M., McDuffie, R. S., Jr., Elliot, R. B., Chase, H. P. Prevention or delay of Type 1 (insulin dependent) diabetes mellitus in children using nicotinamide. *Diabetologia*, 1991; **34:** 362–5.

Scott, R. S., Brown, L. J., Darlow, B. A., Forbes, L. V., Moore, M.P. Temporal variation in incidence of IDDM in Canterbury, New Zealand. *Diabetes Care*, 1992; **15:** 895–9.

Shield, J. P. H., Baum, J. D. (eds). *Clinical Paediatrics: Childhood Diabetes*, Volume 4, No. 4, WHO multinational project for childhood diabetes. Baillière Tindall, 1996.

Skyler, J. S., Marks, J. B. Immune intervention in type 1 diabetes mellitus. *Diabetes Review*, 1993; **1:** 15–42.

Vadheim, C. M., Rimoin, D. L., Rotter, J. I. Diabetes Mellitus. In *Principles and Practice of Medical Genetics*, (Emery, A. E. H., Rimoin, D. L., eds), 2nd Edition, Churchill-Livingstone, Edinburgh, 1990: 1521–58.

Verge, C. F., Howard, N. J., Irwig, L., Simpson, J., Mackerras, D., Silink, M. Environmental factors in childhood IDDM: a population based, case–control study. *Diabetes Care*, 1994; **17:** 1381–9.

WHO DIAMOND Project group. Childhood diabetes, epidemics, and epidemiology: an approach for controlling diabetes. *American Journal of Epidemiology*, 1992; **135:** 803–16.

Yip, P. S. F., Bruno, G., Tajima, N., Seber, G. A. F., Buckland, S. T., Cormack, R. M., Unwin, N. *et al.* Capture–recapture and multiple-record systems estimation II: Applications in human diseases. *American Journal of Epidemiology*, 1995; **142:** 1059–68.

2

The Diagnosis (Practical Issues)

G. R. LAWSON AND I. JEFFERSON

PATHOPHYSIOLOGY

To consider the diagnosis of diabetes in a child one must first understand the basic physiology and biochemistry of the normal non-diabetic state. After a meal the carbohydrate component of ingested food is absorbed from the intestinal tract after being broken down into simple sugars by enzymes. Glucose then enters the circulation and soon reaches the pancreas whose β cells rapidly release insulin. Insulin is a key anabolic hormone with effects on proteins, fats and carbohydrate. The main actions of insulin are summarised below.

1. *Directly reduces blood glucose:*
   - It allows glucose entry into cells, especially muscle and adipose tissue
   - It stimulates glycogenesis through the conversion of glucose into glycogen most notably in the liver (which does not require insulin to allow glucose into its cells).
2. *Inhibits release of stored glucose:*
   - It inhibits glycogenolysis by which glucose can be rapidly released into the circulation when needed
   - It inhibits catabolism of proteins and lipids by which gluconeogenesis would otherwise occur.

The lack of insulin in diabetes prevents glucose utilisation by muscle and adipose tissue as well as the storage of glucose as glycogen in the liver; as a consequence hyperglycaemia results.

Childhood and Adolescent Diabetes. Edited by S. Court and B. Lamb.
© 1997 John Wiley & Sons, Ltd.

In the development of the symptoms of diabetes (Table 2.1) a sustained elevation of blood glucose leads to an osmotic diuresis. The kidney is unable to reclaim the massive amount of glucose which is filtered out into the urine during this hyperglycaemic phase, and there is an obligatory loss of water with the glucose. This in turn leads to an excessive fluid loss (polyuria) which must be compensated for by an increased intake (polydipsia). If insufficient fluid is taken, or more critically if the child in addition starts to vomit, then dehydration will develop rapidly.

Insulin deficiency also leads to excessive fatty acid catabolism and the production of ketone bodies leading to ketonaemia and ketonuria. The breakdown of fats leads to the production of glycerol which is used for gluconeogenesis. At the same time the ketone bodies (3-hydroxy butyrate, acetoacetate and acetone) are produced which can act as an alternative metabolic fuel. This is the biochemical path upon which all slimmers depend; in the non-diabetic diet-restricted individual a consequence of low insulin production will be the breakdown of adipose tissue to provide energy. However, in the diabetic the insulin deficiency is sustained and the unrestrained biochemical process of fat catabolism that results inevitably leads to weight loss and the development of life-threatening diabetic ketoacidosis (DKA).

The clinical presentation of the later stages of DKA are of air hunger (Kussmaul breathing), a sweet smell on the patient's breath (likened to pear drops) and severe dehydration. DKA carries a significant risk of mortality and the diagnosis should be made if possible before this point is reached. Figure 2.1 represents a clinical and biochemical summary of the effects of insulin deficiency.

THE SIGNS AND SYMPTOMS

'Diabetes mellitus is an easy diagnosis to make if one has it in mind.' Oman Craig.

Table 2.1. Signs and symptoms of diabetes at the time of diagnosis

- Polyuria and polydipsia
- Weight loss
- Appetite — voracious or anorexia
- Lethargy
- Infection, especially genital candidiasis
- Ketoacidosis
  Acidotic breathing
  Abdominal pain and vomiting
  Dehydration
  Depressed consciousness

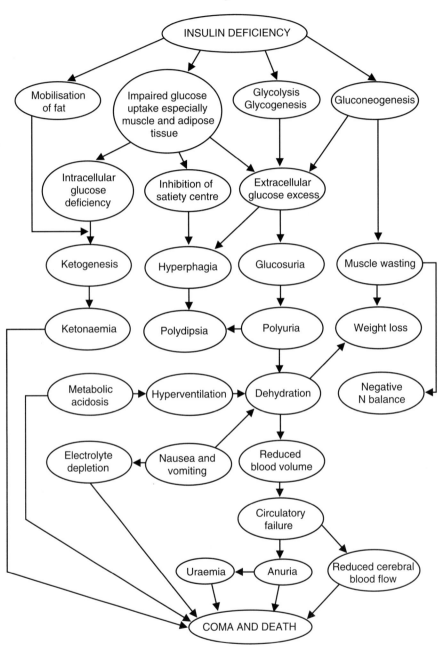

Figure 2.1. The effects of insulin deficiency

Table 2.2. Differential diagnosis of glycosuria

Insulin deficiency
- Insulin dependent diabetes mellitus (>95%)
- Maturity onset diabetes of the young (MODY)
- Secondary
  Chromosomal disorders, e.g. Down's, Turner's, Klinefelter's
  Syndrome, e.g. DIDMOAD, Prader–Willi
  Pancreatic disease, e.g. haemochromatosis, cystic fibrosis
  Post pancreatectomy
  Acute illness, e.g. shock, burns

Insulin antagonism
- Cushing's syndrome
- Steroid therapy
- Phaeochromocytoma
- Thyrotoxicosis

Few asymptomatic children present with a chance finding of glycosuria on routine testing, since the time interval between onset of glycosuria and the onset of clinical symptoms is usually brief. The exception occurs where there is already a diabetic child in the family as the parents often test their other children for glycosuria and hyperglycaemia if at all suspicious. Consequently siblings can present early with few if any symptoms.

In diabetes insulin deficiency occurs in parallel to the destruction of pancreatic β cells. The symptoms which follow become apparent in 60% of children over the ensuing two to six weeks, with 20% presenting before and 20% after this time period. When symptoms occur it is because a critical point has been reached at which insufficient insulin is being produced to keep the blood sugar level lower than the renal threshold. The resultant glycosuria inevitably leads to an osmotic diuresis. Thus the clinical diagnosis of diabetes should not be difficult as the history of obvious polyuria and polydipsia is almost always present (Table 2.3). The first indication may be nocturia or unexpected secondary nocturnal enuresis but the more obvious sign is a raging thirst. Children have been known to drink rain, bath, or other waste water when their parents presumed their polydipsia was attention-seeking behaviour and tried to deal with this by limiting their fluid intake.

Table 2.3. Differential diagnosis of polyuria and polydipsia

- Diabetes mellitus
- Psychogenic polydipsia
- Diabetes insipidus
- Chronic renal failure

Weight loss can become noticeable over one to two weeks. Initially this is more gradual and is caused by the utilisation of protein (muscle) for gluconeogenesis. Together with lethargy these may be the symptoms presented by the child's parent and further specific questions may be needed to come to a correct diagnosis. In retrospect parents may bring to mind episodes in their child's history prior to diagnosis which suggest episodic hypoglycaemia during the prodromal phase. This presumably reflects islet cell instability during the early phase of immunological attack.

A missed diagnosis and presentation in diabetic ketoacidosis only happens for a minority of children (Table 2.4). To reduce the frequency of such presentations requires a wider public knowledge of the significance of early symptoms, and the absolute need for 'same day' referral to a specialist diabetes service. This is important as children are susceptible to diabetic ketoacidosis on a far shorter time-scale than adults and can become severely and rapidly dehydrated over one to two days. The condition of children at the time of diagnosis, level of dehydration, severity of ketoacidosis, level of consciousness and the speed of referral represent means to audit the referral pathway.

In unusual cases, diabetes in children may present with any of the following.

- Acute abdomen — this can mimic acute appendicitis or even pancreatitis
- Cataracts — classically presents after a long prodrome at diagnosis or to ophthalmologists with visual problems
- Necrobiosis lipoidica — this may antedate the classical acute presentation
- Skin sepsis
- Genital and flexural candida infection.

Such presentations are seen by paediatricians almost exclusively as slides or short-answer questions in postgraduate examinations rather than in everyday clinical practice. If any are presenting features of diabetes it is almost certain that the more usual symptoms of polydipsia and polyuria will also be present.

Table 2.4. Differential diagnosis of acidosis

- Diabetic ketoacidosis
- Salicylate poisoning
- Septicaemia
- Severe respiratory distress: asthma, pneumonia

Where a child has the disease's classical symptoms (Table 2.1), along with glycosuria and non-fasting ketonuria, then the diagnosis of diabetes mellitus is confirmed by demonstrating a random blood glucose greater than 11 mmol/l (venous or capillary whole blood). With simple equipment a fingerprick test of blood glucose can put the diagnosis beyond reasonable doubt. In the child who is not well this can be all that is necessary prior to the beginning of treatment with insulin. In rare circumstances the diagnosis may need to be confirmed with a fasting blood glucose of >6.7 mmol/l. A raised glycosylated haemoglobin (HbA) level where this is three standard deviations above the normal mean confirms impaired carbohydrate handling over a long period and has high specificity for diabetes mellitus, but is not as yet an accepted biochemical standard in diagnosis.

DELAYED DIAGNOSIS

Usually the diagnosis of diabetes is simple to make, but there are a number of reasons why delay occasionally occurs.

1. During infancy. Diabetes is very rare in this age group and babies normally have a high fluid intake anyway. Polyuria may not be obvious in an infant who is wearing nappies. Wasting and failure to thrive are important clinical signs.
2. In older pre-school children. The incidence is still uncommon. Parents and primary health-care workers may not recognise or may misunderstand the symptoms, e.g. a diagnosis of urinary tract infection may be made because of polyuria or enuresis. Acidotic breathing may be mistaken for severe asthma or pneumonia.
3. Intercurrent illness. Children can present with other major illness including pneumonia where rapid breathing is expected. *All* ill children should have a blood glucose measurement performed.
4. In the adolescent. This age group may simply ignore or conceal their symptoms from parents and peers. In an older child the symptoms of acidotic breathing and glycosuria may also be attributed to the stress of other illness. Weight loss in adolescents may be seen as desirable, particularly if obesity has been a problem.
5. Where referral is made by letter (as is common practice for new referrals for diabetes in adults) there is great potential for delays. A telephone call to the diabetes service is far more appropriate.
6. Occasionally the diagnosis is considered and the right investigations ordered, but the results are delayed or not checked. Again, if the diagnosis of diabetes mellitus is considered *in a child*, they should be seen that day by a specialist diabetes service for confirmation and immediate management.

OTHER CAUSES OF GLYCOSURIA

It is unusual for a child with diabetes to present only with isolated glycosuria. There are circumstances where glycosuria is a transient phenomenon or secondary to another medical problem (Table 2.2).

Stress-induced Glycosuria

Transient glycosuria can follow hyperglycaemia secondary to the stress of major illness such as pneumonia, meningitis and seizures and is also a well documented feature in infantile gastro-enteritis. The stress of illness leads to an increased production of stress hormones, adrenaline, cortisol, glucagon and growth hormone which in turn raise blood glucose levels above the renal threshold to as high as 15–20 mmol/l. Very rarely the hyperglycaemia seen with gastro-enteritis in pre-school children may be severe and prolonged enough to require insulin therapy. These children may be very sensitive to insulin and a low-dose insulin infusion is probably the safest method of treatment, which is rarely needed beyond 36 hours.

Urinary Tract Infection, Salicylate Poisoning and Fabrication of Illness

Glycosuria can also be detected in children with a urinary tract infection but it is not known whether this is due to a stress-induced hyperglycaemia or a temporarily reduced renal threshold. Salicylate poisoning can lead to glycosuria, but this is now rare following the introduction of childproof containers and avoidance of the routine use of aspirin in children. Another rare circumstance that should be considered is factitious illness syndrome. Glucose may be added to urine in order to confuse medical staff, because of psychological illness in the patient or parent.

Pancreatic Disease

Any destructive disease of the pancreas damages the islets of Langerhans and leads to insulin deficiency. Acute pancreatitis may cause prolonged hyperglycaemia and glycosuria whilst chronic pancreatitis, such as seen in cystic fibrosis and thalassaemia, can lead to the permanent development of insulin dependent diabetes.

Renal Disease

Any condition which alters the renal threshold for reabsorption of filtered glucose can result in glycosuria. An example is Fanconi's anaemia in which there is also a generalised amino aciduria.

Other Endocrine Disease

Although rare, other endocrine disorders can lead to glycosuria and even diabetes. Situations of adrenocorticoid excess such as Cushing's syndrome and disease may show glycosuria, although the commonest cause of steroid excess in childhood is secondary to steroid treatment of illness such as acute severe asthma and nephrotic syndrome.

Maturity Onset Diabetes of the Young (MODY)

MODY will also present with hyperglycaemia and glycosuria. It is best described as a non-insulin dependent form of diabetes occurring before 25 years of age. It is inherited most frequently as an autosomal dominant disease and is rare in Caucasians. Diagnosis depends on having a high index of suspicion, especially with a strong family history of Type II or maturity onset diabetes. As young adults with MODY can develop severe complications it is important to make an early diagnosis. It is *not* a mild form of diabetes.

GLUCOSE TOLERANCE TEST

There is rarely any doubt about making a diagnosis of diabetes when the typical symptoms, glycosuria and ketonuria, are present, but occasionally isolated glycosuria may be found. This may be in the context of steroid treatment for acute asthma, for example, or other illness, and when this is associated with borderline elevation of blood glucose levels it may lead to difficulties of diagnosis. When children present with temporary glucose intolerance the only generally recognised test for confirming the diagnosis of diabetes is the oral glucose tolerance test. An abnormal glucose tolerance test is a late phenomenon in the development of childhood diabetes as it does not become positive until β cell destruction and insulin deficiency are well advanced.

Although various suggestions have been put forward for glucose tolerance testing, the best method probably remains that agreed by the WHO in 1980[1], which has the advantage of being relatively straightforward to perform. An oral glucose load is given: 2 g per kg up to three years, 1.75 g per kg up to 10 years to a maximum of 50 g, and 75 g as a total dose thereafter. Blood glucose is measured before and two hours after the glucose load. The technique used to measure blood glucose is very important when interpreting the results. For the same sample whole blood glucose measurement gives lower results than plasma, and venous blood gives lower values than capillary blood. The blood glucose values for a diagnosis and impaired glucose tolerance are given in Tables 2.5 and 2.6.

Table 2.5. Blood glucose values and the definition of diabetes[1]

	Whole blood glucose (mmol/l)		Plasma glucose (mmol/l)	
	Venous	Capillary	Venous	Capillary
Fasting	⩾6.7	⩾6.7	⩾7.8	⩾7.8
Two hours after glucose load	⩾10.0	>11.1	>11.1	>11.1

Table 2.6. Blood glucose values and the definition of impaired glucose tolerance[1]

	Whole blood glucose (mmol/l)		Plasma glucose (mmol/l)	
	Venous	Capillary	Venous	Capillary
Fasting	<6.7	<6.7	<7.8	<7.8
Two hours after glucose load	6.7–10.0	7.8–11.1	7.8–11.1	8.9–12.2

There are three possible outcomes: diabetes confirmed, impaired glucose tolerance and negative. It is often difficult to have absolute confidence in an abnormal result or results and circumspection as to the significance of an isolated result should certainly be employed. Thus the greatest value of the glucose tolerance test is when it is negative!

PRACTICE POINTS

☞ Polyuria and polydipsia are almost always present at diagnosis.
☞ Telephoned referral to paediatrician on the day of diagnosis is mandatory.
☞ Diagnosis can be confirmed by glycosuria and a high blood sugar (random more than 11mmol/l) with or without ketonuria.
☞ Glucose tolerance tests are rarely needed and difficult to interpret.
☞ If the child is not vomiting at the time of diagnosis, the management can comprise subcutaneous insulin and an oral intake of food and fluid.

REFERENCE

1 WHO Expert Committee on Diabetes Mellitus. *WHO Technical report series, No 646*. Geneva, 1980.

FURTHER READING

Baum, J. D. *Metabolism in Clinical Paediatric Physiology*. Oxford: Blackwell, 1979.

Kelner, J. H. (ed.). *Childhood and Adolescent Diabetes*. London: Chapman and Hall, 1995.

Saunders, E., Chambers, T. Delay in treating diabetes in childhood. *BMJ* 1982; **285:** 1395–6.

3

Diabetes — Management of the First Few Weeks

IAN JEFFERSON AND MOHAMMED KIBIRIGE

INTRODUCTION

There can be few medical diagnoses that have such a potentially devastating acute and long-term effect on a child and its family as insulin dependent diabetes mellitus. The management of the disease, the education, empowerment and support of the child and family at the time of diagnosis, and in the first few weeks and months of treatment, can and do have long-term effects on the family's acceptance of the diagnosis and their skills and enthusiasm in its management. It is important, therefore, to optimise this period of management for a condition that touches every aspect and minute of the child's subsequent life.

With increased public and general practitioner awareness, the suspicion of diabetes and a finding of glycosuria are often early events, and thus fewer children present with severe symptoms or diabetic ketoacidosis. More are diagnosed with only mild symptoms (possibly just polyuria) and when still feeling extremely well. In childhood the diagnosis of insulin dependent diabetes rarely requires more than the documentation of a single raised random blood glucose test. Thus, convincing the child and the family that they have a potentially life-threatening and life-long disease requiring 'painful' treatment and monitoring and a 'special' diet can be difficult and can lead to questioning of the diagnosis and the need for treatment after a few weeks, especially if there is a pronounced 'honeymoon period' of low insulin requirements.

Childhood and Adolescent Diabetes. Edited by S. Court and B. Lamb.
© 1997 John Wiley & Sons, Ltd.

The mainstay of management is a team approach, where the child and family are central to that partnership and the professionals tailor their approach and final details of management to the individual needs, resources and capabilities of the child and the family. Explanation and education particularly must be tailored to the individual, for while the basics of diabetes management may seem relatively straightforward to the professional, they are nearly always outside the experience of the family. There are, however, a few essential pieces of information that are a requirement of all children (according to age) and their families at diagnosis, and these are outlined below.

1. A simple explanation of the aetiology of the disease, pointing out that it is really a combination of 'bad luck' superimposed upon a genetic susceptibility. It is really a question of 'the right person being in the wrong place at the wrong time'. Although many environmental factors have been implicated, there is no clear causation; the most important message to get across to the parents and the child is that really no one is to blame, since at this stage there is often a good deal of guilt and searching for someone or something to blame for the child's illness.
2. Unfortunately, despite what they might hear to the contrary, once you have diabetes it does not go away.
3. Again, despite what they may hear to the contrary, diabetes can really only be treated with injections of insulin.
4. Despite the popular conception of injections equalling pain, the modern disposable insulin syringe or injection device and needle are so sharp and so fine that the injections are almost 'painless'.
5. Although it will all seem extremely complicated and confusing to start with, they will quickly learn the essentials of diabetes management.
6. Although it would clearly be much nicer if the child did not have diabetes, life goes on — essentially there is nothing that the child does now that they will not be able to do in the future.
7. Although the word 'diet' might sound daunting it is really only a question of healthy eating, and with luck the whole family will end up healthier because of the diagnosis.
8. That there are lots of rules to do with having diabetes but only two of these are absolutely unbreakable:
8.1 Never stop your insulin.
8.2 Always carry glucose sweets or their equivalent for treatment of hypoglycaemia.
The other rules are open to negotiation!
9. It is not advisable to visit the local library or listen to neighbours and friends over the garden fence or in the supermarket — the former will

almost certainly be out of date and the latter have an almost universal tendency to spread worrying misinformation interspersed with much doom and gloom.

10. Finally, despite all this apparent bad news, the ongoing management is a team approach, with the hospital Diabetes Team and the family forming an important alliance. By working together a healthy life can continue very much as previously.

HOSPITAL VERSUS HOME MANAGEMENT

The philosophy of independence of self-management has to be encouraged in all children with diabetes. The decision to manage a child either at home or in hospital, however, is dependent on the manpower available locally. Other factors include the general condition of the child and social circumstances of the family. The decision should always be made in the best interests of the child. We feel that the intelligence and ability to grasp new ideas of the carer are major factors.

The guidance from the St Vincent's Declaration and Consensus Management[1] outlines the ideal manpower requirements. In practice, however, not all hospitals have been able to recruit the necessary personnel. Therefore resources are stretched for those who do not have a Diabetes Specialist Nurse or a designated Diabetes Team, but fortunately these are few[2].

There is some controversy as to whether or not a child should be managed in hospital soon after diagnosis. Knowledge acquired by the carers in the first few days and weeks is crucial. It may influence long-term management of the individual child and therefore decisions should not be taken lightly. The diagnosis of diabetes mellitus, the demands, anxieties and uncertainties of its course and treatment can be devastating for parents. Family life adjustments are required when this happens. Rapid adjustments help the care of the child but in some situations obsessive behaviour may result. Delayed adjustment may be the result of denial and therefore compromise the care. Parents need support and advice from the Team. This will be dealt with in more detail later in this chapter under 'Support in Hospital and at Home'.

A well co-ordinated team approach is highly recommended, for it builds confidence in the child and the carer. If a child has to be admitted to the hospital the whole Team must be well versed with the overall picture of handling the situation. This entails imparting the practical knowledge for 'survival' to the child and carer without causing system overload.

The family disruption and emotional disturbance should not be taken lightly as it may result in behavioural problems in either the index child or siblings. It is therefore important that when a decision is made to admit a child to the ward the length of stay is minimised. This caters for immediate support being accessible, optimises education, reduces degree of dependence on professionals and allows parents to manage their child at home as soon as possible.

There are other factors which dictate that a child be admitted to hospital: a child who is in diabetic ketoacidosis requiring either intensive care or high dependency care, a child who may have other life-threatening illness associated with or precipitating diabetes, or a child who lives at too great a geographical distance from the Diabetes Team for secure management. Social circumstances, such as a single parent or spouse working away from home or lack of a telephone, may dictate that the parent is unable to cope on their own. The availability of the Diabetes Team at the time of diagnosis is a crucial factor in determining the length of stay. The Diabetes Specialist Nurse and the Paediatric Diabetologist/Endocrinologist have the biggest impact on the service. If either or both of them were away at the time of diagnosis then it would be impossible to supervise the child's care at home.

It is our practice to admit the child for a short period of stay on the ward when the full Team is available and the patient is well. This usually means two or three days. We find that this is sufficient time for the parents to learn enough practical detail to allow them to leave hospital. Parents are given initial information and some time to digest it. They are given instruction on practical procedures and then perform them under supervision, knowing that their child will not be in danger if they make a mistake. We also find that parents use this opportunity to stay away from the child for a short period and grieve out of sight of the child. In the majority of our patients this procedure works very well. For the older age group and young adults, the children themselves learn much faster, sometimes faster than their parents, and it is not necessary to stay for as long as three days.

When the Diabetes Specialist Nurse is on holiday the length of stay may be more than three days, but it is unusual for it to be more than two weeks. The overall aim is to get the families home as soon as possible in order to reduce the culture of dependence in decision-making, which is commonly associated with long stays in hospital.

A decision to manage the child at home puts a lot of pressure on the parents, the child and the Diabetes Team. The parents need to learn very quickly and they must have support at all times. It is essential that they have a telephone. Home management encourages the philosophy of independence and the understanding that diabetes is a condition and not an illness, and emphasises the ambulatory nature of care. The older age group and young adults are very amenable to this approach. The biggest worries are the fear of insulin injection and blood glucose monitoring. The first tests and injection may be done in hospital or soon after returning home by a member of the Diabetes Team. It is, however, better that they are done by either the child or parent under supervision. Even then subsequent practical procedures need to be supervised to ensure that everything is being done correctly. This is advantageous in that there is little interruption from other hospital staff and the training is consistent.

The team that uses this approach needs to set aside a great deal of time. There must always be somebody available for telephone consultation, and a team member needs to be available to provide a physical presence as required in the first 48 hours. It means freeing themselves of many other commitments during this time and this may be difficult in a district general hospital set-up.

Children with significant diabetic ketoacidosis cannot be managed at home under the current guidelines from the British Society of Paediatric Endocrinology and Diabetes. Schneider in 1983 reported results of his out-patient approach in the United States of America[3]. He reported that 6% of children newly diagnosed with diabetes mellitus needed hospital care. The main influencing factors were metabolic decompensation, social circumstances such as the lack of a telephone in the house, and parental satisfaction. Most parents were relieved not to experience the trauma and expense of hospitalisation. The parents felt that they were directly involved in the care of the child at home. This reduced their anxiety in spite of a traumatic first night.

There are some practical points to be taken from Schneider's work which can be adapted to managing individual children in other parts of the world. Where hospitalisation may lead to financial ruin a decision not to admit should be explored. The levels of understanding must be very good to ensure rapid communication and safety. The paediatrician in charge must be available and should be ready to change his/her mind.

Drash[4] outlined management guidelines in the USA, and an ambulatory care programme was developed and shown to be safe and effective in a well organised Diabetes Therapeutic Team. Unfortunately such teams tend to be restricted to the main teaching centres, and district general hospitals in Britain are unlikely to achieve them in the immediate future. However, ambulatory management in the USA and other parts of the world has become acceptable.

In summary, most children with insulin dependent diabetes mellitus are managed as out-patients by the Diabetes Team. The authors recommend a short stay but where financial ruin is likely an effort should be made to use the ambulatory service sooner rather than later after diagnosis.

Children with diabetic ketoacidosis and those with metabolic decompensation should be managed in an intensive care or high-dependency unit. Education should be given to all to enable them to cope and to minimise their length of stay. Future management is discussed as necessary.

Psychologists and behavioural scientists are involved in evaluation and for long-term support as this is an essential component in successful management.

INSULIN TREATMENT

Clearly all children with newly diagnosed insulin dependent diabetes mellitus need to be started on a regimen of subcutaneous insulin injections. If there is no evidence of significant ketosis or decompensation then there is no immediate rush to institute treatment as long as the child is under medical observation. It must clearly be understood, however, that at this point the child is on a knife-edge and it takes very little in terms of additional metabolic stress to tip them into potentially life-threatening ketoacidosis. Hence the need for same day telephone referral from primary care through to the hospital Children's Diabetes Team as soon as the diagnosis is suspected.

The first injection is a major hurdle in the management at the time of diagnosis. With careful management by experienced personnel the hurdle can be cleared easily, and is then a major milestone in the confidence-building exercise of self-management.

The age at which a child can be expected to undertake his or her first injection is obviously very variable and dependent on the individual child; however, it is not uncommon for a child of five to seven years to undertake this first injection successfully and painlessly under supervision. Certainly over this age self-injection should be encouraged.

It is my personal practice to sit quietly and explain to the child and its parents that modern insulin needles are so sharp and so fine that nine times out of 10 the injection is in fact painless. I explain to them that when I first stuck an insulin needle in my leg to find out what it was like I did not believe this either! Having sat there long enough and plucked up courage, when I eventually did push the needle into my leg, much to my surprise I found it to be painless. I explain to them that I really do not expect them to believe me, but that for the time being they are going to have to take my word for it and afterwards they can tell me who was right and who was wrong. I explain that the 'block' to giving an insulin injection is in their minds rather than down where the needle meets their leg, and that if they can only get past this first injection they will see what I mean. This is often aided by me sticking an insulin needle in my own leg whilst I am explaining things to them and saying that I really would not do it if it hurt. Parents who are going to undertake injections on small children can often benefit from putting a needle in their own legs and proving to themselves that it does not hurt so that they know they are not 'inflicting great pain on their child'.

It is also important to be completely honest at the outset and explain that occasionally the injection will hurt, if one is unfortunate enough to hit a nerve ending. I explain that eight out of 10 injections will probably be virtually painless, one out of 10 they will feel a bit, and one out of 10 will feel like a definite pinprick but should be no worse than that.

The personnel supervising and supporting the child and parent at the time of this first injection are all-important and should really be restricted to members of the Team who are experienced in this and good at it. This first injection can certainly set the scene and make all the difference to subsequent insulin management.

- " The initial insulin regimen is open to debate. If there is clear evidence of ketosis then initial soluble insulin may be necessary subcutaneously once or twice six-hourly to control initial hyperglycaemia and ketonaemia, but it is usually possible just to start on the projected twice-daily insulin regimen. The older approach of days on six-hourly sliding scales of soluble insulin to establish insulin requirements really has very little to recommend it and unnecessarily increases the trauma to the child. Many, if not most, Units choose an initial regimen of twice-daily fixed-mixture insulin, the commonest ratio being 30% soluble to 70% medium-acting. While 'do-it-yourself' mixtures of soluble and medium-acting insulin are conceptually attractive to the physician, they are unnecessarily complicated to the child and parent and any gain in 'fine-tuning' is usually lost in the well documented inaccuracy of mixing the cocktail.

It should be remembered that initial ketosis will increase insulin resistance and therefore increase the dosage of insulin that might be required. Conversely, the absence of ketoacidosis, particularly in the very young child, often makes them very insulin-sensitive at diagnosis, particularly to soluble insulin. For these reasons in the very young child it may be appropriate to choose to use just an intermediate-acting insulin with no soluble component at the outset. For the same reason, and because of the long overnight fast in the young child, some people will choose to use once-daily 'before breakfast' insulin in small children as long as this produces acceptable control.

There was a feeling that initial tight control and achievement of normoglycaemia was important to avoid complications and maintain β-cell reserves; however, there is little to support this and my personal practice is to initiate a regimen that will achieve safety by avoiding ketoacidosis and abolish the symptoms of polyuria and polydipsia, and then work on tightening control and fine tuning over the first few weeks or months. The production of troublesome hypoglycaemia in the first few weeks of management does nothing to build confidence in the child or family. "

There used to be a habit of practising injection techniques on oranges. As far as I can see this teaches you nothing but how to inject an orange with insulin, a skill for which I have yet to find a use. We have abandoned this practice.

Opinion varies as to whether children at diagnosis should be started on a standard, size-appropriate, disposable insulin syringe and needle or be introduced directly to one of the 'pen injection devices'. It is my personal practice to start all children using a standard syringe and needle for a period of six months to a year; this reassures me that they become used to, and understand the use of, this most basic therapeutic tool which may be necessary in the future in case of breakage, loss or failure of the more complex injection devices. The physical act of drawing up a certain volume of insulin also aids in grasping the concept of variation in dosage and of a certain volume of insulin having a particular effect.

Despite the undoubted convenience of the injection pen devices and their initial popularity other factors should be borne in mind. Many of the 'pens' are very heavy compared to an insulin syringe and needle, and small hands do not always cope well with the weight and the pressure required to push down the plunger. Syringes on the other hand (particularly the volume-appropriate 30 unit and 50 unit syringes) are small and light, and the plunger is easily depressed with minimum pressure. It is my practice after six to 12 months using standard syringe and needle to show and demonstrate the various injection pen devices to the patient and offer them the choice of how they wish to proceed. Having said this, some diabetes teams now only issue pen injectors and do not teach syringe techniques at all.

Finally, we have also abandoned attempts to produce controlled hypoglycaemia in the hospital setting. In most people's hands this is a frustrating exercise since the usual scenario is that the child is given his insulin before his breakfast but is then denied breakfast, mid-morning snack, lunch and mid-afternoon snack and is still waiting for his hypo at teatime, by which time he is feeling very disgruntled and hungry and wondering if these doctors and nurses really do know what they are talking about! Hypos on the whole tend to be unpredictable events and what is really needed is a careful explanation to the child and its carers about the likely symptoms, the likely causes and how to react under those circumstances.

MONITORING

Monitoring is an important and integral part of diabetes. This must be done accurately using the appropriate equipment to minimise trauma to the child and parents. The equipment may appear innocent and slick to the Diabetes Team but the first experience will always be remembered vividly by the child. 'I saw the huge, horrifying needle from the corner of my eye and the thought of making a hole in my finger gave me butterflies in my stomach' is how a 12-year-old recalled her experience three years after the diagnosis. This was in reference to a fingerprick to allow blood glucose monitoring and diagnosis.

"Blood glucose monitoring is used routinely and we recommend monitoring before each meal and before bed in the first few days. This is done to assist with insulin adjustments as well as highlighting the changes that take place from day to day. Most parents usually settle on a twice-daily monitoring routine, except in the very young where monitoring varies from once a day at different times of day to more frequently if the child is unwell.

The grids of the diary record books are also designed to assist parents in interpreting the results. We advise parents to monitor more frequently in all children if the children are unwell. We train the parents and their children to start with visual reading of blood glucose strips to ensure proficiency. This also ensures that the parents would be able to use this method in case of reflectance meter failure.

We recommend that parents purchase blood glucose meters for use at home. It is not standard practice to test for colour blindness, although this must occasionally be considered. When parents have been instructed on blood glucose monitoring we stress that the clinical state of the child is more important than the reading on the meter. If there is a discrepancy between the readings and the condition of the child then the condition of the child takes priority. This ensures that children are not given Hypostop or Glucagon because the reading shows hypoglycaemia in an otherwise well child.

Blood glucose monitoring in other situations, such as at school, physical education, lessons and other relevant activities, is usually discussed at a later stage.

Parents are instructed on urine testing for ketones to be used when the child is either unwell or has an elevated blood glucose. Urine testing as a measure of blood glucose really has no place where capillary blood glucose testing is available.

Recording of results is very important for retrospective analysis of blood glucose and determining the course of action. The authors normally recommend that results are recorded in the diary to assist parents and children whenever necessary. If results are only stored on a meter with a memory this application should assist transfer of information into the diary rather than replace it. The diary presents a pattern of blood glucose to the child, parents and the Diabetes Team. A series of numbers on the meter does not give you a visual picture. This is crucial to all children, and specifically to those involved in sport and other physical activities. "

FOOD

The management of diabetes is dependent on manipulation of insulin doses based on blood glucose monitoring, ingestion of food and exercise. A normal healthy balanced diet is recommended to all our children with diabetes. It is a relief to all parents when they learn that they do not have to adjust their budget to accommodate their child's diabetes. The main carers have the greatest relief in knowing that cooking habits only have to adjust to healthy eating, unless the family have wayward dietary patterns. The authors do not recommend 'a diabetic diet' because they do not believe in its existence, but the concept of exchanges is used and recommended in our practice. Calculating the carbohydrate content of equivalent foods is a difficult concept to understand and exchanges are a tool that facilitates this understanding by allowing direct comparison of different foods (see Chapter 10). This concept is best explained where possible in the child's home after assessing the social and normal eating habits of the family. This reassures the parents that they can use their home menu instead of trying to copy what they saw in hospital.

This concept is also helpful to the School Meal Services. A visit to the school by our Diabetes Specialist Nurse and Dietitian is standard practice; they accompany the parent when the child returns to school. This visit gives them the opportunity to see and discuss the school menu. The concept of carbohydrate exchanges helps in giving appropriate advice in the management in sport, exercise and hypoglycaemia. We also recommend that long-acting carbohydrates are eaten after the appropriate management of hypoglycaemia. Long-acting carbohydrates are also recommended for exercise.

In summary, within the first 48 hours, we recommend a healthy diet dependent on the child's appetite using sugar-free foods and a normal eating pattern. The Dietitian and Diabetes Specialist Nurse will visit the home and the school.

HYPOGLYCAEMIA/HYPERGLYCAEMIA

As outlined above, it is not the authors' practice to induce controlled hypoglycaemia in the ward setting. This is usually a frustrating exercise which unnecessarily prolongs the hospital stay and adds little to the successful management of the child.

It is of course important to give information on hypoglycaemia, its likely causes and ways of anticipating those causes, and on how best to avoid severe symptomatology. The likely symptoms should be explained to both the patient and the carers, together with its management by administration of rapidly absorbed carbohydrate orally and/or the use of Glucagon if the child is deeply unconscious or fitting. It is important to explain that hypoglycaemia can come on quite quickly (within minutes), hence the importance of one of the two unbreakable rules of diabetes, i.e. always to carry glucose or its equivalent on one's person. It is perhaps worth informing the parents at this stage that if hypoglycaemia is severe then a convulsion may occur. This can be done in a matter of fact way without engendering undue anxiety. I usually point out that this information will not stop them panicking under these circumstances but somewhere at the back of their mind will be the knowledge that I told them that 'things would be all right'. I usually point out that, fortunately, in children with diabetes, they have a 'self-saving mechanism' since their very brisk and healthy counter-regulatory system will put the glucose back to normal via release of cortisol and adrenaline in addition to the therapeutic manipulations by the parents. It is our policy to ensure that all families have a supply of Glucagon at home for use either by themselves or any attending doctor or paramedic in the case of such an emergency.

Hyperglycaemia also needs to be explained. The family need to realise that the symptoms of hyperglycaemia are likely to come on much more slowly (over hours or days) but the complications of this are potentially much more serious. It should be explained that if the insulin injections are administered correctly and regularly then severe diabetic ketoacidosis is extremely unlikely.

SUPPORT IN HOSPITAL AND AT HOME

PURPOSE OF DIABETES TEAM

The main purpose of the Diabetes Team is to support and educate the child and family. The constitution of the Team is outlined in the *Principles of Good Practice for the Care of Children and Young People with Diabetes* (BDA)[1] and all Health Services should strive to achieve that goal, otherwise it is impossible to give the necessary support. Where possible a Psychologist and Social Worker should be involved very early in the care of the child, and all members of the Diabetes Team should present themselves to the family during the initial short stay.

The family will be devastated on learning the diagnosis, the child will be frightened and bewildered. The blood glucose monitoring and insulin administration give rise to added anxiety. A child in ketoacidosis makes both the parents and staff anxious, but support must be given to the parents immediately in hospital and other support to cope at home. The authors recommend that children be admitted for a short period during which this initial support can be given on a 24-hour basis. The ward where such children are admitted should be able to provide consistent advice identical to that given by the Diabetes Team. The Social Worker will also look quickly at the family's needs. Parents are also given the addresses of the local Parents' Support Group and British Diabetic Association, although it is very rarely that they have to use those services immediately.

Diabetes Nurse Specialist

The Diabetes Nurse Specialist (DSN) plays a double role of hospital and home support and acts as the main link between the family and other supportive agencies. The DSN will visit the school, the home, and contact the primary care team and any other relevant agency. We recommend that telephone facilities be made available to those families who may not already have them. There are no statutory guidelines in this country for financial support for families whose children develop diabetes but we recommend that the families do apply for financial help.

Parents are shown the Children's Out-Patient Department before going home, and especially for single parents the telephone number of the Parents' Support Group is made available. The majority of parents and their children need and appreciate this level of support.

COMPLICATIONS

It is clearly important that children and their carers are aware of the acute complications of hypo- and hyperglycaemia before discharge from hospital, and although one does not want to engender undue anxiety it is essential that they understand the importance of insulin administration and the potentially severe consequences of ketoacidosis. There is little point in going into the details of the long-term complications associated with diabetes with the parents at or soon after diagnosis. Many of them, however, will have this as a specific question and it may be necessary to outline some details. The essential message needs to be one of optimism, and that modern childhood diabetes management includes a very close watch for the early signs of these complications so that they can be detected at a time where early intervention should avoid any major problems. It should also be emphasised that modern diabetes control is by and large much more efficient than the diabetes control that was available 10 or 20 years ago to those people with diabetes now experiencing complications. It is important for the family to realise that this is a subject at the forefront of the minds of the managing Team.

As outlined above, it should again be emphasised not to listen to the neighbours or relations who say 'my uncle Johnny had that and he went blind and both legs dropped off'—I am constantly amazed by that facet of human nature that delights in spreading doom and gloom.

PSYCHOLOGICAL SUPPORT

As previously mentioned, the diagnosis of insulin dependent diabetes in a child has a huge emotional impact on all members of the family. Potentially it has a major effect on family dynamics, exacerbating existing dysfunctional features and producing new pathology in its own right. For these reasons there are now clear guidelines that the Paediatric Diabetes Team should include a person with experience in clinical psychology who also has a sound understanding and experience of diabetes in childhood and its ramifications. Ideally this person should be introduced to the child and family as soon after diagnosis as possible. This not only enables them to be available to help with emotional issues soon after diagnosis but also, in the future, allows them to be perceived as a regular member of the Team and not as someone you go to see when you are not coping. Psychological and emotional support for the child and its family comes, of course, from other directions, not least the Diabetes Specialist Nurses who have the most contact with the family and who can receive advice (and support themselves) from the Clinical Psychologist. The Parents' Support Group of the British Diabetic Association, which is active in many areas, can also provide invaluable lay support and encouragement to newly diagnosed families.

SUMMARY

In summary, the diagnosis of insulin dependent diabetes in childhood is potentially devastating physically to the child and emotionally to the child, family and extended family. The aim of management in the first few days and weeks is to minimise the trauma associated with the event, to provide initial prompt and safe treatment and to support the child and family through the initial, very steep slope of the learning curve. Early messages must be clear and simple, with enough information to cope with the basics of management and to deal with the misinformation that abounds outwith (and occasionally within) the hospital walls. Once the child is out of hospital there must be initial close and frequent support from members of the Diabetes Team in the form of Out-Patient Clinic visits, home visits and support to continue the education process.

Clearly, different clinics will have slightly differing approaches and resources available. One message, however, remains clear: optimum diabetes management can only be achieved with a dedicated Specialist Children's Diabetes Team comprising a Paediatrician with a special interest in diabetes, Paediatric Diabetes Specialist Nurses or Diabetes Specialist Nurses with a special interest in childhood diabetes, a Dietitian with paediatric and diabetes experience and an appropriately experienced

Clinical Psychologist. The other part of the Team is of course the child and its family. It is only by working together, including close liaison with the family's general practitioner, and by providing a uniform and consistent message of advice and education, that we will achieve good diabetes control and a healthy future for the child, both physiologically and emotionally.

REFERENCES

1   *Principles of Good Practice for the Care of Young People with Diabetes.* British Diabetic Association, 1996.
2   Lessing, D. N., Swift, P. G. F., Metcalfe, M. A., Baum, J. D. Newly diagnosed diabetes: a study in parental satisfaction. *Archives of Diseases in Childhood*, 1992; **67:** 1011–13.
3   Schneider, A. Starting insulin therapy in children with newly diagnosed diabetes. *American Journal of Diseases of Children*, 1983; **137:** 782–6.
4   Drash, A. L. Management of the child with diabetes mellitus, clinical course, therapeutic strategies and monitoring techniques. In *Paediatric Endocrinology* (Lifsuitz, F., ed.), 1990; **2:** 681–700.

4

Diabetes in the Under-Fives

CAROLINE McCOWEN

INTRODUCTION

Diabetes occurring in children under five years of age offers a significant challenge to all carers. Although numerically small, comprising only 8–10% of the total paediatric clinic population at any one time, nearly half of the paediatric diabetic population are diagnosed in this age range. Evidence (see Chapter 1) is accumulating that insulin dependent diabetes mellitus (IDDM) in the under-fives forms a distinct sub-group, with onset more influenced by genetic than environmental factors, and with a more sudden and aggressive initial course. Management of these very young children poses particular problems, both practical and psychological. This chapter offers some practical advice for the diagnosis, management and support of these children and their families.

PRESENTATION

It is likely that the onset of the disease in the very young is more rapid, with a shorter period of recognisable symptoms and a higher proportion presenting in ketoacidosis and requiring IV insulin infusion[1]. Furthermore, the initial diagnosis of IDDM in children less than two years old may be difficult to make, since the classical symptoms of thirst and polyuria may not be obvious. In babies particularly it is likely that these early signs will be missed and the child may be admitted in ketoacidosis with a mistaken diagnosis of pneumonia or severe asthma. This illustrates the importance of routine ward testing of urine on all admissions.

Childhood and Adolescent Diabetes. Edited by S. Court and B. Lamb.
© 1997 John Wiley & Sons, Ltd.

The experienced paediatrician will recognise the difference between the conditions. Important points to emphasise are:

—history of recent weight loss
—evidence of dehydration
—deep, laboured breathing (air hunger) with subcostal and intercostal recession, the 'Kussmaul' breathing of acidosis (compared with panting, shallow breathing of pneumonia and the prolonged expiratory phase of asthma)
—smell of 'acetone' on breath
—alteration of level of consciousness.

The estimation of blood glucose as well as blood biochemistry is essential in the investigation of any ill child, however young, in order not to miss this crucial diagnosis. Caution is needed, however: the diagnosis should not be made too readily, since many infants stressed by illness, particularly meningitis or severe gastro-enteritis, may have transiently high blood glucose levels. When in doubt it is important to be sure the blood glucose measurements are persistently high and require insulin to correct them.

PRINCIPLES OF MANAGEMENT

The diagnosis of diabetes has a major impact on parents and families, and in general the younger the child, the more serious the diagnosis is perceived to be. The element of shock and psychological trauma should be borne in mind at the time of diagnosis and suitable support and reassurance given. The initial teaching should involve, if possible, both parents and any members of the external family who take part in the child's care. It should allow for the practical difficulties, such as giving insulin injections to a lively toddler, imposing blood tests on a self-willed two-year-old and regulating the diet of a three-year-old who is already a fussy eater. The overall aim should be to make the management as simple and as stress-free as possible.

The siblings must not be forgotten, since their needs will inevitably take second place to the newly diagnosed young diabetic. Co-ordinated working between the ward staff, the Diabetes Nurse, the Dietitian and the Paediatrician is particularly important, both during the child's admission and after discharge.

Ideally the diagnosis should be confirmed by a consultant paediatrician who should set aside at least an hour to talk to the family before discharge to give them an opportunity to express their fears and feelings as well as to make sure they understand the bare essentials of managing a child with diabetes. They should always be given a 'hot line' number and a home telephone should be installed if they do not have one. Early and frequent visits from the Diabetes Nurse Specialist are essential and an early review with the Paediatrician is also very important. If possible, the Psychologist should see the family at an early stage to counsel them on acceptance of the diagnosis. If a Social Worker is attached to the department their help can be valuable in arranging practical support for the family.

INSULIN MANAGEMENT

INSULIN DOSAGE

The standard dosage of insulin of 0.8 u/kg/day is a rough guide to the insulin requirements of the pre-school child, although in the early months after diagnosis the required dose may be less than this and a significant minority need less than 0.5 u/kg. Dosages of more than 0.8–1.0 u/kg should be looked at critically, even if control is imperfect, as it is unlikely that increasing the dose beyond this level will improve control and may well drive the child towards obesity. Look carefully for other underlying problems that may have a negative effect on control.

REGIME

"The standard twice-daily injection of a pre-mixed insulin delivered through a pen device is usually a suitable regime for young children. The 30:70 mixture (30% short-acting:70% long-acting) is a good starting point, though this may need to be changed in the light of experience. Very young children appear to need less short-acting insulin (say 20:80 or 10:90 mixtures) or they may be better controlled on an intermediate-acting insulin alone (e.g. an Isophane insulin). This can be a satisfactory regime for babies who are still being fed very frequently. Sometimes young children in the months after diagnosis can be well controlled on a single daily dose."

INJECTION SITES

From the very first the parents and child must accept *that having an injection is not negotiable*, though where to have it might be. Always check that the finest possible needles are prescribed. Parents often find that the easiest site to use in a young child is the buttock. The child can be placed over the parent's knee to achieve some degree of immobility. The other favoured sites are the thighs. Pain from the injection can be reduced by applying ice to the skin before injecting. Parents should always be encouraged to rotate the injections, sometimes using the upper arms if possible, and to spread out the site of injections in each area to avoid fat hypertrophy. Young children should be encouraged from the outset to take an active role in their injections by, for example, pressing the plunger on the syringe. It is surprising how quickly children accept insulin injections when they realise that they are inevitable.

MONITORING

Parents should be taught the techniques and the underlying principles of both blood and urine testing and should ideally rely on a mixture of the two for good monitoring, though a flexible approach, to encourage the parents to use what they are most comfortable with, will always be best. Interestingly, most parents seem to prefer blood tests, as these give more precise information and are easier to interpret.

Either blood or urine should be checked once a day at varying times before meals and at bedtime, as a routine. If urine tests are the daily routine, a series of blood tests should be done about once a fortnight. These tests give the basic information as to whether the regular insulin dose is correct. Parents should be taught to look at trends and to adjust the insulin if blood tests are consistently above or below the normal range, or if urine tests are positive for glucose. It is important that the insulin affecting the blood glucose at a particular time of day is adjusted, i.e. the evening insulin affects the morning blood glucose and vice versa.

Parents should be encouraged to check a blood glucose whenever practical if the child appears to be hypoglycaemic, to make sure that they are interpreting the symptoms correctly.

An 'illness regime' should be given to parents, to encourage frequent (4–6-hourly) blood glucose monitoring whenever a child is unwell, with urine testing for ketones, so that appropriate adjustments to the insulin dosage can be made, see Figure 4.1.

DIET IN UNDER-FIVES

The key principles of dietary advice in this age group are flexibility and a relaxed approach.

QUANTITY

For children with a good appetite who will eat anything put in front of them, there is no problem in regulating the amount of carbohydrate (CHO) intake for each meal. Children with small and erratic appetites who are already very choosy about what they eat can pose a real problem in

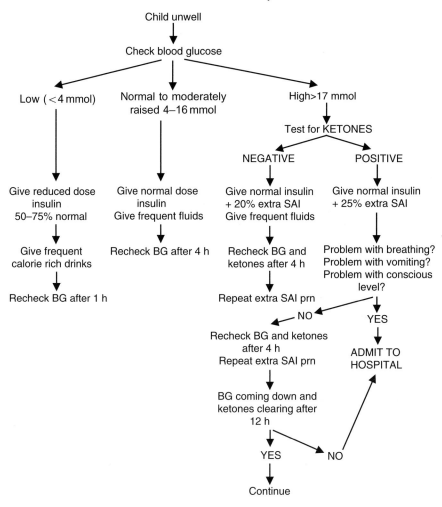

SAI = Short-acting insulin (Actrapid/Humalog); BG = blood glucose

Figure 4.1. Intercurrent illness — a flowchart

management. Parents should be reassured that if the child does not eat the full amount of CHO they should not worry unduly. It is very important that the young child is not put under pressure to eat, or, worse still, force fed. This is likely to lead to food refusal. Try to educate the parents to take a relaxed approach and allow the child to eat as much as he/she wants to. If the child has a hypoglycaemic attack, that can then be treated, and the child will learn from the experience.

QUALITY

The standard advice of high CHO, high fibre, low fat and low free sugar needs modification in the very young child to meet their dietary requirements — for example a moderate intake of fat is recommended, including full-cream milk.

A very high-fibre diet is unsuitable for children under two, and can be difficult even for the child under five to eat and digest. A more relaxed approach, therefore, to free sugar in the diet is appropriate, in order to achieve a high carbohydrate diet. (See Chapter 10.)

ACTIVITY, DIET AND INSULIN

Activity in young children is very variable and unpredictable. It is, therefore, usually not practical to suggest altering the insulin dosage in advance of a period of increased activity. The only way, therefore, to compensate for variation in activity is by alteration in dietary intake, and in a young child, as we have seen, even this may not be easy. Because of these factors it is usually very difficult to achieve tight control in a young child. A compromise needs to be reached where the diet is flexible and the insulin dosage one that achieves reasonable control without an excess of hypoglycaemic attacks.

MANAGEMENT OF INTERCURRENT ILLNESS

Young children tend to be more vulnerable to infectious disease than older children. Most febrile illnesses increase the body's demand for insulin, though an episode of gastro-enteritis can have the opposite effect by reducing the calorie intake.

Parents need to be taught that whenever their child is unwell they need to be monitored with at least 4–6-hourly blood glucose measurements (see Figure 4.1). If the blood glucose rises, extra short-acting insulin should be given, in the form of Actrapid® or Humalog®, in addition to the normal dose of mixed insulin. A suitable initial dose is 20–25% of total normal dose. The urine should be checked for ketones and if present the insulin dose should be more generous. Extra insulin should be given regularly until the blood sugar falls and the ketones disappear. If the ill child with high blood sugar and ketones starts vomiting they should be brought to hospital immediately. In reality, most parents will need the reassurance of visits from the Diabetes Nurse, or at least regular phone calls, in order to maintain the young child safely at home during a significant intercurrent illness.

Some intercurrent illnesses, e.g. gastro-enteritis and migraine, reduce the requirement for insulin due to loss of appetite and vomiting, and this can be recognised by a low blood glucose on testing. In this situation the normal dose of insulin needs to be reduced, though never below 50% of normal. Close monitoring is essential and if a satisfactory blood glucose cannot be maintained the child may require admission.

Many young children go through a period of recurrent infections, often of the nose, ear and throat, and this is usually accompanied by difficult control of the diabetes. Sometimes longer term antibiotics, or the intervention of an ENT surgeon can improve the situation. Parents need reassurance that the child will grow out of the phase and the control will then improve. "

MANAGEMENT OF HYPOGLYCAEMIC ATTACKS ('HYPOS')

'Hypos' are difficult to avoid in very young children, since their eating patterns are often erratic and their activity very variable. It is, therefore, almost inevitable that in most children mild hypos will occasionally occur even though the child is adequately controlled. There is some evidence to suggest that admissions to hospital for hypoglycaemia are more frequent in this age group. Of greater concern is the suggestion that frequent severe hypos in pre-school children may result in a degree of intellectual impairment. Severe hypos should be avoided in the young child. Parents and nursery teachers need reassurance and guidance on how to manage them, and the child should always carry glucose and biscuits.

RECOGNITION

Very young children are unable to recognise for themselves the symptoms of hypoglycaemia. These can vary in the young child, from the classical pallor, sweating and unsteadiness, to more subtle signs, such as deterioration in behaviour. These signs need always to be confirmed by a blood test: it is very important not to reward every temper outburst with some sweets unless the hypo is genuine! Most parents get to know the particular pattern of symptoms that their child exhibits.

Severe hypos can occur in young children, usually during the night, and may give rise to hypoglycaemic fits. It is of great importance that parents are warned about this at the time of diagnosis and given Glucagon with clear instructions on how to use it. They should be strongly reassured that this is not epilepsy and that even severe hypoglycaemic attacks are very rarely harmful.

TREATMENT

1. Mild hypo — give glucose or drink containing sugar+food, e.g. biscuit or sandwich.
2. Moderate hypo (child not co-operative):
   — give Hypostop (glucose gel) into side of mouth, or drink of glucose
   — when partially recovered give food, e.g. biscuit.
3. Severe hypo (child unconscious, fitting) — give Glucagon, half dose followed by second half if no response after 10 minutes and blood glucose still <3 mmol/l; drink and food as above when consciousness recovered.

Unfortunately many children vomit after a severe hypo (probably due to the hypo as well as to the Glucagon) and may need hospital admission if an adequate blood sugar cannot be achieved at home.

PSYCHOLOGICAL ASPECTS OF DIABETES MANAGEMENT IN THE VERY YOUNG

It has been shown that the diagnosis of diabetes is a psychological trauma to the child and the family; the younger the child the greater is the psychological impact and the higher the level of associated anxiety. This must be recognised by the professional team and full and sympathetic support given from the outset.

Parents may benefit from counselling in the initial phase to help them through the grief reaction associated with the loss of their normal child. If a clinical psychologist or psychiatrist is part of the Diabetes Team it is very helpful for them to meet the family before discharge and follow them up afterwards. As well as helping them through the initial shock, it serves as a good moment for introduction, should psychological intervention be appropriate later.

Practical support to the family immediately after diagnosis and in the following months and years is provided by the Diabetes Nurse Specialist, Dietitian and Paediatrician. Parents need a point of telephone contact which is always available. This can be provided by a mixture of the Nurse, Paediatrician, and the Children's Ward, depending on the local set-up.

A healthy psychological environment for the young child with diabetes is the most important factor in terms of the long-term outcome. The child who is psychologically robust stands a good chance of becoming a responsible adult who takes care of his condition.

Time should be spent with the parents in discussion over this aspect of management. Advice at an early stage may avoid the establishment of patterns of behaviour that will prove damaging in the long term. Children with diabetes, like all children, need a firm framework within which to function; they need consistency of approach without too much restriction. They need to develop their independence from an early age. Above all, they need warmth and affection and time spent in positive and enjoyable activities. These may seem obvious, but in a child with diabetes they are sometimes difficult to achieve.

Diabetes is the ideal weapon with which a very young child can manipulate his parents. It is important that parents are made aware of this danger and take early steps to avoid it happening.

Many children hate their diabetes; this is partly a reflection of their parents' attitude to it and partly a feeling that diabetes is a punishment. Yet in order for them to manage it properly as adults they need to accept it, to take it on board as part of their lives without resenting it, and to learn to live in harmony with it. At this very early age the pattern for their future attitude towards it may be set. It may be possible to modify the parents' and, therefore, the child's attitude to his diabetes by early discussion. This sets the scene for the gradual process of the child taking over the responsibility and ownership of the diabetes for himself, within the framework of family support.

THE ROLE OF THE PROFESSIONAL AND THE DIABETIC CLINIC

It is now generally accepted that all children with diabetes should be managed by a dedicated team which includes a Diabetes Specialist Nurse with an interest in childhood diabetes, a Dietitian with experience of paediatrics and diabetes, a Paediatrician with a special interest in diabetes and a Clinical Psychologist or Psychiatrist.

The role of the professional in the very young child can be summarised as follows.

1. Advice and support to parents over management.
2. Education of parents, family and child about diabetes.
3. Monitoring of condition and feedback.
4. Direct management of crises.
5. Counselling, psychological support and intervention.
6. Support for family in wider community — nursery, school, Social Services.

These elements, together with clinic structure and management are discussed in more detail in Chapter 7. It is more difficult managing the very young child with IDDM, and strict management prescriptions for diet, insulin, etc. are impractical. When faced with the inevitable problems brought to the clinic or by telephone contact perhaps the best approach is to identify the key problem and devise a strategy for dealing with that. For example, consider a child who hides and screams at injection time. The parents need support in maintaining that injections have to be given. They can use negotiated rituals to help — 'Teddy gets it first' — but they must not allow these to create enormous delays. Even toddlers can accept deals. Another problem is where a toddler will refuse to eat. One solution is to give their injection after they have eaten. However, the toddler must not be allowed to have freedom of choice over his diet. This is an area where parent support groups can be helpful.

PARENT SUPPORT GROUPS

Parents who are going through the trauma of having a young child diagnosed as diabetic can gain enormously from the support of other parents who have been through, or are going through, a similar experience. Age-banding the clinics allows parents to react and to get to know each other, and often they will form their own parent support group with little or no encouragement from professionals.

THE FUTURE

Children diagnosed under the age of five years form a significant proportion of paediatric diabetics. By the time they reach adulthood they will already have had diabetes for at least 15 years. There is at present no evidence to indicate that this cohort are particularly subject to long-term complications. Therefore it seems reasonable to aim to encourage a framework of safe management and good control within the context of a healthy psychological environment for the child and family. With the advent of Paediatric Diabetes Specialist Nurses and ambulatory paediatricians it may in the future be possible to provide almost all the care for these children within the context of their home and local community, thus minimising the disruption and trauma of the family.

REFERENCE

1   Jefferson, I. G., Smith, M. A., Baum, J. D. Insulin dependent diabetes in under 5 year olds. *Arch Dis Child* 1985; **60**: 1144–8.

5

Five to Ten and the Start of Puberty

MICHAEL SILLS AND ALAN ENGLISH

INTRODUCTION

The period of middle childhood seems, for many, an age when diabetes is relatively straightforward, when children have a school routine, are growing steadily and are to a large extent under the control of their parents. Once the remission phase has passed, with stable insulin requirements few major problems seem to arise.

Professional staff who have struggled to understand and cope with the many and different problems which can arise for children with diabetes and their families have learnt not to underestimate the power of diabetes to destabilise and undermine equilibrium, confidence and self-esteem. Certainly this is not merely a time to relax before the testing years of adolescence, but a time to invest for the future and learn to know and understand individual families and their children. We can also help by giving the support and encouragement which they need now and for the years ahead by keeping the lines of communication open, and by not confusing a desire for independence with the ability to cope.

It is essential that medical, nursing and other staff remember the individual needs of children and their parents in creating a supportive network of professionals who may look at the problems of diabetes from different perspectives. It is important to have access to staff with not only experience and expertise of diabetes itself, but also the ability to understand the effects of a chronic condition in childhood on the family, and the

Childhood and Adolescent Diabetes. Edited by S. Court and B. Lamb.
© 1997 John Wiley & Sons, Ltd.

psychological dimensions and the stresses and strains of daily life and growing.

THE HOLISTIC APPROACH

Some clinics have been lucky enough to forge individual partnerships between children's physicians interested in diabetes and clinical psychologists with an interest in the families who have children with diabetes, and have attempted to develop a 'holistic approach' to diabetes in young people that enshrines the principles of children- and family-centred care.

This approach has enabled all staff to be reminded that children at this age are developing in subtle ways. They are developing concepts of self, are learning to understand the world, are exploring their relationships with peers and parents and gradually working towards independence. Some will need the security of their families for some time to come, but others will be 'streetwise' and start to go their own way much earlier. The self-esteem they need to help them towards more reliable independence may very easily be affected by illness and the attitude of peers and family. There are a number of times when this approach is important.

AFTER DIAGNOSIS

The effect on the family created by a child developing a chronic childhood illness can be immense, and parents especially may need to grieve a little so that they can come to terms with their loss and accept that they no longer have a 'perfect' child. When diabetes is diagnosed there is an instant need to 'do something' and for a lot of action, usually by 'experts'. Before too long it is time for the family to cope on their own. How well they manage will depend a little on the stability of the diabetes but maybe more on their own experience and perception of illness, their ability to cope with unusual situations, on how much they believe 'being and staying healthy' matters, and how good a relationship they develop with the specialist diabetes professionals in their own area.

An important issue is consistency of advice. Confidence in one or a team of professionals can be a very potent force in helping families. If different experts say different things, however well meant, this can cause confusion at the least and may lead to mistrust. At times this can drive families to seek more distant opinions which, however caring and competent, will not have the benefit of local perspectives and may be difficult to access quickly in times of sudden need.

Children with diabetes want to be children first, they do not want to be different, they do not really want to have diabetes, and many hate the illness which seems to cause so many difficulties in their lives. They do not understand why it should have happened to them, they feel anger and resentment, although not always initially. These feelings can lie dormant, repressed when first diagnosed by their loyalty to their parents and 'the experts' who have helped them through, to emerge at a later time expressed directly or indirectly through behaviour disturbance, unhappiness or rebellion. Poor blood sugar control is often the end result of these feelings. The parents also do not really want their child to have diabetes and in addition to anger and resentment they may display guilt and self-blame. Many mothers especially will feel they must put off things in their own lives to see their child's diabetes is kept in best balance — perhaps to make up for their guilt in allowing their child to develop diabetes in the first place! How terrible parents can feel when a child starts to grow up and no longer wants all the attention and supervision, wishing to grow and experiment for themselves with a probable deleterious effect on blood sugar control. We can almost hear them saying: 'How dare you do this to us after all we have done for you to keep your diabetes in best balance'.

However, the carer of a young child with diabetes has a genuine need to create or preserve some routine in a child's life, at least so that food and insulin can be given regularly and consistently. This will inevitably lead to more control being exerted over the child's life. This can be healthy, and many young people with diabetes develop some sense of self-control early in life which is of considerable benefit to them later on. If the control is too great, or the parents want to regain too much, this can set up a paradox for the child where being safe becomes a welcome or unwelcome alternative to developing self-confidence and growing towards independence.

A responsible and well motivated parent will quickly realise that their child's long-term health depends on their achieving consistently satisfactory blood sugar readings, and this goal will be encouraged and underwritten by the caring and knowledgeable 'expert' who is aware of evidence attesting to the benefit of good long-term control. This situation will often lead to the parent exerting even more control over the child's life, which in many cases children will accept. However, unless this is managed skilfully there can be short- to medium-term problems with children regressing (staying home with Mum), becoming frightened of new and difficult situations (school trips and holidays), and perhaps becoming sad and missing out (peer friendships). In the long term the child's failure to develop towards independence, perhaps due to a 'well meaning parent's' desire to continue to remain in control so that the child does not suffer potential long-term damage, will set up conflicts for the future. Previously compliant children can rebel, with very difficult consequences, or children may agree to allow their parents to control them, thus putting off their own adolescence and causing problems later due to their failure gradually to develop an individual and confident personality.

Children at this age, although often appearing resilient, are sensitive to atmosphere and emotion. They can and do cope with many experiences and have less difficulty in coping with issues about their diabetes, if these are approached openly and in a calm and confident manner. However, anxiety in a carer can easily be communicated and cause reaction in the child:

- Do they run away and hide if it is all too confusing or distressing?
- Can they continue to trust that their carers and the experts really still know best?
- Do they reverse roles and act to support their carers in their hour of need?

All this can and often will have an effect on a child with diabetes and can affect blood glucose regulation — perhaps by chemical or hormonal mechanisms. The child's hard won self-confidence and self-esteem can also be threatened. The interaction of physical and psychological factors may continue to further destabilise the 'diabetes' in unpredictable ways.

WHEN THINGS START TO GO WRONG

When things start to go wrong, it can be difficult to decide what has happened. Inevitably the concern and anxiety levels of carers and experts may increase and this itself may make things worse for the child. Expert and carer becoming increasingly convinced there is some serious physical problem and it is then a matter of professional pride and honour for the 'expert' to solve this.

Experts with a strong medical background can become increasingly confirmed in the view that there is a physical–medical solution, and the child and family will continue to trust the expert's knowledge. In such a situation the temptation will increase to change the insulin, change the time of injections, change the delivery system and even consider bringing a child into hospital. Often this does not bring about a resolution but, in such a situation, attention to the psychological environment can be very powerful. If people can be convinced that there is nothing inherently wrong with the diabetes, this can help them to relax, give up blaming the insulin, begin to calm down and gradually feel more at ease with having a child with diabetes in the family. This can help the vicious circle to subside. It is not unusual for the lead physician in the team to admit to his own self-esteem taking something of a tumble when this humble approach produces an improvement where the medical magic bullets had failed.

CASE HISTORIES

For professional staff wishing to learn about diabetes and its effects on children and families, there can be no better grounding than exposure to the problems that can arise, at either first or second hand. Certainly this has helped to form and refine our own clinical approach, and a review of our own experience has helped underpin the general philosophy of management in our clinic. It might therefore be helpful at this point to consider some brief case histories in an anonymised form before considering the nature and origins of our approach.

Case 1

A staff member was involved with a child aged about eight years, who was referred on account of poor growth and who had had diabetes for several years. The child was admitted to hospital for tests. Shortly after arrival in the late morning this doctor was summoned by the child's articulate and caring parents to explain to them why we had proposed to give their daughter lunch when she had sugar in her urine (these were the days before widespread home blood glucose monitoring had been fully taken up), and the family explained that if she had sugar in her urine they would never let her eat because that would make the diabetes worse. It seemed the family had obviously adopted the strategy of reducing food intake when the blood sugar levels were high, which would then have proved successful as her diabetes was better controlled. However, by putting blood sugar control at a premium a situation had almost certainly arisen where the child was undernourished and on close evaluation this proved to be a major component of the growth difficulties. However, it did prove extremely difficult to persuade the family to adopt different strategies towards management of her diabetes.

Case 2

A similar incident occurred when a staff member was consulted about a family with a child of about 10 years, who had developed diabetes some three to four years previously. This child had high blood sugars and was not growing; on close investigation it transpired that the child was still taking the same dose of insulin and the same amount of food as had been advised when the child had been discharged from hospital after diagnosis. The family were extremely pleased and proud that they had been able to control the situation and keep the diabetes under control just as they had been asked. They also felt they had been able to prevent the diabetes getting worse as the insulin dose had not risen and they felt almost certainly if the child were to eat more, the situation would deteriorate. Again, it was very difficult to persuade the family that the child should be allowed more to eat in order to grow and also more insulin to facilitate growth, since the belief in their seemingly successful strategies to date had been immense.

These two cases from times now past show how misunderstandings about the role of food in diabetes could occur. Hopefully in these enlightened times things are different. They also illustrate how seemingly strange coping tactics can become a vital component of the way families manage with a difficult, chronic illness. Both these families felt they had been very successful in controlling the diabetes, which they had felt was the most important thing for their child. However, the fact that they failed to understand the wider needs and that perhaps these had not been fully explained would nowadays give rise to some concern.

Case 3

The mother of a child who developed diabetes at the age of two years, decided she must do the best for her son. Up until the age of five years, she could account for almost everything he had eaten. His blood sugar control and glycated haemoglobin results were impeccable. He then developed increasing problems with behaviour, although his biochemical control remained very satisfactory. However, difficulties within the family built up to the extent that psychological intervention was thought appropriate. The family was persuaded to be a little less restrictive with him, and for a while the situation improved as regards his behaviour. However, his blood sugar control worsened. The family responded by learning to watch his blood sugar very closely and monitor blood tests very frequently, they learnt to give extra insulin if he showed any tendency to high blood sugar and when he developed episodes of ketosis or hypoglycaemia they became adept at treating this at home with high quantities of insulin, high quantities of fluid and a large amount of calories. His diabetes became increasingly brittle, leading to the frequent need for hospitalisation, and throughout this period blood sugar control was considerably less than desirable. Eventually, during a stay in hospital, this child, by then bordering on adolescence, was confronted by the medical perception that he might not always have been giving his insulin as frequently as we and his parents perceived. He was given extra support and encouragement to do well with his diabetes, the episodes of ketosis disappeared dramatically and control gradually reverted to his previous good norm.

Case 4

A child of 12 years, who had had diabetes for two years and initially achieved very good levels of control with the help and support of his parents, suddenly started developing high blood sugars which did not respond to seemingly very high doses of subcutaneous insulin. He became very difficult and abusive to his parents and at times would stuff chocolate bars into his mouth deliberately in front of his mother. Eventually he was persuaded that this situation could not continue and he agreed to come into hospital and accept help. He became very sheepish and quiet after the suggestion was made that he might be injecting his insulin into his mattress rather than his leg and he eventually agreed to accept help on the understanding that he manage his diabetes himself without his parents' intervention. From this point on he achieved extremely good control of his diabetes and went on to fulfil his potential as a high achiever.

These two cases perhaps illustrate the child's lack of acceptance of diabetes—if the child feels hemmed in by it they may well rebel. The full force of this may fall upon the parents, whom the child may, in some subtle way, blame for their plight. For the parents who have been trying so very hard to do the right thing this can be very difficult and in bright, wilful children who are potential high achievers the situation can be worse. These cases emphasise the need to begin to hand over some control of the diabetes to children at an early point so that confrontations of this nature can be avoided.

Case 5

A happy, self-willed young lady developed diabetes at the age of five years. Her whole family worked hard to manage and contain the condition and her mother put off developing her own career. Her blood sugar levels were always prone to swing up and down, causing considerable concern, and there was often friction between herself and her mother. After a particularly long and difficult period of persisting high blood sugar levels, we felt the need to intervene. Initially we thought the fault must lie with the diabetes but changes of insulin type, dose, timing and delivery system made little or no difference and admission to hospital produced only a transient improvement. When we elected to adopt a more psychological approach and the medical experts in our team could be persuaded that there was no inherent physical difficulty with the diabetes, the situation began to resolve. As the family were helped to feel more at ease with her diabetes and accept her as a person in her own right, control improved, swings in her blood sugar became less vicious and to a certain extent the relationship between mother and daughter was repaired.

Case 6

A boy of seven years of age developed diabetes. He and his family seemed to take very little time to come to terms with the problem and initially wanted very little help. For 18 months blood sugar control seemed reasonable. However, it then became apparent that blood sugar levels had been steadily rising, and changes in insulin did not improve matters significantly. His parents tried very hard to bring the situation under control and felt very threatened by the problem, almost as though it were their fault, and for a while they were almost keen to hide the full situation from us. Timely intervention of a psychological nature in the clinic enabled the boy to talk through his feelings about having diabetes and externalise his distress, and his family were able to understand more what he was going through. Following attempts to diffuse the feelings of guilt and blame and with increased support and encouragement things improved. At the same time the boy was persuaded to ask for and was given a new pen delivery system, which perhaps symbolised a new start, and since that time his control has improved, his parents have allowed him more freedom and licence to make decisions about his diabetes and control at home is more of a team effort rather than a parent-centred activity.

These cases serve as a reminder that, although many children at this age will seem to achieve good control easily, problems with adjustment can arise at a later date which can lead to deterioration in blood glucose regulation. The cause for this is not necessarily physical and the well-meaning concern of family and expert can sometimes make it less easy for the child who requires space and time to come to terms with their own condition in their own way. In solving these problems, somebody with an understanding of the emotional and psychological world of the child, and who is perhaps not a regular member of the expert team, can sometimes be a potent force for resolution and change.

SUMMARY

Children at this age and stage of development, with or without diabetes, need help and support if they are to grow as individuals and gradually become more independent within a family and develop the confidence to move more away from their parents and to face the problems of the world with the support of their families. Parents too need help and guidance to recognise that, whereas they have a duty and responsibility to control their child's environment initially, as the child grows they will need gradually to allow their child to take increasing responsibility for areas of their own lives. They may need help to give their children permission to move on and experiment. Parents need to embark on the process of letting go some time before the start of adolescence.

This process can be easily disturbed when a child in a family develops diabetes and well-meaning strategies can, if not well handled, create increasing difficulties as the child progresses. It is harmful for children and parents alike to impair this natural process, and if parents seek to continue to assert excessive control over their children into adolescence, great difficulties can be set up for the future.

HYPOGLYCAEMIA

It is important and relevant to emphasise at this point that hypoglycaemia itself can also be a serious cause of long-standing anxieties and difficulties with control. Most clinicians feel it desirable that children experience mild hypoglycaemia from time to time so that they keep on their guard and become aware of the warning symptoms. Regular mild hypoglycaemia also provides proof positive that the blood sugar levels are being kept as low as is practicable. Certainly this seems to be wise, but in some circumstances excessively tight control results in children swinging rapidly from low blood sugar to high blood sugar with rebound hyperglycaemia being produced, similar to that described by Somogyi[1].

From a family point of view, the possibility of hypoglycaemia can be very frightening and can cause a lot of anxiety. The recurrence of regular mild hypoglycaemia, however, tends to diminish these feelings and improve the confidence of both parents and child in their ability to cope. Nevertheless, when a child suffers sudden and severe hypoglycaemia, especially if this is unexpected and occurs fairly soon after diagnosis, it becomes very worrying for all those involved in looking after the child and can lead to excessive measures being taken to ensure there is no recurrence. The child's lifestyle can be restricted, sometimes parents may be reluctant to let them go and play with friends, to go on school trips or even to school itself, and family activities can be altered to avoid risks. All this is obviously in no one's best interests. Children want to live life normally and they wish their parents to allow and encourage them to tackle age-appropriate activities. Having diabetes is difficult enough without feeling that those who care for you are being over-restrictive, and if not addressed this can lead to increasing resentment by the child of the parents' overcontrolling approach.

If severe hypoglycaemia occurs at night this can be devastating for the parents and can produce a lot of guilt and anxiety. Certainly, most parents, once they begin to understand diabetes, increasingly realise and worry that hypoglycaemia may occur at night, and often seek further information and ask questions. It is certainly appropriate to reassure parents, to try to put their fears to rest and to remind them that severe hypoglycaemia at night is extremely rare and, although frightening, almost certainly not life-threatening — and they believe this! The problem is that once this happens, especially to a young child, the parent is rarely off guard again. In their determination to ensure that they do not put their child at risk again, extra food is often given (but not often admitted to) at night and extra blood sugars are performed. Many parents do not sleep well, the child's morning blood sugars are invariably high following the extra food and even during the daytime parents may insist on other restrictions. It is often the mother that takes on her own shoulders the guilt and responsibility for having subjected the child to such a frightening and potentially dangerous occurrence, and sometimes this has profound effects upon on her, her partner and the child's brothers and sisters.

CASE HISTORIES

For the clinician these situations can be difficult. Families may not easily admit to what is happening — perhaps for fear of criticism or worry that their own fears about night time may not be understood or acknowledged. The good doctor's response to high morning blood sugars would logically be to suggest an increase in long-acting insulin delivered in the evening.

Case 7

A young child with diabetes, aged between four and five years, was admitted on two occasions following severe night-time hypoglycaemia, and on both occasions the child presented with a hemiparesis that proved transient and not associated with any abnormality on cranial imaging. For four or five years after this the mother hardly slept, admitted to getting up to check her daughter's blood sugars up to three times a night and made sure her daughter had plenty of food before bed to keep her sugar levels up. This mother was intelligent, well motivated, had some insight into the problem and recognised that she was over-reacting, but found it very hard to bring herself to change her tactics because of a very real fear of her child suffering again. Blood sugar control did suffer for a while, but eventually with encouragement and support the mother was able to address the situation in her own time and at her own speed and again achieve a reasonably satisfactory level of control.

Case 8

In another family, assessments of blood sugar control were poor for some time despite reasonable levels of blood sugar recording during the day, sometimes performed under the control of clinic staff. Eventually it was discovered that the child had experienced quite severe episodes of night-time hypoglycaemia fairly soon after diagnosis. His mother had learned to take evasive action herself which continued for many years; this included ensuring plenty of food was taken at bedtime. It was very difficult to encourage change and his control only improved once he left school and empowered himself to take full responsibility for his own diabetes.

However, the true origin of the morning hypoglycaemia is not understood, and this may only encourage increased clandestine feeding at night. This perpetuates the problem and enables the family to take the view that even the expert does not know best, as their strategy has not worked. Alternatively, sometimes parents may falsify or omit high morning blood sugar readings to avoid being put under pressure to change.

A proactive approach to minimise the risk of overnight hypoglycaemia can be helpful, along with a sympathetic response to parents' fears and anxieties. It is also disconcerting to see how long it can take some parents to come to terms with and accept severe episodes of low blood sugar, especially at night, and perhaps only those who have witnessed children having severe episodes of night-time hypoglycaemia can begin to understand. For the parents the terror has been real and they may very well feel that in some way they let their child down by allowing it to happen, however illogical this may seem.

SCHOOL

School is, of course, a very important part in a child's life and one they very readily separate from their lives at home. A child with diabetes needs experiences of education, socialisation and development of self-esteem, just like any other child. Perhaps because of their condition, their need to establish a secure concept of self and self-image is even more important.

However, it is so easy for everything to seem to be against them. Suddenly, they can be whisked away — often into hospital — raising curiosity and interest. They return with 'diabetes' and they are 'different' — different foods, different mealtimes and being required to eat snacks enlarges this difference. Anxiety from school staff can be considerable. Added to this there is increased interest in school matters by the parents, and extra attention from the school nurse and school doctor. It can be difficult for the child to settle back into school because of a climate of overinterest, overconcern and overprotection. All this can lead to difficulties with friends and activities in school as well as outside it. Too often they can be given much more attention than before, albeit for very good reasons.

It is essential that clinic staff allay fears of family and school, encourage normality and minimise the sense of being different. School staff need to be reminded that the child is still the same, their general needs have not necessarily changed, but in order for them to continue successfully in school, some minor adjustments and appreciation may be required. Strategies and what to do in emergencies can be openly discussed with staff, and if the child and teacher alike are given open and free access to 'hypo-stopping' foods then much anxiety can be removed. Activity needs to be encouraged, with the child involved fully, and the child needs to be encouraged and empowered to eat extra to allow for the activity. Explanation, education and support should militate against the need to indulge in overprotection as a response to a new problem. In addition, peers and friends can be encouraged and taught to look for, and in some cases treat, episodes of hypoglycaemia. Through all this the child's right to take a full part in school life can be upheld.

It is perhaps wise for the physician not to aim for very tight blood glucose control initially, especially in younger children, to avoid scaring the school staff if sudden unpredicted blood sugar swings occur. Once the child, parents and school have gained confidence then blood sugar control can gradually be tightened in the knowledge that significant hypoglycaemia will seem unlikely and even if it occurred, there will be no problem in identifying and dealing with it. Obviously the effect on the school of a child experiencing severe hypoglycaemia soon after return could be considerable.

Schools, like parents, need to gain confidence and can be destabilised and distracted by some unexpected and untrained for events!

Generally most schools are very receptive to the needs of children with diabetes. Some school staff have anxieties and respond to visits and reassurance. Some, however, appear overconfident, especially if they have had similar children in the past. It is a reflection of a child's individual worth and value that any new situation should be taken seriously by schools. For each individual the particular circumstances need to be understood and catered for in a way which keeps the child very much at the centre of activities. Developing diabetes can be quite damaging to self-image and anything schools can do to encourage and repair this will help the child be accepted as an individual and to continue the journey which will lead in time to independence. There needs to be an emphasis on the importance of giving due attention to a child's needs without seeming to give them special attention or spoil them in any way.

It is important that the school nurse and school doctor know about individual children with diabetes, as this ensures that the school under-stands the situation and has effective strategies in place for emergencies. At times the child with diabetes may need an advocate in school, and the school nurse or school doctor can perform this role. In addition, they can perform an early warning function by alerting the clinic team about any problems that might be occurring at school or at home. On occasions the school may need specific advice about diabetes and, where necessary, a member of the clinic team can be involved. However, it is not recommended that school-aged children with diabetes be singled out for individual attention by being called for extra medical examinations or interviews in school.

EMOTIONAL AND PSYCHOLOGICAL FACTORS

As mentioned in an earlier section, the 'holistic approach' to the management of childhood diabetes recognises the complex links between physical, psychological and social well-being. Whilst there has been a great deal of theoretical research into psychological aspects of childhood diabetes, there has been rather less in looking at the application of psychological knowledge to day-to-day management. Having a clinical psychologist attached to the clinic team can help to achieve this.

In our own clinic at Huddersfield, prior to the involvement of a clinical psychologist, as with many clinics, the emphasis was on tight biochemical control as a primary objective. However, an increasing number of problems arose, to which discussions suggested that our management strategies might be contributing. In addition, a number of children developed prolonged episodes of hypoglycaemia with physical symptoms persisting several hours after the restoration of normoglycaemia. We began to wonder whether good control might come at a price, and whether this was really in the best interests of the children we were seeing, or if other strategies could achieve similar ends.

The clinical psychologists undertook some structured work in the clinic to investigate some of these factors. At the same time, enquiries were being made into the success of diabetes control in a number of clinics in our region. Both parents and children were given a number of questionnaires to complete, and some of the results were presented as an MSc thesis by Karin Westeman (unpublished).

The initial results of these studies suggested strongly that good biochemical control (glycated haemoglobin) was not related to knowledge about diabetes by either parent or child but was more likely to be influenced by the beliefs and attitudes of the parents. The Health Belief Model[2] had been useful in helping to clarify some of these issues and the questionnaires which were devised used the ideas presented in this model. The results indicated that parents who perceived diabetes to be a 'severe' condition were more likely to recognise the importance of health issues, were better at problem solving and had children who exhibited better biochemical control.

Consideration was then given to the emotional and psychological well-being of this 'good control' group in relation to the rest of the clinic population. It was discovered that the children who were perceived to be in good control were more likely to have emotional rather than behavioural problems reported by their parents. Furthermore, there was a definite trend for these children to rate themselves as having more depressive symptoms on a short depression scale designed for their age group[3].

Following these studies, the clinic team were led to ask the question 'Good control at what cost?' A gradual change of emphasis emerged in the clinic, considering the well-being of child and family as being a primary objective, helping them to succeed in life and use a problem-solving approach to resolve difficulties posed by diabetes. Good blood sugar control was still recognised as being important, but not to the extent that it outweighed efforts to help families function at their best level. Emphasis was given more to individual needs and to encouraging well motivated families to achieve control of the diabetes to the best of their abilities. Families responded well to this change, and it may be that this was what many of them had quietly learned to do for themselves.

After a few years using this more 'holistic approach' it was decided to check whether this change could be having an effect on overall control, to avoid being seen to condone suboptimal control, which could have obvious later consequences for the health of children with diabetes. Further review of blood glucose control within the clinic together with a number of other parameters was carried out (Table 5.1). This revealed that, although the

Table 5.1. Comparison of clinic statistics between 1986 and 1990

Year	Clinic size	Male/female	Age range (years)	Range HbA1	Mean HbA1
1986	31	19/12	7.25–16.0	8.0–19.8	12.82
1990	50	31/19	5.0–19.4	5.9–22.7	12.32

clinic had grown and the average age perhaps increased, the level of overall control as assessed by mean glycated haemoglobin had, if anything, fallen slightly during the period of concern. In addition, it appeared that not only was blood glucose regulation not obviously adversely affected but there was evidence that the self-esteem of children in clinic had increased, depression scores were down, there were fewer emotional problems and episodes of prolonged hypoglycaemia were no longer being encountered.

Continuing efforts are made to help families to manage diabetes in their child at the highest level and it is now our opinion that the best route to good control is not necessarily through education, instruction and coercion, but by encouragement, empowerment and support, teaching problem-solving skills and encouraging families to apply different strategies to the various problems until they find the best solution for them as individuals.

CONCLUSION

The 'holistic approach' is essential to achieve child- and family-centred care, in that it accepts the child's needs as paramount, and that these needs are not just those created by the diabetes. Well informed families are more likely to make sensible choices and to be motivated to regard the achievement of good control as an important continuing goal.

The school age journey starts when the child is still fully under the control and influence of the parents and ends when the child achieves a reasonable amount of independence yet still acknowledges their parents' interest in their well-being, and this journey needs to be reflected in the way clinics function.

Early consultations involve talking mainly to the parents, while the children stay in or play outside. After a little while the child needs to be involved and encouraged to stay in by directing some questioning to them, involving them in some problem-solving and decision-making, and encouraging them to ask questions. Gradually the majority of the discussion is directed at the young person, decreasingly involving their parents. Eventually the point is reached where not only is the young person happy to come into clinic alone, but the parents are also happy to wait outside knowing that they have not been excluded from this continuation of a natural process. Different families proceed along this route at different rates and it is not possible to insist on achievement at any age as long as the process is ongoing. However, in the main it appears that from the age of 14 years the parents are happy to take a back seat, and many are happy to let children talk to us alone at a slightly younger age.

In summary, the best way to help children with diabetes and their families appears to be, first, to understand the role and concerns of parents/guardians and the child's varying needs for support from them. Secondly, one must avoid saying or doing anything which might frighten or overload families who have obviously had a great shock and not only need time to come to terms with this but also need to assimilate a great deal of information. Thirdly, many parents are very hungry for information, and if not given it at a rate appropriate to their needs they may obtain misinformation from elsewhere, which can potentially create difficulties and conflict. Fourthly, parents and professionals need to be encouraged to believe that there may be no single right way of doing things, and that individual solutions to individual problems are needed. Finally, experts involved with diabetes must understand that they need not only to safeguard children from the complications of diabetes, which may occur many years in the future, but also to help them to lead good and fulfilling lives today and not to be frightened to take their diabetes with them.

REFERENCES

1   Somogyi, JC, Elmadafa I, Walter, P. New aspects of nutritional status. *Bibl Nutr Dieta* 1994; **51:** 100–4.
2   Rosenstock, IM. Why people use health services. *Millbank Memorial Fund Quarterly* 1966; **44:** 94–127.
3   Birlson, P. The validity of depressive disorder in children and the development of a self rating scale, a research report. *Journal of Psychology and Psychiatry* 1981; **22:** 73–89.

6

Diabetes in the Older Teenager and Young Adult

C. J. THOMPSON AND S. A. GREENE

INTRODUCTION

Adolescence defines the period of physical and emotional maturation between childhood and adulthood. There is little consensus on the time of departure from adolescence; as the remit of this chapter is to discuss the older adolescent and young adult, we shall use an arbitrary upper age limit of 25 years. As the term adolescent is often perceived, particularly by those to whom it refers, to be judgmental and derogatory, we shall use the terms teenager or young adult in this chapter.

The teenage and young adult years are physically and emotionally eventful; the successful negotiation of the physical changes of puberty, and the social and emotional changes such as school examinations, experimentation with sex, alcohol and increasingly, drugs, starting work and leaving home is fraught with difficulties without the added burden of diabetes. The resentment of discipline and authority which is a normal part of the passage through these years often translates into rebellion against the restrictions imposed by good management of diabetes. Glycaemic control typically deteriorates throughout the late teenage years and the frustrations that many physicians develop with regard to missed injections and appointments can develop into confrontation which leads to default from the clinic. In this chapter we shall discuss the problems of living with diabetes and, based on our clinic experience of managing young adults with diabetes, suggest strategies for the management of diabetes in this age group.

Childhood and Adolescent Diabetes. Edited by S. Court and B. Lamb.
© 1997 John Wiley & Sons, Ltd.

EPIDEMIOLOGY

A detailed discussion of epidemiology can be found in Chapter 1, but how does this relate to clinical practice? The age distribution of insulin dependent diabetes mellitus (IDDM) in Tayside is shown in Figure 6.1, and Figure 6.2 demonstrates that for a catchment population of 500 000 the typical district hospital can expect to see 150 young people between 15 and 25 years, though an average-sized general practice would contain only one to five such patients. Almost all patients in this age group have Type I diabetes, though a small proportion may have maturity-onset diabetes of youth (MODY), or, rarely, unusual syndromes such as the Wolfram or DIDMOAD (Diabetes Insipidus, Diabetes Mellitus, Optic Atrophy and Deafness) syndrome[1].

Most teenagers present, therefore, with the classical symptoms of Type I diabetes — polyuria, polydipsia, nocturia, weight loss, easy fatigue during exercise — but with greater public awareness of diabetes, fewer now present with ketoacidosis. In Tayside only 5% of new cases of teenage diabetes require hospitalisation for ketoacidosis[2], although in the USA, 25–40% of young patients present with this condition[3]. The vast majority of teenagers and young adults, therefore, can be managed initially as out-patients and do not require admission for stabilisation or education.

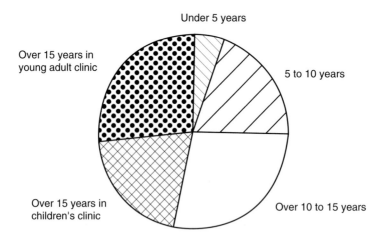

Figure 6.1. Age distribution of young people attending diabetic clinics in Tayside

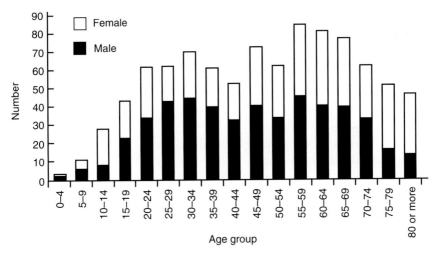

Figure 6.2. Prevalence of insulin-treated diabetes mellitus in Tayside, 1993

METABOLIC ASPECTS OF PUBERTY
AND YOUNG ADULT LIFE

There are profound alterations in the metabolic milieu as a result of the physiological adaptations to puberty and the passage towards adulthood, which commonly manifest as a deterioration of glycaemic control during late teenage years. The onset of normal non-diabetic puberty is characterised by the development of insulin resistance[4], but glycaemic control in teenagers with diabetes is not substantially improved by increased total daily insulin dosage[5]. An excessive increase of insulin dosage during this period of insulin resistance can cause unwanted weight gain[6]. An adjunctive role for IGF1, in addition to insulin, has been proposed as a method of overcoming poor glycaemic control, particularly at night, and has been reported to have short-term success[7], though long-term data are as yet unavailable.

Although there are well documented hormonal and metabolic abnormalities which contribute to poor glycaemic control during the teenage and young adult period, the primary reasons for control difficulties are social and psychological, and it would be a mistake to expect a purely mechanistic or physiological solution to poor glycaemic control.

MANAGEMENT OF DIABETES DURING ADOLESCENCE

A consensus on the management goals for teenagers and young adults with diabetes has recently been considered in Scotland following the original publication of the St Vincent Declaration[8]. This has been incorporated into a document from the Scottish Office and the Scottish Royal Colleges advising physicians and Health Boards on the most appropriate management strategies[9]. In summary, they include the following:

- Promotion of physical and psychological well-being
- Normal growth and development
- Avoidance of hospitalisation, by preventing ketoacidosis and severe hypoglycaemia
- The achievement of good glycaemic control, to prevent long-term microvascular complications
- Adequate screening for the detection of complications
- Integration of the patient into the normal school, social and working life of people in their age group.

MANAGEMENT AT DIAGNOSIS

Confrontation with the diagnosis and the reality of lifelong insulin injections is the single most cataclysmic event in the life of a person with insulin dependent diabetes. For an individual in the psychological maelstrom of the teenage years, where rejection and denial are common emotions, it can be even more difficult to accept the diagnosis and management. The experience of an inexpertly or unsympathetically handled period at diagnosis can lead to denial of the diagnosis and recidivist attitudes which can last for many years. It is essential, therefore, that the initial management is conducted in a sympathetic and supportive manner.

Patients with ketoacidosis should of course be admitted to hospital, but where possible initiation of insulin therapy and education is best conducted as an out-patient, or in the individual's own home.

INSULIN REGIMENS

Once-daily insulin regimens are not appropriate for teenagers and young adults as they can neither achieve the degree of glycaemic control necessary to prevent long-term complications, nor confer the flexibility to accommodate a hectic teenage lifestyle. Most teenagers manage happily with twice-daily injections of soluble and isophane insulins prior to breakfast and the evening meal, with mixing of the insulin in the syringe. Although there has been some resistance in the past to the use of pre-mixed insulins in young people, on the basis that they do not allow the independent adjustment of soluble and isophane insulins, they can be used without deterioration in metabolic control, even in young children, and have the advantage of convenience and patient preference[10]. In practice, many of our patients opt for a multiple injection regimen, despite the more frequent injections, as this allows greater freedom in meal times (and portion sizes) and spontaneity in joining in sport or other recreational activities. Although improved glycaemic control was reported in some early studies with the multiple injection regimen[11], the clinical experience has been disappointing, with little impact on glycaemic control in the long term. Although many teenagers prefer the freedom of the multiple injection regimen, the flexibility to increase insulin dosage to accommodate extra meals and high-calorie foods, such as pizzas, can lead to weight gain, particularly in young women[5]. In practice, the insulin regimen should be individually tailored, according to preference and lifestyle, as there is little to choose between different regimens in terms of glycaemic control. A regimen using three injections a day has achieved popularity, particularly in European countries. Our experience of this type of regimen is limited, and again it does not appear to improve long-term control during the teenage years[12]. We do not use continuous subcutaneous insulin infusion pumps in young adults because of the possibility of rapid onset ketoacidosis if malfunction occurs.

The insulin requirements of young adults vary considerably, with an increase in daily insulin dose at the time of puberty, falling again thereafter. For post-pubertal older teenagers, insulin dosages greatly in excess of 1.0–1.2 u/kg usually represent over-insulinisation, with the risk of hypoglycaemia, rebound overeating and consequent weight gain and elevated glycated haemoglobin concentrations; it is worthwhile attempting gradual supervised reduction in insulin dosage in these individuals.

We routinely start all newly diagnosed patients on human insulins. Although reduced hypoglycaemia awareness has been reported on changeover from animal to human insulins[13], there seems to be no such difficulty in patients who are starting insulin *de novo*, and loss of warning for hypoglycaemia seems to be predominantly a problem of patients with long disease duration whose control was intensified at the time of changeover of insulin species[14].

MONITORING

Routine home urine testing is rarely undertaken on a regular basis by the majority of teenagers in monitoring glycaemic control; they report finding the procedure messy, embarrassing and an interference with everyday life. We feel that measuring urine glucose has no place in the management of young people with diabetes. Measurement of urinary ketones is useful during intercurrent illness, but self-monitoring of blood glucose is the method of choice for assessing day-to-day glycaemic control. Our philosophy has been to stress that blood tests are primarily for the benefit and education of the patients so that they can monitor and manage their diabetes effectively. While the patients are encouraged to perform eight tests weekly, and to record results in a log book, the log book is not routinely examined at clinic appointments, and we avoid turning blood results into an area of confrontation with the patient. Many teenagers have a deep dislike of blood monitoring, even those who will happily give four insulin injections daily, and a heavy-handed approach to blood monitoring can lead to conflict, loss of trust and clinic non-attendance. At the clinic, we spend more time discussing the glycated haemoglobin result, which is available at the time of consultation. We have adopted a clinic policy of discussing the results of the Diabetes Control and Complications Trial (DCCT)[15] and the way in which glycated haemoglobin measured in the patient relates to the results of that study. Blood glucose results are only reviewed at the request of the patient, or if there seems a particular problem with glycaemic control.

DIET

A structured distribution of carbohydrate intake throughout the day is a necessary prerequisite to good glycaemic control. Although a reduced intake of unrefined carbohydrate is preferable, most teenagers have a sweet tooth, and it is often advisable to agree a contract where chocolate or sweets are allowed at certain times of the day, such as prior to exercise. Complete bans on sweets tend to be ignored and it is better to acknowledge that almost all youngsters will eat sweets irrespective of health issues, and deal with the reality sensibly. Teenagers have a very high energy expenditure, particularly if they participate regularly in sport, and adequate calorific intake should be advised.

Eating difficulties are extremely common in teenagers and will be dealt with in more detail later in the chapter. Eighty per cent of non-diabetic teenagers binge on food, and in the diabetic teenager, this can readily lead to weight gain, particularly if total insulin dosage is increased to maintain glycaemic control[5].

SPORT AND EXERCISE

Sport and exercise are the central features of daily life for many teenagers, and diabetic teenagers should be encouraged to participate actively in regular exercise. There is good evidence that exercise increases insulin sensitivity in people with diabetes, but this does not lead to improved glycaemic control[16–18], probably because of increased calorific intake[17]. However, regular exercise does improve cardiovascular fitness, lower cholesterol levels and reduce the long-term risk of vascular disease (Table 6.1). Just as importantly, it provides a medium for mixing with peers, gaining self-esteem and attaining a sense of belonging and achievement.

The vast majority of sports are open to people with diabetes, although some sports, such as boxing, do not allow insulin-treated diabetics to participate, and others, such as martial arts, have some restrictions based on insurance coverage. A full list is given in Table 6.2, and the British Diabetic Association provides comprehensive up-to-date information on all sports, which they readily make available to members. Many individuals with insulin dependent diabetes have competed to international standard, and such professional footballers as Danny McGrain (Celtic and Scotland), Gary Mabbut (Tottenham Hotspur and England) and Alan Kernaghan (Manchester City and the Republic of Ireland) provide high-profile role models for young men with diabetes.

The major disadvantage of sport and exercise in the eyes of young people with diabetes is the tendency to hypoglycaemia, and the avoidance of hypoglycaemia does require extra preparation and care which in some cases can discourage participation (Case History 1). The likelihood of hypoglycaemia depends on many factors, including the pre-exercise blood glucose and free insulin concentrations, the timing of exercise in relation to

Table 6.1. Benefits of exercise in young people with diabetes

- Increased cardiovascular fitness
- Increased insulin sensitivity
- Increased well-being and self-esteem
- Feeling of belonging and achievement
- Lower cholesterol levels
- Reduced long-term cardiovascular and cerebrovascular risk

Table 6.2. Sports with exercise restrictions on participation for insulin dependent diabetes (reproduced courtesy of the British Diabetic Association)

Participation banned	Restrictions on participation
Bobsleigh	Ballooning
Boxing	Gliding
Flying	Martial arts
Horse racing	Parachuting
Motor racing	Paragliding
	Powerboat racing
	Rowing
	Scuba diving

the previous insulin injection and carbohydrate intake, and the duration and intensity of the exercise. The huge variation in sports, individual levels of fitness and exertion, and carbohydrate preference means that general recommendations on how to adjust insulin or diet around the time of exercise are less appropriate than individualised recommendations for treatment modifications[19]. Once individual advice has been given, the confidence to experiment develops rapidly. One specific area to address in the avoidance of hypoglycaemia, is the fall in blood glucose which occurs after exercise has been completed; hypoglycaemia can sometimes occur up to 24 hours after vigorous exercise[20]. This is particularly common if exercise has been sustained over several hours, such as a hillwalk or a long-distance run, and individuals may have to double or even treble their evening carbohydrate intake when on diabetic camps or activity holidays or reduce their daily insulin dose by as much as 50%.

Case 1

A 17-year-old schoolboy, who played soccer with a local semi-professional side, was diagnosed to have insulin dependent diabetes. He started treatment as an out-patient with twice-daily insulin and was doing well until he played his first game of soccer in a highly competitive match. Just before half-time he became hypoglycaemic and disorientated, which contributed to the loss of a crucial goal. He was substituted and, as a disciplinary measure, his club banned him for two matches. In embarrassment he gave up soccer; four years later he does no sport and has gained 11 kg in weight.

Our advice to young people with diabetes who are undergoing planned exercise is to reduce the dose of whichever insulin covers the period of exercise and take extra carbohydrate immediately prior to exercise; the type of carbohydrate depends on the personal preference of the individual and the quantity will be determined by prior experience. We also advise that individuals should have ready access to carbohydrate during exercise and that team mates, fellow participants or referees are aware of the diagnosis of diabetes. We discourage solo long-distance runs, hill walks or mountaineering, and indeed, participation in some sports, such as underwater swimming, is only allowed in the company of a non-diabetic 'buddy'.

We feel that exercise is a very important adjunct to healthy living in diabetes and encourage participation wherever appropriate. However, not everyone likes sport, and in a study of 50 diabetic children and 50 non-diabetic children in our own clinic, we found that diabetic children played fewer team sports, took part less often in parties and made fewer friends than non-diabetic controls[21]. Encouragement to exercise must therefore be very much given on an individual basis.

OUT-OF-CLINIC ACTIVITIES

Out-of-clinic activities have become increasingly recognised to have a useful supporting role in the management of young people with diabetes, though a recent UK postal survey found only one centre in four provided such facilities[22]. Young diabetic groups are often difficult to maintain at a local level, as they depend on the enthusiasm and efforts of both patients and carers. However, although local groups wax and wane, the Youth Diabetes Project, started in 1983, has flourished with the active participation of young people with diabetes from throughout the UK[23]. As well as an annual national conference it runs a variety of courses and camps. Camps are another useful out-of-clinic activity. The Firbush project, run until recently by Dr Ray Newton of Dundee and now supervised by Dr Alan Connacher in Perth, continues to provide an annual adventure camp for 16–22-year-olds on Loch Tay in Perthshire, and the British Diabetic Association runs regular camps for all ages. Further information on the YD Project can be obtained from Novo Nordisk UK Ltd and the Youth Diabetes Group, British Diabetic Association.

ALCOHOL, SEX AND DRUGS

Most young people with diabetes use alcohol to much the same extent as their non-diabetic counterparts, and this can have serious consequences. In the long term, alcohol excess can lead to weight gain and deterioration in glycaemic control but in the acute situation alcohol can have profound effects. Alcohol excess is now the commonest identifiable cause of ketoacidosis in male teenagers, and possibly females, and is second only to abnormal insulin treatment behaviour in young people under the age of 25 years[24]. It is also a major cause of hypoglycaemia and has been implicated in sudden unexplained nocturnal death in young people — the 'dead in bed' syndrome[25]. Although alcohol intake is very much a reflection of the prevailing culture in this country, and thus a complete ban is likely to be ignored, it is important to give sensible advice about intake (Table 6.3). Little is known about the effects of recreational drugs on diabetes, although the feedback from camps and young adult clinics suggests that drug use is just as prevalent in diabetics as in the general population. Anecdotal reports do not suggest acute perturbations in blood glucose following the use of most drugs, although the appetite-stimulating effects of marijuana can lead to binge eating and deviations in blood glucose. 'Ecstasy' (MDMA) is associated with symptoms in teenagers with diabetes mimicking diabetic ketoacidosis: dehydration, hypotension acidosis and hyperglycaemia[26]. Drug misuse is more likely in people with psychological disruption, who

Table 6.3. Advice on alcohol consumption in diabetes (see also 'Alcohol and you' appendix to Chapter 10)

1. Never drink and drive.
2. The safe upper limits for alcohol intake are 21 units/week for men and 15 units/week for women, with two to three alcohol-free days per week.
3. Do not miss meals when drinking alcohol; be sure to have a carbohydrate snack before going to bed if you have been drinking during the evening.
4. Low-sugar 'pils' beers and lagers are very high in alcohol and are therefore best avoided because of the risk of hypoglycaemia. Check low-alcohol lagers for sugar content as some varieties are rich in sugar.
5. It is illegal to sell alcohol to persons under the age of 18 years.
6. Long-term alcohol consumption leads to weight gain.

are at higher risk of 'brittle diabetes'. The combination of poor control and Ecstasy may be lethal. Despite the absence of evidence to suggest specific deleterious effects of drugs in diabetes we routinely advise against their use.

Teenagers are sexually active at an increasingly young age, and although awareness of AIDS has increased the use of barrier contraceptives, unwanted pregnancies still occur regularly in young diabetic females as in the non-diabetic population. Because the effects of poor glycaemic control increase the rate of major congenital malformations, it is essential to prevent unplanned pregnancies in young diabetics. The progesterone-only 'mini-pill' is safe to use in diabetes, although the rate of pregnancy while fully compliant is higher than with a combined preparation. There is continued debate about the effect of the combined oestrogen/progesterone pill on cardiovascular risk, but in non-smokers who have no family history of thrombosis, the low-dose oestrogen combined pills are probably safe. We routinely discuss the issue of contraception and pregnancy with young females with IDDM who attend our 'young adult' clinic; unplanned pregnancies often occur against a background of chaotic glycaemic control with potentially disastrous consequences for fetal development and we feel that adequate counselling and contraceptive advice should be available to men and women at the clinic.

ACUTE COMPLICATIONS OF DIABETES

KETOACIDOSIS

Diabetic ketoacidosis remains the commonest cause of death in young people with diabetes in the UK, and although the mortality rate from ketoacidosis is low amongst young patients[27], the majority of episodes of ketoacidosis do occur in the under-25 years age group[28]. In a recent retrospective survey of all cases of ketoacidosis admitted to Ninewells Hospital in Dundee, younger patients (15–25 years of age) had higher preceding glycosylated haemoglobin concentrations, were more likely to have had recurrent admissions in the preceding five years, had less severe acidosis and dehydration, and were more rapidly stabilised and discharged from hospital than older (>25 years of age) adults[24]. In addition, fewer patients had an underlying organic precipitant to ketoacidosis; the major cause of ketoacidosis in the young adults was abnormal insulin treatment behaviour (Table 6.4). Most clinicians now recognise that omission of, or intermittent compliance with, insulin is the commonest precipitant of ketoacidosis in young adults, and it is almost invariably the cause of recurrent admissions with ketoacidosis. Almost all young people using insulin omit insulin for variable periods of time; and in a minority this manifests as recurrent ketoacidosis. At the extreme end of the spectrum

Table 6.4. Causes of diabetic ketoacidosis (DKA) in a three-year survey in Dundee[28]

Causes of DKA	Patients <25 years (n=52)	Patients >25 years (n=75)
Infective	Gastro-enteritis (n=2) Hepatitis A Viral pericarditis Conjunctivitis (n=5) (Total n=9)	Urinary tract infection (n=14) Pneumonia (n=6) Septicaemia (n=6) Bronchitis (n=2) Tooth abscess Sub-acute bacterial endocarditis Gastro-enteritis (Total n=31)
Others	Alcohol (n=6) Oesophagitis (Total n=7)	Pancreatitis (n=6) Myocardial infarction (n=5) Alcohol (n=5) Haematemesis Ischaemic bowel Hypothermia Carcinoma of the lung Self-poisoning (Total n=21)
Insulin error or manipulation	20	8
Not known	14	10
New diagnosis	2	5

manipulation of insulin dose, as a result of complex social and psychological factors, produces the syndrome of brittle diabetes, where life is constantly disrupted by episodes of metabolic decompensation and frequent hospital admission[24].

Treatment of the acute episode of ketoacidosis differs little in teenagers from the standard management of adult ketoacidosis. Cerebral oedema is far less of a management problem than in young children, and is rarely seen in people over 20 years of age unless large amounts of sodium bicarbonate are given to treat acidosis. Although most cases of ketoacidosis are caused by insulin omission or dosage reduction, underlying illness should be sought; in practice, however, very few investigations yield positive results[24]. A highly important aspect of ketoacidosis management is good education in the convalescent stage, in methods to prevent further episodes. It is rarely helpful, even with incontrovertible evidence, to confront a teenager with the diagnosis of insulin omission, though recurrent admissions should raise suspicion of psychological difficulties with the diagnosis of diabetes, which may benefit from counselling or formal psychological intervention.

HYPOGLYCAEMIA

Hypoglycaemia is an extremely common complication of everyday life for a young person with diabetes. Although most episodes of hypoglycaemia are mild and easily dealt with, severe hypoglycaemic attacks are highly unpleasant and potentially serious complications of insulin treatment. In a recent survey of the attitudes of young people with diabetes to the results of the DCCT, fear of more frequent or more severe hypoglycaemia was the principal reason given by people who were not persuaded to improve their glycaemic control, and was the major concern of those individuals sufficiently encouraged by the result of the study to attempt better control[29]. Episodes of severe hypoglycaemia can also lead to poor glycaemic control in order to avoid further hypoglycaemia (Case History 2, opposite), and hypoglycaemia is greatly underestimated as a cause of behaviour and attitudes which lead to chronic hyperglycaemia.

CHRONIC COMPLICATIONS

It is quite clear that microvascular complications of diabetes are seen frequently in the context of teenage and young adult diabetic clinics. In one longitudinal study of retinal changes in young people with diabetes up to the age of 32 years, fluorescein angiography identified retinopathy in 47% of individuals[30]. The main risk factors for retinopathy were poor glycaemic control and longer disease duration[31]. In a recently published paper in a

---

Case 2

As a young teenager, Ms X had excellent glycaemic control with glycosylated haemoglobin values almost in the non-diabetic range, and her frequent home blood glucose tests, which were supervised by her caring, though over-protective, parents, ranged between 4 and 7 mmol/l. She had frequent mild hypoglycaemic attacks which she dealt with efficiently, with the help of her family. During her first term at University she had stayed up late after a party during which she had drunk more alcohol than usual, and developed a grand mal seizure during an episode of severe hypoglycaemia which was witnessed by several other students. She was rushed to hospital, where X-rays revealed fractures of the second and third lumbar vertebrae. Her determination to avoid further hypoglycaemia led to a marked deterioration in glycaemic control; within four years she required vitrectomy for vitreous haemorrhage from new vessels at the optic disc, but despite this she was registered blind at the age of 24 years.

---

younger cohort (range 10.4–20.6 years), stereoscope fundus photography identified background retinopathy in 41% of a cohort of 203 adolescents[32]. Although some studies have found lower prevalence of retinopathy the message is that a significant proportion of the patient population of a typical clinic will have clinically significant retinopathy. The main adverse risk factors for development and progression of retinopathy are long diabetes duration and poor glycaemic control[31,32], although it has been suggested that the contribution of the pre-pubertal years to the risk of retinopathy is minimal[33]. Interestingly, recent evidence has suggested that depressive illness in young adults may be a marker of risk of retinopathy, with longer duration of depression associated with larger risk of retinopathy[34]. Proliferative retinopathy is, however, uncommon in teenagers and good longitudinal data on the rate of progression from background to proliferative retinopathy are limited. It is clear from the results of the DCCT, however, that good glycaemic control is effective in preventing the progression of background retinopathy to vision-threatening forms[15].

Only a small proportion of patients with IDDM develop clinical nephropathy, and there is some evidence from Denmark that the incidence of nephropathy is declining[35]. However, microalbuminuria, which is an important predictor of renal disease[36], has been reported in 10–20% of post-pubertal teenagers with diabetes[37,38]. In Dundee, 18% of patients attending our young adult (<22 years) clinic have persistent microalbuminuria. Given the powerful predictive value of microalbuminuria in identifying those patients at risk of declining renal function it would seem reasonable to target those with persistent microalbuminuria for intensive input. The DCCT has clearly shown the benefits of tight glycaemic control[15], and our own data show that young adults are particularly inclined to respond favourably to the results of the DCCT[29], so there seems little question that tight glycaemic targets should be set for individuals with microalbuminuria. Aggressive treatment of concomitant hypertension is also accepted to slow down the decline in glomerular filtration rate[39]; debate continues, however, over the role of treatment of normotensive microalbuminuria with angiotensin-converting enzyme inhibitors, which has been shown to slow the rate of decline of renal function[40]. Part of the difficulty lies in establishing what exactly represents normotension or hypertension. Although the World Health Organisation definition of hypertension is 160/95, diagnostic parameters have been redefined by a variety of organisations, such as the American Diabetes Association, as being 140/90 for insulin dependent diabetes. However, a blood pressure of 135/85 may represent significant hypertension in a 16-year-old, particularly if their blood pressure was stable at 110/60 prior to the development of microalbuminuria, and many physicians now intervene with ACE inhibitors at much lower blood pressure readings than traditionally recommended. The concern with this approach remains the issue of drug side-effects, and particularly the teratogenic potential of ACE inhibitors if prescribed to sexually active young women. Our current practice is to treat normotensive microalbuminuria if there is clear evidence of an increase in blood pressure after the development of microalbuminuria. If the patient is female, the need for adequate contraceptive precautions is emphasised.

Although clinical neuropathy is uncommon in this age group, subclinical sensory, motor and autonomic abnormalities can be demonstrated in teenagers, even those with short disease duration. Young and his colleagues in Edinburgh found abnormal electrophysiological tests in 72% and abnormal tests of cardiac autonomic function in 31% of a series of 79 teenage patients[41]. The abnormal results were particularly associated with poor glycaemic control. One of the commonest forms of clinical neuropathy in young people is painful neuritis, usually of the feet, which is usually associated with poor glycaemic control, especially against a background of missed insulin injections. Painful neuropathy has also been described in association with anorexia nervosa[42], and in our experience neuritis can be a troublesome feature of both anorexia nervosa and bulimia, which is often resistant to conventional treatments such as tricyclic antidepressants and carbamazepine. Symptoms usually persist until good glycaemic control is attained, which typically depends on resolution of the underlying eating disorder.

EATING DISORDERS

Young females with IDDM are more likely to be affected by eating disorders than would be expected by chance; in one series, 7% of a large cohort of Scottish females with IDDM, under the age of 25 years, were shown to have a clinically significant eating disorder[42]. This seems to be largely a problem of young females, though males are affected occasionally. When the same workers in Edinburgh used the well validated and objective Eating Attitudes Test (EAT), they found male patients with IDDM score similarly to non-diabetic males, but young diabetic females had higher EAT scores than female controls or either of the two male groups[43]. The underlying factors which lead to eating disorders are complex, including insulin omission to control weight, a background of poor glycaemic control, abnormal attitudes to the change in body image soon after starting insulin therapy and low self-esteem, and all contribute to the psychological milieu which allows the development of eating disorders[42-45]. Patients require flexible and individualised management strategies, which should incorporate a relaxed clinic atmosphere that promotes honest discussion of food intake, glycaemic control and eating attitudes. Psychiatric or psychological support is occasionally valuable, though some patients are resistant to psychiatric interventions. It is important to recognise that patients with eating disorders commonly have microvascular complications, particularly severe retinopathy but also nephropathy and neuropathy, and regular screening for complications is essential.

ORGANISATION OF DIABETES CARE

The transfer of diabetes care from a closely knit, familiar paediatric service to a larger, less personal, adult diabetes service can be traumatic. Adult clinics are perceived as cold, overcrowded and authoritarian, and dissatisfaction often leads to default from the clinic. Equally, teenagers who attend an adult service from the time of diagnosis often feel intimidated by the older population of the typical diabetes clinic, some of whom may be blind, wheelchair-bound or amputees.

We believe that because of the complex physical and emotional changes which occur in the older teenage years, a specific clinic for young people provides the optimum medium for delivery of diabetes care. Many centres now run 'adolescent' or young adult diabetes clinics, with input from both paediatricians and adult physicians, as well as nursing staff, dietitians, chiropodists and, in some cases, psychologists. Enrolment to the young adult clinic is at the discretion of the paediatric staff, who make a judgement based on physical and emotional maturity, as well as the ability to manage diabetes independently of parental control; most patients move 'up' at age 14–16 years and stay until transfer at the age of 22 years.

In Dundee our Young Adult Clinic takes place in a relaxed setting, with coffee-making facilities available in the waiting areas; patients are encouraged to socialise and discuss diabetes amongst themselves. Although patients are free to choose which of the diabetes team they see at each visit, the aim is to screen everyone annually for complications from enrolment with dilated fundoscopy, measurement of blood pressure and micro-albuminuria, and examination of feet and injection sites. The default rate from this clinic is significantly lower than that for young adults who elect to attend the standard adult diabetes clinic. We regard the low default rate as an important attribute of the young adult clinic in view of the high complication rates in chronic clinic defaulters.

Out-of-clinic activities can be extremely valuable adjuncts to a diabetes service. Many teenagers respond well to the opportunity to meet socially with other young people to discuss diabetes and develop their own support structures. Teenagers are often more receptive to the experiences and advice of their peers than to what they may perceive to be the authoritarian dictates of the clinic staff, and young diabetes groups are an important source of support and information for them.

Although most physicians are well disposed towards the concept of out-of-hours activities, time constraints limit the extent to which many are able to contribute. In the USA, study leave and continuing medical education (CME) credits are available for attendance at camps and education holidays, and it may be that the adoption of a similar policy in the UK would lead to more widespread participation in out-of-clinic activities.

Formal diabetic camps have been run by the British Diabetic Association since 1936 and have provided activity holidays for over 100 000 children and teenagers. The Firbush Outdoor Activity Centre on Loch Tay in Scotland provided the venue for a novel camp which sought to harness the powerful benefits of association between teenagers with diabetes to enable them to provide support for those struggling to adjust to life with diabetes[46]. The success of this camp led to the formation of the Youth Diabetes (YD) Project, a nationwide network of young people who meet to share experiences of diabetes. This has acted as a conduit for their opinions on how diabetes services should be styled to best meet the needs of teenagers and young adults. Over the years the YD Project has become an increasingly influential voice within the British Diabetic Association and has made many important contributions to the development of the principles upon which services for young people with diabetes are based.

REFERENCES

1   Drash, A., Lifshitz, L. (eds). *Diabetes Mellitus in the Child; Classification, Diagnosis, Epidemiology and Etiology.* New York: Marcel Dekker, 1996: 555–65.

2   Newton, R. W., Greene, S. A. Diabetes in the adolescent. In *Childhood and Adolescent Diabetes* (Kelnar, C. J. H., ed.). London: Chapman and Hall, 1995: 367–74.

3   Santiago, J. V., White, N. H., Pontious, S. L. Diabetes in childhood and adolescence. In *International Textbook of Diabetes Mellitus* (Alberti, K. G. M. M., DeFronzo, R. A., Keen, H., Zimmet, P., eds). Chichester: Wiley, 1992: 1025–58.

4   Hindmarsh, P. C., Matthews, D. R., Silvio, L. D. I. Relations between height velocity and fasting insulin concentrations. *Arch Dis Child* 1988; **63**: 666.

5   Mortensen, H. B., Hartling, S. G., Petersen, E. E. A nationwide cross-sectional study of glycosylated haemoglobin in Danish children with IDDM. *Diabet Med* 1988; **5**: 871–6.

6   Gregory, J. W., Wilson, A. C., Greene, S. A. Obesity among adolescents with diabetes. *Diabet Med* 1992; **9**: 344–7.

7   Dunger, D. B., Cheetham, T. D., Holly, J. M. Does recombinant insulin-like growth factor (IGF1) have a role in the treatment of insulin dependent diabetes mellitus during adolescence? *Acta Paediatr* 1993; **388**: 49–52.

8   Diabetes Care and Research in Europe: St Vincent Declaration. *Diabet Med* 1990; **7**: 360.

9   Petrie, J. (ed.). *Scottish Intercollegiate Guideline Network (SIGN)*. Edinburgh: Royal College of Physicians, 1996.

10 O'Hagan, M., Greene, S. A. Pre-mixed insulin delivered by disposable pen in the management of children with diabetes. *Diabet Med* 1993; **10**: 972–5.

11 McCaughey, E. S., Betts, P. R., Rowe, D. J. Improved diabetic control in adolescents using the penject syringe for multiple insulin injections. *Diabet Med* 1986; **3**: 234–6.

12 Mortensen, H. B., Hougaard, P., for the Hvidore Study Group on Childhood Diabetes. Comparison of metabolic control in a cross sectional study of 2873 childen and adolescents with insulin dependent diabetes from 18 nations. *Diabet Care* 1997; (in press).

13 Berger, W. G., Althaus, B. U. Reduced awareness of hypoglycaemia after changing from porcine to animal insulins in IDDM. *Diabet Care* 1987; **10**: 260–1.

14 Gerich, J. E. Unawareness of hypoglycaemia and human insulin. *BMJ* 1992; **305**: 324–5.

15 Diabetes Control and Complications Trial Research Group. The effect of intensive treatment of diabetes on the development and progression of long term complications in insulin-dependent diabetes mellitus. *N Engl J Med* 1993; **329**: 977–86.

16 Wallberg-Henriksson, H., Gunnarsson, R., Henriksson, J., DeFronzo, R., Felig, P., Ostman, J., Wahren, J. Increased peripheral insulin sensivity and muscle mitochondrial enzymes but unchanged blood glucose control in Type 1 diabetics after physical training. *Diabetes* 1982; **31**: 1044–50.

17 Zinman, B., Zuniga-Guadjardo, S., Kelly, D. Comparison of the acute and long term effects of exercise on glucose control in Type 1 diabetes. *Diabet Care* 1984; **7**: 515–19.

18 Landt, K. W., Campaigne, B. N., James, F. W., Spending, M. A. Effects of exercise training on insulin sensitivity in adolescents with Type 1 diabetes. *Diabet Care* 1985; **8**: 461–5.

19 Campaigne, B. N., Wallberg-Henriksson, H., Gunnarsson, R. Glucose and insulin response in relation to insulin dose and caloric intake 12 hours after acute physical exercise in men with IDDM. *Diabet Care* 1987; **10**: 716–21.

20　MacDonald, M. J. Postexercise late-onset hypoglycaemia in insulin dependent diabetic patients. *Diabet Care* 1987; **10:** 584–8.

21　Greene, S. A., Thompson, C. Exercise. In *Childhood and Adolescent Diabetes* (Kelnar, C. J. H., ed.). London: Chapman and Hall, 1995: 283–93.

22　Thompson, C., Greene, S. A., Newton, R. W. Diabetes and adolescence. *Diabet Rev Int* 1995; **4:** 2–6.

23　Davies, R. R., Newton, R. Progress in the Youth Diabetes Project. *Pract Diabet* 1989; **6:** 6–8.

24　Thompson, C., Cummings, F., Chalmers, J., Newton, R. W. Abnormal insulin treatment behaviour; a major cause of ketoacidosis in young adults with type 1 diabetes. *Diabet Med* 1995; **12:** 429–32.

25　Tattenall, R., Gill, G. Unexplained deaths of type 1 diabetic patients. *Diabet Med* 1991; **8:** 49–58.

26　Seymour, H. R., Gilman, D., Quin, J. D. Severe ketoacidosis complicated by 'ectasy' ingestion and prolonged exercise. *Diabet Med* 1996; **13:** 908–9.

27　Barn, A., Close, C. F., Jenkins, D., Krentz, A. J., Nattrass, M., Wright, A. D. Persisting mortality in diabetic ketoacidosis. *Diabet Med* 1993; **10:** 282–4.

28　Elleman, K., Soerensen, J. N., Pedesen, L., Edsberg, B., Andersen, O. O. Epidemiology and treatment of diabetic ketoacidosis in a community population. *Diabet Care* 1984; **7:** 528–32.

29　Thompson, C. J., Cummings J. F. R., Chalmers, J., Gould, C., Newton, R. W. How have patients reacted to the implications of the DCCT? *Diabet Care* 1996; **19:** 876–9.

30　Burger, W., Hovener, G., Dusterhus, R., Hartmann, R., Weber, B. Prevalence and development of retinopathy in children and adolescents with type 1 (insulin-dependent) diabetes mellitus — a longitudinal study. *Diabetologia* 1986; **29:** 23–9.

31　Weber, B., Burger, W., Hartmann, R., Hovener, G., Malchus, R., Oberdisse, U. Risk factors for the development of retinopathy in children and adolescents with type 1 (insulin-dependent) diabetes mellitus. *Diabetologia* 1986; **29:** 23–9.

32　Bonney, M., Hing, S. J., Fung A. T. W., Stephens, M. M., Fairchild, J. M., Donaghue, K. C., Howard, N. J., Silink, M. Development and progression of diabetic retinopathy; adolescents at risk. *Diabet Med* 1995; **12:** 967–73.

33　Kostraba, J. N., Dorman, J. S., Orchard, T. J., Becker, B. J., Ohki, Y., Ellis, D., Doft, B. H., Lobes, L. A., La Porte, R. E., Drash, A. L. Contribution of diabetes duration before puberty to development of microvascular complications. *Diabet Care* 1989; **12:** 686–93.

34　Kovacs, M., Mukerji, P., Drash, A., Iyengor, S. Biomedical and psychiatric risk factors for retinopathy among children with IDDM. *Diabet Care* 1995; **18:** 1592–9.

35　Kofoed-Enevoldson, A., Borch Johnsen, K., Kreiner, S. E. Declining incidence of persistent proteinuria in type 1 (insulin-dependent) diabetic patients in Denmark. *Diabetes* 1987; **36:** 205–9.

36　Mogensen, C. E. Microalbuminuria as a predictor of clinical diabetic nephropathy. *Kidney Int* 1987; **31:** 673–89.

37　Mathiesen, E. R., Saurbrey, N., Hommel, E., Parving, H. H. Prevalence of microalbuminuria in children with type 1 (insulin-dependent) diabetes mellitus. *Diabetologia* 1986; **29:** 640–3.

38　Dahlquist, G. L., Rudberg, S. The prevalence of microalbuminuria in diabetic children and adolescents and its relation to puberty. *Acta Paediatr Scand* 1987; **76:** 795–800.

39 Parving, H. H., Anderson, A. R., Smidt, U. E. Early aggressive antihypertensive treatment reduces rate of decline in kidney function in diabetic nephropathy. *Lancet* 1983; **ii:** 1175–9.

40 Marne, M., Chatellier, G., Leblanc, M *et al.* Prevention of diabetic nephropathy with enalapril in normotensive diabetics with microalbuminuria. *BMJ* 1988; **297:** 1092–5.

41 Young, R. J., Ewing, D. J., Clarke, B. F. Nerve function and metabolic control in teenage diabetics. *Diabetes* 1983; **32:** 142–7.

42 Steele, J. M., Young, R. J., Lloyd, G. G., Clarke, B. F. Clinically apparent eating disorders in young diabetic women: associations with painful neuropathy and other complications. *BMJ* 1987; **294:** 859–62.

43 Steele, J. M., Young, R. J., Lloyd, G. G., MacIntyre, C. C. A. Abnormal eating attitudes in young insulin-dependent diabetics. *Br J Psychiatr* 1989; **155:** 525–31.

44 Stancin, T., Link, D. L., Reuter, J. M. Binge eating and purging in young women with IDDM. *Diabet Care* 1989; **12:** 601–3.

45 Steele, J. M., Link, D. L., Lloyd, G. G., Young, R.J. *et al.* Changes in eating attitudes during the first year of treatment of diabetes. *J Psychosom Res* 1990; **34:** 313–18.

46 Newton, R. W., Isles, T., Farquhar, J. W. The Firbush Project–sharing a way of life. *Diabet Med* 1985; **2:** 217–24.

7

The Point and Purpose of the Clinic — Personnel and Practical Aspects

KEN ROBERTSON AND BILL LAMB

POSITION OF THE OUT-PATIENT CLINIC IN THE 'CARE MODEL'

Historically, children with newly diagnosed diabetes were admitted to hospital for stabilisation and education, discharged home after one to two weeks, and then seen regularly in out-patient clinics by general paediatricians with little contact between visits. This model of care is now unacceptable.

Outcomes are known to be better where specialist children's diabetes clinics operate, and both the British Paediatric Association and the British Diabetic Association have issued guidance on minimum standards of care.

The 'clinic' should be staffed by a multidisciplinary team including at least a diabetes specialist nurse, a paediatrician with a special interest in diabetes and a dietitian experienced in diabetes and paediatrics. Ideally, there should also be a child psychologist/psychiatrist with sessional commitments to the diabetes service. Access to a social worker and chiropodist is also helpful.

Where a community-based approach is not possible the diabetes service necessarily revolves around the clinic visit, but a minimum of 24-hour telephone support is required. In an audit of Scottish clinics, however, only 50% were offering this service. The nature of the disease for most patients is that things run relatively smoothly but punctuated by crises, and families

Childhood and Adolescent Diabetes. Edited by S. Court and B. Lamb.
© 1997 John Wiley & Sons, Ltd.

must feel confident that they can reach reliable advice, preferably from someone that they know. Access to a ward nurse or doctor is better than nothing but often parents feel, usually correctly, that they know more about their child's diabetes than such a professional, so telephone support is best provided by experienced members of the Diabetes Team. Practically, this can be provided by a combination of electronic paging devices, mobile phones and a reliable 'on-call' roster held by a central switchboard so that families need only phone once.

THE CLINIC

For most families who have a child with diabetes, the 'clinic' remains the point of contact with medical carers, and it is the responsibility of those carers to ensure that the families benefit from the limited clinic time available. Reasonable clinic aims include support, education, monitoring of control and helping to promote physical and mental well-being. To achieve this, clinics must be effective and flexible in meeting the needs of children and their families. What individual clinics offer depends upon the resources available both physically and personally. The frequency of visits should reflect the needs of families, take account of travelling time, family and school commitments or other activities and be flexible enough to cope with crises. People prefer to have reliable appointment times, become irritated by pointless 'double-booking' but are understanding if more time is needed to solve problems. The norm in the UK is four 30-minute clinic visits a year, one of which is an annual review. Asking patients how clinics can be improved is important but must include all families to avoid the vocal few imposing their own views.

When full community support with visits and telephone advice can be offered, the clinic becomes the opportunity to take an overview of control, assess the usual medical parameters and tie up loose ends, rather than another tiny window of opportunity to stuff as much education down the family's throat as possible. The former approach goes a long way towards reducing family anxiety about coming to the hospital to see 'the consultant' and offers better opportunity to structure the clinic process.

PRE- AND POST-CLINIC TEAM MEETINGS

Preparation produces better results—this is as true in the diabetes clinic as elsewhere. If possible the team should meet briefly before the clinic to discuss known or anticipated problems, for example, excessive weight gain, rising HbA1c results, family strife, problems at school, etc. Patients can then be allocated more rationally and specific issues flagged. At the end of the clinic, the opportunity to discuss problem patients, strategies for change and possible interventions is of benefit to all. Later enquiry by the family to any of the professionals is then less likely to be met with conflicting advice. This is also the time to discuss the follow-up of defaulters.

AGE BANDING OF THE CLINICS

In all but the very smallest centres there will often be sufficient numbers in different age groups to justify segregating the clinic. There are several advantages in this approach. Older children in particular resent having to share the waiting area with difficult toddlers, whose parents in turn may find a surly, leather-jacketed adolescent a little disturbing. The parents also have an opportunity of sharing the experiences and problems that are common to different age groups of children. The size and age distribution of the groups depend upon the size of the clinic but pre-school, primary school and secondary school age groups should be possible.

Pre-school

Children under five years of age are particularly difficult to shoehorn into routines and those with diabetes are no different. The advantage of a supervised diet is offset by the disadvantage that they are often faddy eaters. Parents can be driven to distraction chasing wilful toddlers around the house with carbohydrate that they 'must eat', and allowing similarly afflicted families to meet and exchange strategies is valuable.

Primary School

These children will be at school and taking on more responsibility for their diabetes. Where possible, they can be divided into a younger and an older age group. The five- to 10-year-olds attend primary school and, generally, the routine there is predictable. They will usually have one class teacher per year who can get to know them and how to recognise and manage hypoglycaemic attacks. Children of this age tend not to be away from home much without their parents other than to an occasional British Diabetic Association holiday, Cub Scout or Brownie camp.

The older group, from 10 to 12 years, are on the brink of big changes. They are usually beginning to take on more of the day-to-day management of their diabetes and need support to do this safely and confidently. The girls, in particular, are often beginning to enter puberty, with all the physiological turmoil that this can bring to their blood sugar control. In addition, at 12 years most children are moving into secondary education with big changes to their routines. The effort to pre-empt problems at this stage can be valuable and splitting the age groups aids in this. For example, skills testing and discussion can be group-based rather than one-to-one.

The Over-12s

Teenagers are commonly regarded as the most difficult to manage group of young people with diabetes. There are, of course, many physiological and psychological reasons for this and, if no other age banding occurs, it is at least useful to separate this group from the rest. It will often be best to see the patient without parents, at least at the beginning of the consultation, to allow discussion about broader issues such as alcohol, sex and smoking. This can prove difficult and may have to be deliberately engineered by the team, distracting the parents while the child sees another team member.

It is better to pre-empt these situations by discussion and to set a contract for the next visit. This is also an opportunity to test the diabetes knowledge and skills of the young person. It is often apparent that children who have been diagnosed young and whose diabetes has, of necessity, been managed entirely by their parents for many years, have a poor understanding of the disease. This has been shown to be the case in the Royal Hospital for Sick Children in Glasgow. Recognition of this fact leads to the targeting of education towards those most in need. It is especially important to see such patients alone for some time otherwise the accompanying parent may, from habit, dominate the discussion, leaving the impression of good knowledge and family harmony. It is generally recognised that the teenage years of increasing independence are also difficult for parents, and when the teenager has diabetes this adds to parental anxiety. Efforts have to be made to ease the transition to adulthood and to give sound practical advice about late nights, staying away from home, alcohol, etc. It is a good tactic to get parents to discuss anxieties about adolescent behaviour separate from diabetes and then to give practical advice where diabetes care may be affected.

Transfer to Adult Clinics

At some stage the children become adults and can no longer be looked after by a children's diabetes service. They need to be formally handed over to an adult service, but the age and manner of the transfer will be dictated by local circumstances. A convenient milestone may be the end of secondary schooling. Often there are enormous differences between the way paediatric and adult clinics are run and the culture shock could result in the patient attending no clinics at all. There have always been GP-run diabetes clinics for adults and this may be one option, but these vulnerable patients must not simply be cast adrift because, by the time they seek medical advice again, some of them will have developed microvascular complications. Some units run a special adolescent or 'young adult' clinic with a paediatrician and adult diabetologist consulting together. Smaller units may share the nurse specialist with the adult service and they can act as the common link. Care should be taken to ensure that all relevant information is available and this is facilitated where patient-held records are used. University students can present problems (although many will delay clinic attendance until they are home for holidays) and liaison should be established with their base clinics. Patient-held records may be especially valuable in such circumstances.

GEOGRAPHY OF THE CLINIC

Sadly, the physical environs in which we deliver care to our out-patients are not normally within our control. None the less, something can be done to make the average clinic area more conducive to the purpose. All of us will have experience of the typical clinic geography: a dull waiting area, a receptionist who changes daily and a series of closed doors behind which the consultants sit in their ivory towers. Patients and parents wait, without the inclination or opportunity to converse with others, until they are called. Having seen the doctor, they make an appointment and leave.

THE WAITING AREA

If one professes a special interest in diabetes then patients with this disease are special and deserve to be treated as such. Efforts should be made to provide educational material in a variety of formats. The British Diabetic Association has produced many leaflets and magazines for all ages that cover a variety of issues. Some clinics will also have their own written material covering such matters as adjustment of insulin doses and management of illness. Several centres are lucky enough to have room for educational games to be set up for patients and some, such as Newcastle upon Tyne, have published pamphlets detailing these.

   Since the majority of children are now aficionados of computer games, it is only right that this format should be available for help in diabetes education. Several packages are available (e.g. *Captain Novo*) and can be run on a Personal Computer in the clinic.Videos are another familiar medium for the delivery of information and some clinics have a video playing while families wait. Most companies concerned with diabetes produce a selection of videos that are freely available upon request.

WEIGHING, MEASURING, BLOOD TESTING
AND CONSULTATION

Patients deserve privacy for weighing, measuring and blood testing. Other considerations aside, it is against the guidelines for the treatment of laboratory animals to allow them to watch other animals being bled, so we should treat our patients at least as well. Privacy is also extremely important in the consultation. A minimum of people, other than the family, should be in the room, allowing for the occasional need for students etc. to attend. When other people are sitting in they should be introduced at the outset and permission to attend sought from child and family. There may be times when visitors should be asked to leave.

PRACTICAL MECHANICS

Whatever philosophy underlies a clinic visit, certain practical and house-keeping tasks must be undertaken and some thought should be given to their value and execution.

WEIGHT AND HEIGHT

Auxology is important in the management of any child with a chronic disease and diabetes is no exception. Poor longitudinal growth (which should be measured at least annually) as an indicator of poor glycaemic control is quite unusual but deviations from the centiles should be plotted and the significance considered. Weight (measured at each visit) is a more sensitive indicator — excessive gain associated with overtreatment and loss with poor control. Hypothyroidism or coeliac disease may be suggested by a fall on the centile charts. Measurement is worthless unless accurate and should be performed using suitable equipment by a trained clinic assistant or auxologist.

HbA1c — INSTANT VERSUS DELAYED

It is now inappropriate to manage any child with insulin dependent diabetes mellitus without regular assessment of glycaemic status by haemoglobin A1c estimation. To be of any value this must be viewed in the context of a local paediatric reference range and not simply the manufacturer's quoted range, which will have been established on a non-paediatric population.

All those involved in the care of patients, young and old, with diabetes are agreed that having the current value in front of them when they see the patient has transformed the consultation. We have all played the game of guessing the HbA1c for patients at the time of the clinic, only to find how wrong we were when the results return from the laboratory a few days later. We then have the problem of how best to convey the news (usually bad) to the patient and parents. Many centres now have 'instant' analysis so that assays are performed in the clinic. Where this cannot be justified it is possible to arrange for patients to send samples by post. Capillary blood may be collected onto blotting papers[1] or in a capillary tube[2] and sent to the laboratory in time to provide results for the clinic.

URINE TESTING

There is little value in assessing glycosuria in the clinic. The child may have produced the specimen in the clinic, after a long journey punctuated by a snack. There may be considerable anxiety relating to the clinic visit, and thus a raised blood sugar with spill-over into the urine. There may have been genuine pre-prandial hyperglycaemia — a fact which should be obvious from the blood sugar results and HbA1c.

A check for protein or albumin excretion by stick testing may precipitate a check for urinary tract infection. Ketonuria, except in those obviously unwell, can usually be inferred from the HbA1c and blood sugar results.

The main value of urine testing is screening for microalbuminuria. This should be done on a first morning specimen of urine and positives followed up by timed overnight collections[3].

CLINIC PRACTICE

SHOULD PATIENTS ALWAYS SEE A DOCTOR?

This question lies at the heart of the philosophy of the Diabetes Team. In a team that functions well as a unit and has regular meetings to discuss policies and individual patients, the answer to this question could reasonably be 'no'. This is not to say that each team member does not possess unique knowledge and skills, but is simply recognition of the fact that most patients do not have too many problems most of the time. For them a meeting with the dietitian or diabetes nurse specialist together with feedback on HbA1c levels are all that is required. A structured clinic document will ensure that the appropriate information is gathered. Consistency of approach by all involved will help to strengthen the impression of a well organised team.

The situation is different where there is no community support and the only interaction with the professionals is at the clinic; in this case the doctor should be involved with each patient.

CO-MORBIDITY

Many children will have other illnesses as well as diabetes. These can be medically significant, such as cystic fibrosis, severe asthma or migraine — particularly difficult when vomiting is a feature. They can all affect diabetes control and need managing. Even minor ailments such as warts, sore throats, etc. will be brought to the clinic and, while encouragement to attend the GP is appropriate, the patient and family will still expect intervention by the clinic doctor.

RECORDING THE VISIT

A clearly laid out clinic sheet goes a long way towards ensuring consistency of approach and also hugely facilitates the collection of data for entry into a computer system (see Chapter 12). Each clinic will have its own preferred format but it is the dataset that is critical and not the layout. The best sheets will allow the perusal of several visits at once and require a minimum of free text. It should be immediately apparent who saw the patient on their last visit and what, if any, specific tests, such as retinal examination, are required this time.

WHO OWNS THE BLOOD SUGAR BOOK?

Clinic visits which revolve around the blood sugar book are a breeding ground for problems. This method of delivery of care is not holistic and is geared towards the punishment and reward ideology. For patients who are doing well (perhaps because of the honeymoon period) the overall impression of the visit will be positive. This is not so for those who are finding the going a bit tougher. For them the clinic becomes a huge blot on the landscape, which they first dread then weather the inevitable storm. The natural consequence is to make sure that the results in the book match everyone's expectations. This is managed by either complete fabrication or by only doing tests when the child knows that they will have a good result. The record book then loses any value it may have had.

Despite these comments the record of blood sugars remains important for the management of diabetes. Of course the clinician should view the results if they are proffered and may even ask to see the book, but only the most inexperienced will ask for this immediately the patient enters the room. In turn, beware the patient who enters the room holding the record book in front of them. This is certain to be someone who believes that, in the eyes of the professional, their results are more important than themselves. Now that HbA1c results are readily available, the value of the results book is in offering advice on practical issues such as changing insulin dose or type, meals and exercise.

PATIENT-HELD RECORDS

Some clinics have experimented with patient-held records in a variety of formats. One of us has used such a system for several years, modelled on the Pre-school Parent Held Record. These booklets hold a complete copy of the hospital diabetes records, including the results of all investigations, records of hospital admissions, annual reviews, and a mirror of the clinic flowchart. In addition there are places for the child or family to record 'hypos' and illness. Most children bring their books regularly and some are clearly well used and often referenced. Others 'lose' the book, and some bring it as a ritual of no personal value. It does act as a source of information for other health professionals and has proved useful for some holiday-makers, and university students who may not always register with the university or other health service.

INFORMED CHOICE VERSUS PATERNALISM

Modern medicine is moving towards giving patients and parents a greater say in their care. Little will be gained in terms of family confidence when statements are made at diagnosis about 'becoming their own doctor' if the professionals then encourage a dependent attitude. Clearly, the education process should be geared towards providing enough knowledge of the principles of diabetes management that safe decisions can be made, independently of the Diabetes Team. This situation can be achieved through a combination of one-to-one teaching and the provision of clear, practical written guidance.

This approach has a profound effect upon the running of the clinic. How many of us have shuddered to hear the words, 'We knew we were coming to the clinic, so we didn't want to change anything', and this four or five weeks after control began to deteriorate?

Furthermore, families who can reliably be left to their own devices and who know when to seek help can safely be left a little longer between visits, so freeing up more time for those with problems. Once more, adequate community provision supports this targeting philosophy.

The teenage years are often difficult, when patients seem uninterested in everything and especially their diabetes. It is essential to keep them coming to the clinic and not to alienate them by constant lectures about diet and blood tests. The teenager will know their importance as well as the doctor, and the essence of success is compromise to tide them over the bad spell.

TRANSFER OF SKILLS/RESPONSIBILITY
FROM PARENT TO PATIENT

There is no ideal time for a child to start participating in the care of their diabetes. Some three-year-olds will wish to fire the blood lancet and press the plunger on the syringe or pen, while a few 12-year-olds would rather have everything done for them. Clearly, these are extremes, with most children wishing to learn about injections and testing at around seven or eight years, coinciding with opportunities to spend nights away from home with friends or organisations such as school, the Brownies or Cub Scouts. The offer of certificates or other recognition from a team member can be a powerful incentive for some children.

For the Diabetes Team, the usual role is simply to support the family in the way they choose to devolve responsibility. Occasionally, however, a more proactive role is called for when too much is being expected of a young child. More often an older patient of 11 or 12 requires the encouragement of the team to take a more active part in his/her management. The problem may be an uninterested child, but more frequently it is overprotective parents who, having meticulously followed every instruction for years, have to be persuaded to begin the handover process. It is a common mistake to assume that because the patient has had diabetes for years, they will know all about it. Such children may have to be regarded almost as new patients in terms of the education process, with the added complication that they will most probably have developed ingrained habits.

Such families will require considerable support and often encouragement to stop overprotecting their child and let them find their feet, just as they did years before. It must, of course, be a gradual process of transfer of responsibility, and there will be times, such as during illness, when a reversion to dependency is entirely appropriate.

DISCUSSION

In an environment tailored towards diabetes, and especially if the patients attending are age banded, it is reasonable to hope that families will engage in useful informal conversation. The role of the facilitated group discussion is difficult to evaluate and sometimes even more difficult to get going. None the less, it can be very useful, provided it does not deteriorate into a tutorial by the professional. The wealth of experience amongst parents of diabetic children should be tapped for the benefit of others who may be less experienced or confident. The professional's role in this situation is to act as chairperson and referee. It may not always be appropriate to try to trigger discussion or there is a risk that longstanding parents will become bored and disinterested.

SEX, DRUGS, SMOKING AND ALCOHOL

Sex, smoking and alcohol have long been issues in diabetes. More recently, recreational drugs have presented a growing problem. In the past, adult diabetologists have criticised paediatricians for not addressing these difficult issues, but many children's clinics now have a policy of discussing them before transfer to adolescent or adult clinics. This must be the correct approach, in the light of clear evidence in the United Kingdom that more children are sexually active under the age of 16 and that the prevalence of smoking is actually increasing in young people, especially girls. It is not the role of health professionals to be judgmental about social practices and morals although, clearly, on health grounds alone, it is right to discourage dangerous practices. The anti-smoking campaigns of the 1970s and 1980s proved that scaring people with pictures of black lungs and stories of lung cancer was ineffective. A calm, practical and well informed approach to the issues may be more successful. Remember, many of the patients have learnt to say 'no' to their peers already in response to offered sweets and may find it easier to refuse cigarettes and drugs. Children with diabetes are known, as a group, to be more health-conscious.

Choosing the moment to discuss these topics can be difficult. The odour of smoke, albeit parental, on a patient's hair when examining their optic fundi provides a suitable opportunity to emphasise the risks of cigarette smoking in diabetes. Rather like the dietetic approach to changing a whole family's eating habits, it may be an opportune moment to suggest that parents give up smoking.

Few parents will object to discussion of smoking but sex and drugs may be a different matter. In Glasgow we have been explicit at British Diabetic Association meetings and elsewhere that we will discuss these issues with our patients, and we have met with no hostility. We begin talking about sex when girls reach menarche as the practicality of managing blood sugars during periods provides an opportunity to talk in simple terms about pregnancy and the importance of planning. It is more difficult with the boys, but both boys and girls who are regularly out at discos and raves are at particular risk from exposure to drugs and sexual activity. In some areas, recreational drugs such as Ecstasy, temazepam and LSD are available in schools, so local knowledge will dictate when and what discussion are appropriate. Many Health Authorities and other bodies produce excellent leaflets on the individual properties and dangers of these drugs. Such material should be available in the clinic — and read by the professionals!

When so much effort may have gone into providing integrated family support for a patient's diabetes over many years, it is a clever feat to instil in a young person the confidence that they can bring worries over such matters to the diabetes clinic in the knowledge that their revelations and questions will remain confidential. This realisation is critical to the development of individual responsibility.

THE MEMBERS OF THE TEAM

DOCTOR'S ROLE

Traditionally, the doctor is the leader of the Diabetes Team. The principal reason is medico-legal, with a named physician being responsible for the patients. With the expanding role of Nurse Practitioners, including Diabetes Nurse Specialists, this may change. Democracy is fine but there is a requirement for leadership in any organisation and patients, parents and staff feel more comfortable when this is apparent. It will be clear that the 'doctor' in this context is the consultant paediatrician. There must be a place in the clinic for doctors in training, but efforts should be made to ensure that they follow the ethos and philosophy of the team. The diabetes clinic is probably one of the easiest medical clinics to drift through with neither understanding nor useful contribution because families do so much for themselves. However, it is insulting to experienced parents and patients to subject them to the musings of innocents who may attempt to cover their ignorance with arrogance — and who of us has not been guilty? It is here that the 'Battle of the Blood Sugar Book' is most often waged. Junior doctors should sit in with the consultant for several clinics before being allowed to see patients alone and, even then, they should report back to the consultant or Diabetes Nurse Specialist before despatching the family.

Practically, the doctor should act as the hub of the clinic — a focus for those problems that cannot easily be solved by the other team members. Every clinic has challenging patients and it is with these that the consultant can most usefully spend time. Some problems may be related to diabetic control but, more commonly, the difficulties with diabetes are merely symptomatic of chaotic lifestyle and social deprivation. It is critical that, in those rare cases where parental neglect is responsible for problems, the consultant takes the lead in any child-protection proceedings. There may be other medical concerns, as in those patients with co-existing problems such as hypothyroidism, asthma or epilepsy. Very often, other members of the team will present a patient's problem together with the solution and all that the doctor has to do is concur.

The doctor will also have the main role in formulating policy on drugs and equipment as company representatives may target any member of the team. Regarding insulin, most clinics use a relatively small range of products so that they acquire familiarity and therefore, as in any other area of medicine, new products must offer clear benefits.

DIABETES NURSE SPECIALIST'S ROLE

Diabetes Nurse Specialists (DNS) often run the service and are essential. They are in continuous contact with patients and develop close relationships with the families. This gives insight and understanding rarely shared by the doctor unless the team communicates effectively. Given that diabetes is so sensitive to social and emotional turmoil, these factors must be weighed in reaching management decisions. The DNS will often see patients alone in the clinic, and this is entirely appropriate. It would, after all, be odd to allow professional development of the role out of hospital only to expect a subservient attitude in the clinic. With her intimate knowledge of family, social and school circumstances the DNS is able to present difficult problems to the doctor in such a way that solutions are suggested. Moreover, she will know what further support will be required to implement change and can arrange home and school visits as appropriate.

DIETITIAN'S ROLE

Children with diabetes should all have access to the skills of a dietitian, preferably one with a special interest in diabetes and paediatrics. Few centres will have enough patients to justify a dietitian dedicated only to diabetes, but efforts should be made to ensure continuity with one or two individuals identified to provide the service. In the average children's clinic there will be toddlers, young schoolchildren, teenagers and perhaps even one or two babies. Their dietary needs and habits are poles apart and beyond the experience of adult dietetics. Theory must bend to practicality and there is no place for the standard lecture based on 'Thou shalt not have...!' Where a community service is provided, the dietitian will see the family's and patient's diet in the context of home circumstances. This crucial insight begs a pragmatic approach. Annual Reviews apart, the dietitian should attend the clinic and space should be provided for her to see families alone when detailed advice is required. Sometimes she may accompany the doctor and/or the DNS in a consultation, particularly for a new family's first visit to the clinic.

PSYCHOLOGIST'S ROLE

The majority of children's diabetes clinics will not have a clinical psychologist attending. However, most now have access to the service by referral. The benefit is greatest where the psychologist has a special interest in diabetes. While the value of psychology input to the clinic is hard to quantify, it would be a very unusual clinic population that did not contain several individuals from each age group with obvious problems of adjustment to diabetes. Examples include needle phobia, eating disorders and denial of their diabetes. The main advantage of having a psychologist as part of the team and attending clinics is that their formulation and plan can be integrated into the approach of the others. Additionally, it is hugely valuable for the psychologist to sit in with the other team members to provide feedback on their approach to patients and families. A great disadvantage of the pyramidal structure of medicine is that, on achieving consultant/specialist status, doctors can happily consolidate all their bad habits without the moulding influence of critical review. As part of the team, particularly if introduced at the time of diagnosis, seeing the psychologist/psychiatrist is less of a threat to the child and family.

SOCIAL WORKER'S ROLE

Once again, only the largest clinics will have the dedicated services of a social worker and the Diabetes Nurse Specialist often takes on this role. Many of the intractable problems in the diabetes clinic will have a social element. Material and practical help can often make a huge difference to a family's ability to cope with the disease. Identification of a social worker prepared to take a special interest in diabetes is an advantage. Amongst other things, filling out the Disability Living Allowance forms (UK) requires a lot of help and there may be other benefits and grants available, for example funding for provision of a telephone (Rowntree Trust).

In adult practice, when a patient repeatedly defaults from clinics, attempts will usually be made to persuade them to attend but, ultimately, it is their choice. Paediatrics is rather different because of the child protection issue and a more dogged approach, supported as necessary by the Social Services, may be required.

ANNUAL REVIEW

The concept of an annual review is enshrined in most documents on provision of diabetes services. There are, however, a number of ways to achieve the same ends. A separate clinic session may be held periodically to process a batch of patients but this is probably not practical in centres with large numbers. A more *ad hoc* approach is only possible if those seeing the patients always check to see when the last review was performed.

Centres will differ in what investigations are performed, influenced by research interests, etc. The following should be examined at least once a year.

INJECTION SITES AND TECHNIQUE

The injection sites should be examined and appropriate advice given on rotation of sites. Explaining about differing absorption times and the practical implications can act as an encouragement to rotate, as can a reminder of the cosmetic disadvantages of 'lumps'.

BLOOD PRESSURE

Given the growing evidence that raised blood pressure has a role in diabetic renal disease[4], it is justified to begin measurement early in a patient's career. The baseline data are then available later when one is trying to assess whether or not blood pressure is abnormal. This area of monitoring, like assessment of microalbumin excretion, could reasonably be described as research, but large clinics should be participating in projects aimed at elucidating the links between these factors.

FEET

Good habits of foot care learned in childhood may prevent later problems in adults. Simple advice on cutting toenails and referral of any problems, such as verrucae, to a chiropodist can be offered.

EYE EXAMINATION AND MICROALBUMIN SCREENING

There is now ample evidence[5] that the pre-pubertal period is not 'safe' and that duration and control before puberty do matter, but the pick-up rate for retinopathy and microalbuminuria in pre-pubertal patients is certainly very low, even when using the most sensitive techniques.

From a practical standpoint, then, annual checks for microvascular disease can reasonably be delayed until around 12 years of age, and disease duration of four years. Some centres have retinal photography available and screening can be done on alternate years. Eye tests are free to people with diabetes and local opticians may be involved in screening programmes, particularly for adults. It is often reassuring to all for a detailed examination to be carried out by an ophthalmologist after 10 years' duration.

AUTO-ANTIBODIES ETC.

Given the strong association between Type I diabetes and other auto-immune diseases, it is reasonable to screen periodically for evidence of impending thyroid disease by assaying serum T_4 and TSH and looking for anti-thyroid antibodies. Addison's disease is rare (0.03% of IDDM)[6] but will usually be preceded by anti-adrenal antibodies and presents with falling insulin requirements.

Coeliac disease is reported to occur in almost 5% of patients with IDDM[7], so some centres screen annually for anti-gliadin, anti-endomysial and anti-reticulin antibodies. Positive results need confirmation by jejunal biopsy before the enormous burden of a gluten-free diet is imposed.

LIPIDS

Dyslipidaemia is strongly associated with ischaemic heart disease and, diabetes apart, this is a major killer in many parts of the world. Abnormalities in lipid profile have been described in children with diabetes and an association is found with metabolic control[8]. It is perhaps worth screening at least once to exclude familial dyslipidaemias. Clearly, more careful dietetic and/or drug management would be required in those with abnormalities.

DIETARY AND DIABETES NURSE SPECIALIST REVIEW

Where a paediatric dietitian has not been in regular contact with the family during the year, the opportunity to review dietary management is usually welcomed, at least by parents.

Techniques of blood testing and injection should be reviewed, since bad habits are readily acquired. Modern meters which do not require careful timing or stick wiping have made this aspect of care much easier, although poor technique can still lead to major errors in blood glucose estimation. Pen injectors similarly have simplified life for the average patient.

CONCLUSION

The diabetes clinic is quite different from most other medical paediatric clinics. The patients get to know one another, most of them will be in rude good health throughout their childhood, and they have far more influence on the eventual outcome of their disease than any member of the Diabetes Team. None the less, it is vital that families keep coming to the clinic; visits must therefore be made as pleasant as possible and offer more than a pat on the head or rap on the knuckles. Children's diabetes clinics, and those who staff them, should be dynamic, adaptable and receptive to new ideas.

REFERENCES

1 Eckerbom, S., Bergquist, Y. Improved sample collection technique for capillary blood on filter paper for determination of glycated haemoglobin. *Ann Clin Biochem* 1989; **26:** 148–50.
2 Shah, A. R., Challner, J., Elsey, T. S. *et al.* A novel capillary collection method for obtaining current glycosylated haemoglobin levels in diabetic children. *Diabet Med* 1994; **11:** 319–22.
3 Shield, J. P. H., Hunt, L. P., Baum, J. D. *et al.* Screening for diabetic microalbuminuria in routine clinical care: which method? *Arch Dis Child* 1995; **72(6):** 524–5.
4 Gilbert, R. E., Cooper, M. E., McNally, P. G. *et al.* Microalbuminuria: Prognostic and therapeutic implications in diabetes mellitus. *Diabet Med* 1994; **11:** 636–45.
5 Bonney, M., Hing, S. J., Fung, A. T. W. *et al.* Development and progression of diabetic retinopathy: Adolescents at risk. *Diabet Med* 1995; **12(11):** 967–73.
6 Lifshitz, F. (ed.). *Pediatric Endocrinology—A Clinical Guide.* New York: Marcel Dekker, 1996: 725.
7 Sigurs, N., Johansson, C., Elfstrand, P. O. *et al.* Prevalence of coeliac disease in diabetic children and adolescents in Sweden. *Acta Paediatr* 1993; **82(9):** 748–51.

8   Azad, K., Parkin, J. M., Court, S. *et al.* Circulating lipids and glycaemic control in insulin dependent diabetic children. *Arch Dis Child* 1994; **71(2):** 108–13.

FURTHER READING

Johnston, D. I. Children's diabetes clinics. In *Childhood and Adolescent Diabetes* (Kelnar, C. J. H., ed.). London: Chapman and Hall, 1995: 323–30.

8

The Role of the Paediatric Diabetes Specialist Nurse

JEN CANE AND HILARY RICHARDSON

INTRODUCTION

Diabetes is the commonest endocrine disorder of childhood and is a life-long chronic condition. It is now estimated that there are at least 20 000 people under the age of 20 with diabetes in the UK[1]. Recent data suggest that the incidence of diabetes in childhood is increasing and the onset is occurring at a younger age. Therefore the demand for paediatric diabetes specialist nurses is likely to continue in future years.

The Paediatric Diabetes Specialist Nurse (PDSN) is central to the process of responding to the needs of children with diabetes and their families and is the hub of the Diabetes Team. In order to provide and deliver a high-quality paediatric diabetes service, PDSNs, along with other team members, need to consider certain priorities, some of which are listed below.

1. Having a clear philosophy for a team approach.
2. Having guidelines of practice for the clinic and in-patient unit that take account of Royal College of Nursing guidelines[2].
3. Promoting ongoing education involving:
   — the child/family
   — other health professionals in the hospital or community setting.
4. Facilitating and co-ordinating effective care which is also accessible and therefore efficient. This 'priority' involves interpersonal communication skills which will require diplomacy, encouragement, use of specialist knowledge and organisational skills involving a network of people and agencies.

Childhood and Adolescent Diabetes. Edited by S. Court and B. Lamb.
© 1997 John Wiley & Sons, Ltd.

5. Taking responsibility for personal development needs, keeping up-to-date with specific and general health issues, and recognising the value of research-based practice, with the implication of possible improvements to the service[3].
6. Monitoring the service offered by audit, i.e. by measuring the efficiency, effectiveness and economics of the 'service' according to resources available.

BACKGROUND AND HISTORY

The first nurses with specific responsibility for patients with diabetes were instigated in the early 1950s in Leicester by the late Dr Joan Walker, and were known as 'Diabetes Liaison Health Visitors'.

Specialist nurse posts were developed in the 1970s — the majority of nurses entering these posts had previously worked as ward sisters or community nurses. The number of specialist nurses increased rapidly during the 1980s and early 1990s. In 1996 there were approximately 650 Diabetes Specialist Nurses (DSNs) working in the UK[4]. Along with the increase in the number of DSNs who work with adults, there has also been a steady increase in the number of PDSNs.

Every health authority in the UK now has a minimum of one specialist nurse who looks after children as well as adults with diabetes. Of that total number of DSNs (650), fewer than 100 are PDSNs working exclusively with children, and only two-thirds of these will be in full-time employment[5].

There have been similar developments in 'specialist nurse roles' in the USA, Australia and some parts of Europe. Nurse practitioners developed in America in the 1970s and subsequently evolved into specialist nurse educators. In Australia, the first paediatric diabetes educator was appointed in 1978. In some countries, e.g. Germany, the role of the DSN has developed more recently as part of the development of a comprehensive training programme available to both nurses and dietitians[6].

In France the PDSNs are all hospital-based and do not perform any work in the community. Therefore, all newly diagnosed children are admitted to hospital. Once they are discharged home, the PDSNs maintain contact with the families by telephone and by asking them to attend the hospital for further teaching sessions. Interestingly, state child benefit allowances may be affected if families do not attend their local children's clinic for health, growth and development monitoring by the paediatrician — perhaps this is a significant incentive to attend.

In Holland, most children are cared for by DSNs who have a small number of children on their caseload. There are now a few PDSNs, all are hospital-based with community care follow-up responsibilities and with caseloads of 50–75 children. The programme is also developing to care for the children at home at the time of diagnosis.

Doctors and dietitians are the major educators in Sweden, particularly at the time of the child's diagnosis. It is only later that the PDSN becomes involved[7].

TRAINING AND STRUCTURE

There are great variations between different countries in the training of DSNs. In the UK a Royal College of Nursing (RCN) working party reported in 1993[8]. This recognised the importance of teaching and counselling skills as well as general nursing skills for PDSNs. They need to be able to work with children who have diabetes and their families, both at home and in hospital. The Report recommended that nurses caring for children with diabetes should have paediatric, community and diabetes qualifications. The first children's diabetes course in England, however, had been started in Birmingham in 1978 by Janet Kinson. Since 1982 the English National Board (ENB) gave recognition to a diabetes course (ENB 928) that is now available in at least 20 centres throughout England with a comparable course in Scotland. However, these courses provide very little training in the care of children with diabetes. There is only one course currently available in the UK totally dedicated to the care of children, 'The Management of Children's Diabetes' course held at Birmingham Children's Hospital. In the adult field new diploma and degree courses in diabetes have now been established; there are no comparable courses in paediatric diabetes.

Within the UK there are great variations in the numbers of PDSNs in different areas and the way in which they work. In some areas, DSNs working with adults also have a number of children on their caseloads. Despite these small numbers, children and their families require a disproportionate amount of the DSN's time, emphasising the fact that children's needs are very different from those of adults with diabetes. Some PDSNs work part-time with children with diabetes and part-time in another capacity, for example school nursing, ward or clinic work, or with children with other chronic conditions such as asthma and cystic fibrosis.

PDSNs in the UK may be hospital- or community-based. There are large variations in the size of the PDSN's caseload and in the geographical area being covered. A pattern of 70–80 families to each PDSN, however, seems to be emerging as an appropriate goal.

Many PDSNs in the UK are working in isolation, whether they are based in hospital or in the community. In some areas, PDSNs are in an office with adult nurse colleagues, allowing the sharing of experiences and the development of common strategies of care; this in turn facilitates transfer of children to the adult service. In other areas, the PDSN may be part of a team of community paediatric nurses and would have the benefit of peer support, as all would be working with children with varying conditions but similar needs.

National Groups, such as the UK RCN Paediatric Diabetes Special Interest Group, provide support for all nurses involved in caring for children with diabetes. The bi-annual study days organised by this group offer PDSNs from the different regions of the UK the opportunity to meet and to share ideas and working practices.

HOSPITAL AND HOME

It is recognised that children and adolescents with diabetes have very different needs from adults with diabetes. Children and adolescents should be cared for by specialist paediatric diabetes teams[9]. The PDSN is a key player within the paediatric diabetes team, and is the person with whom many of the children and families have the most contact.

Despite the pioneering work carried out in Leicester, where newly diagnosed children have been cared for at home since the 1950s, most centres in the UK continue to admit newly diagnosed children to hospital for their initial stabilisation and education. By admitting children to hospital, the parents are freed from having total responsibility for their child at a time of great stress, medical and supportive care being provided by others. The parents need to be given time to grieve for the healthy child they have lost, and it can be argued that the start of this process can be helped by being in hospital. Alternatively, when a newly diagnosed child is cared for at home, normal routine can be maintained more readily. The family can all be together at home, something which is rarely possible in hospital when there are other siblings to be cared for, as well as the child with diabetes. As it is their own home they are likely to feel more in control of the situation.

In the authors' children's diabetic unit there is one full-time and one part-time PDSN for 132 patients and their families. We cover a large geographical area which includes the City of Newcastle upon Tyne and the mainly rural county of Northumberland (see Figure 8.1). Fifty-eight per cent of the families live in Northumberland, 38% live in Newcastle and the remaining 4% have been referred to the clinic from outside our normal catchment area.

At present it is our policy to admit all newly diagnosed children to hospital for their initial stabilisation and education. This may be for a minimum of two to three days for a child who is well at the time of

NORTHERN REGION

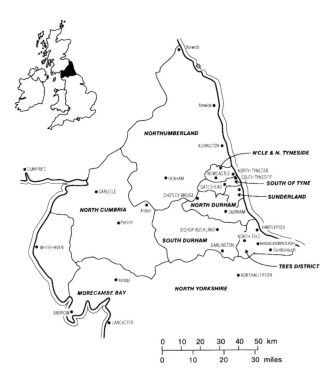

Figure 8.1. Map of the Northern Region

diagnosis, but may be for as long as 10 days if a child presents in severe ketoacidosis, or is young and lives 50–60 miles away. The average stay for the majority of our children is five to seven days.

The child and the family will have the diagnosis of diabetes confirmed by one of the consultant paediatricians. Simple explanations will be given to the family at this time about how we treat diabetes and what to expect in the next few days (treatment by daily injection of insulin, blood and urine tests, and likely discharge date).

It is important for the PDSN to meet the child and family as soon as possible after diagnosis, so that the foundations of a good working relationship can be laid. The PDSN's first meeting with the family must not be rushed. This is not a time for teaching, but a time for introductions and for beginning to get to know each other. It is also a time for listening to the child and the family, allowing them the opportunity to talk about their feelings and fears. Simple explanations may be needed to remove some of the common misconceptions which families may have about diabetes (e.g.

relationship to past sweet eating; no more sweets; the need for a special diet). For most families, the diagnosis of their child's diabetes is distressing but often tinged with relief, often accompanied by feelings of sadness and guilt, particularly if one of the parents has diabetes themselves. Mothers and fathers may manage their feelings of grief in different ways and at different rates[10]. Any information given to them, particularly in the first few days, will need to be repeated, often many times. It is for this reason that we do not begin teaching the families about diabetes for the first 24 hours. Any 'teaching process' can only be effective if the feelings of shock are acknowledged and discussed[10].

Parents can feel guilty over a number of issues.

- Failure to recognise symptoms initially
- Getting cross over the drinking or bed-wetting
- The past diet and the child's sweet consumption
- A family history of diabetes ('it's not on our side').

All these can get in the way. Good counselling skills are needed at this point to eliminate any sense of blame.

It is beneficial for the family to be involved in the practical aspects of the child's care early on. The thought of giving the injection is often much worse than the reality of actually doing it. For the child it is important that their first injection is not too traumatic, and it should therefore be given by the PDSN or an experienced member of the ward staff (the child's named nurse).

INITIAL TEACHING

Sufficient time must be allowed to teach the practical skills of blood testing, urine testing and injections, since good technique is a crucial factor in achieving optimum control. Families will vary considerably in the time they need to master the practical skills.There are no rules dictating the age at which a child should be doing their own blood tests and injections, they will do them when they are ready. Some quite young children see it as a new adventure, they are the centre of attention and may do extremely well in hospital, but the novelty can wear off once at home, and they may refuse to take part at all, preferring Mum and Dad to take the responsibility for practical tasks. Even with older children who are confidently doing their own blood tests and injections, it is still necessary for parents to have these practical skills (for use in times of illness or emergency).

The formal teaching programme can usually begin after the first 24 hours; hopefully the family can start to concentrate and retain new information given to them as they face up to the diagnosis. Initially, the family will have many questions and may bombard the PDSN and the dietitian with lots of them at one session. While it is important to answer all the questions honestly[7], it is very important for the 'educator' to control the teaching session and focus on essentials; more complex questions may need to be laid to one side to be answered after the family have acquired basic information and understanding. Parents should be encouraged to write down questions so that they are not forgotten.

Ewles and Simnet[11] suggest that people learn best when they are actively involved in the learning process and not just passively listening. This is especially true with children. Their need for involvement in the teaching/ learning activities can be as great as that of their adult carers. Children learn through play and are more likely to retain information which is given to them in the guise of 'fun and games'[12] (Figures 8.2, 8.3, 8.4, 8.5 and 8.6).

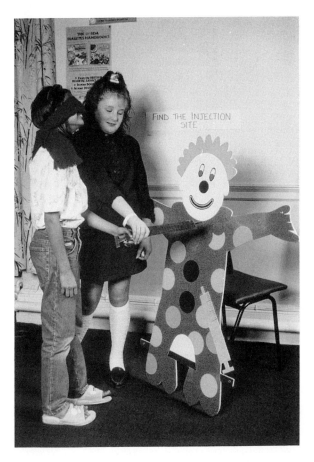

Figure 8.2. Find the injection site. (Reproduced by permission of the University of Newcastle upon Tyne)

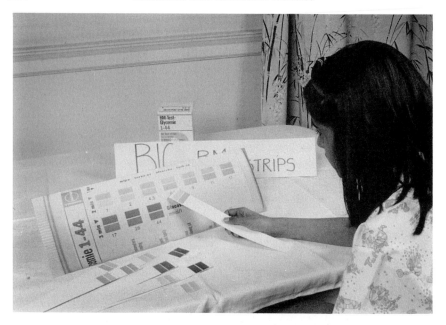

Figure 8.3. Learning to read blood glucose strips. (Reproduced by permission of the University of Newcastle upon Tyne)

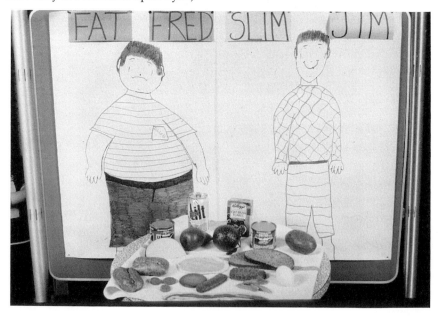

Figure 8.4. Healthy eating! (Reproduced by permission of the University of Newcastle upon Tyne)

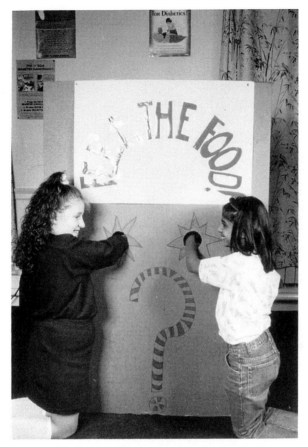

Figure 8.5. 'Feel the Food!' (Reproduced by permission of the University of Newcastle upon Tyne)

Teddies and dolls can be used for demonstrating blood tests and injections; finger puppets can make blood testing time more a 'fun-time' than a painful chore. Encouraging the children to draw pictures of their own body helps when giving simple explanations. It is fascinating to watch a four-year old child draw, along with the parent and PDSN (who guides the 'physiology' lesson). Words and concepts which relate to the picture emerge during the conversation, e.g. tummy, fingers, head, legs, eyes, etc.; this knowledge can be used to good effect, particularly when discussing the relationship between food absorption, glucose levels and insulin. In addition it gives a measure of child and family understanding of biology, i.e. a baseline. Drawing also helps the child understand that there are parts of the body that can be seen, and parts which are not seen ('insides and outsides').

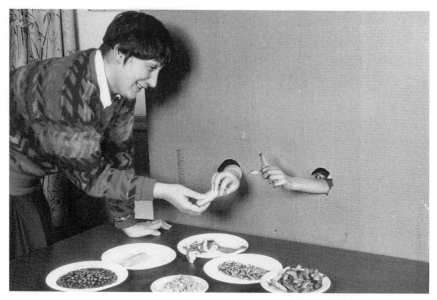

Figure 8.6. 'Feel the Food!' (Reproduced by permission of the University of Newcastle upon Tyne)

With babies and young children, the teaching obviously needs to be directed mainly towards the parents (carers) as they will be responsible for the care of their child's diabetes in both the short and medium term. However, it is still important to involve even young children in the educational process, since it is 'their diabetes'. This age-group can show their awareness of the practical day-to-day skills of their carer by holding the finger in readiness for the blood glucose test, and watching and keeping still during insulin time. It is important for as many family members as possible to be included in the teaching process, including other siblings, who could feel resentful of all the extra attention that the child with diabetes is having. We encourage both parents to be actively involved in the 'teaching sessions'. With single-parent families, it is important for the main carer to have another adult to support or share the responsibility. Grandparents, aunts and uncles may be involved in weekend stays or baby-sitting in a normal family way — this now needs to take account of the necessary diabetes care. The BDA produce a leaflet called *When a Child with Diabetes Comes to Stay*.

Liaison with other members of the Paediatric Diabetes Team, particularly with the dietitian, ensures that the topics discussed, the progress made by the family, and the areas that need further work, are identified. Checklists can be used as a guide but a personalised teaching plan (curriculum) will prove more comprehensive[13].

There is a great temptation to overload families with new and complex information. The duration of the initial teaching sessions must be short, the content simple and focused on the practical, and significant breaks allowed between sessions. Backing up the verbal exchange with written guidance is essential (Figure 8.7). The 'team' approach gives families consistent information and ensures that they are not exposed to conflicting advice.

It is also important to recognise the people who are involved in the child's life. All of them need to have basic education in caring for the child during their time of acting *'in loco parentis'* (Figure 8.8).

PRACTICAL POINTS

Hypoglycaemia is an important topic to discuss, and once the family has grasped the fundamental issues surrounding this, plus the appropriate treatment, they are considered 'safe' to go on trips to a nearby park or shops. This pattern of reintroducing ordinary activities allows families to find their feet, and can show the influence play and exercise may have on blood glucose levels. While 'hypos' are unlikely to occur at this stage, it is important that the families understand:

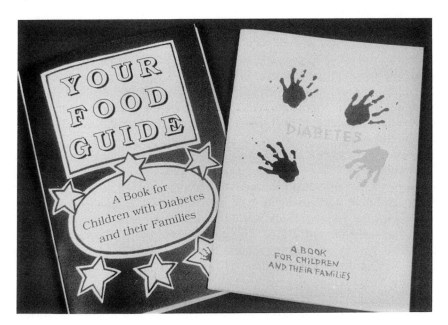

Figure 8.7. A photograph of locally produced leaflets. (Reproduced by permission of the University of Newcastle upon Tyne)

Childhood and adolescent diabetes

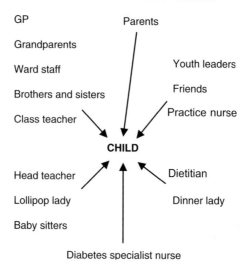

GP
Parents
Grandparents
Ward staff
Youth leaders
Brothers and sisters
Friends
Class teacher
Practice nurse

CHILD

Head teacher
Dietitian
Lollipop lady
Dinner lady
Baby sitters

Diabetes specialist nurse

Figure 8.8. Some significant people in a diabetic child's life

— causation
— the physical symptoms
— the associated feelings
— the treatment.

It is not our practice to produce an artificial hypoglycaemic episode on the ward. We feel it is unpleasant, difficult to achieve, potentially dangerous and disruptive of management at a time when hopefully confidence is emerging. In addition, during the early 'honeymoon phase' hypoglycaemia is uncommon and theoretical knowledge learnt in hospital months before may be forgotten.

We start all newly diagnosed children on a pen system for their injections. Traditionally we have used the BD pop pens, as the ability to make adjustments in single-unit increments is important in the care of babies and young children with diabetes. The children seem to like the colourful patterns on the pen, but there is now a wide choice.

We have a policy of staged discharge home which allows a family a 'protected period' of learning in the home environment before they are finally discharged from hospital. The trip out to town or the park is followed by two more stages.

1. Going home for an afternoon, which will include a blood test, insulin injection and tea at home before returning to the children's ward to sleep overnight.

2. Going home the next day to stay overnight; this would encompass a 24-hour care plan which would be reviewed the next day to sort out any problems encountered prior to the final discharge from hospital.

For each family the actual discharge process is adapted according to their needs and the geographical area in which they live — it would be highly impractical for a family living 60 miles away to follow the above plan.

KEEPING IN CONTACT

The PDSN and the dietitian routinely work from Monday to Friday and generally keep 'office-hours', and this must be remembered if a child is ready to be discharged home at the end of the week. Adequate provision must be made for supporting the family over the weekend.

Before discharge it must be made clear to families how they can make contact with the Diabetes Team, and the kinds of situations where contact is expected (illness, high and low blood sugars, ketonuria). Families must not feel inhibited about making contact at this stage. Specific arrangements need to be made with the family regarding telephone contact times during their initial few days at home. If possible the PDSN should be with the family at the first injection time at home.

During working hours the PDSNs should have an internal hospital 'bleeper', and a radio-pager in order to work effectively in the community, together with a mobile phone; this both enables a rapidly accessible response to family calls and ensures the PDSN's personal safety when travelling alone in remote, sparsely populated rural regions or inner-city areas that may be derelict and dangerous. When nurses are working alone another danger is that of professional 'burnout'. It is therefore important that the work is shared, for example by relieving the PDSN of out-of-hours work, i.e. evenings, weekends and public holidays; these can be covered by a rota-system manned by the medical members of the Diabetes Team, also contactable by a radio-pager. In this way families have access to specialist advice 24 hours a day. This service is also available to other professionals concerned with children with diabetes including General Practitioners, Primary Health Care Team members, baby-sitters, school teachers and youth group leaders. It is important that information about the Diabetes Team service is prominent in the separate literature of those local organisations, particularly schools.

A family's access to 24-hour support would seem to be a cornerstone of the provision of a high-quality service. It is clearly appreciated by families at all stages of their experience and there is little doubt that it, together with the development of the PDSN, has had a dramatic effect on the readmission rates to hospital of children with diabetes. More particularly the families gain in confidence knowing that a 'safety net' is in place. For the smaller clinic this may be difficult to put in place, but it is possible by providing the families with the diabetes consultant's home phone number and by allowing families to phone the children's 'in-patient' ward direct. This can be supported by recruiting one of the acute unit nurses to take a greater interest in diabetes by linking regularly with the PDSN. When a problem is emerging for a particular child it is imperative that effective communication between the different arms of the service is maintained — 'forewarned is forearmed'.

Very regular contact needs to be maintained with the families of newly diagnosed children once they are discharged from hospital. This contact can be in the form of telephone calls, home visits and clinic visits. The families with newly diagnosed children will often initially require frequent home visits. However, this presents difficulties for PDSNs covering large geographical areas, although it should be possible with careful planning to save time by making routine visits to other families in the vicinity. A great deal of PDSN work is done by telephone and this may appear to be more cost-effective in terms of the number of families that might be contacted in the time taken to travel long distances. The telephone, although essential, has limitations; information that has been given to families over the telephone can be misinterpreted. Some families are not comfortable using a telephone, and the nurse needs skill in controlling the conversation while helping the parent or young person convey relevant information in an ordered way at a time of anxiety. Although there may be little time to 'gossip', this can help families relax and prevent them from feeling a nuisance, and help sustain a 'shared-care' relationship. It is important that families do not feel let down by an apparent lack of time for their concerns. For the PDSN, it can be difficult to get the balance between efficient use of time in dealing with problems and education and sustaining the developing relationship. It is important to remember that families are not all the same and may need different approaches. Although there are many ways of recognising the family that is becoming more confident, the reduction in phone calls is one; similarly an increase indicates 'problems'. Logging of phone calls and advice describes this, supports continuity of care and serves as a mechanism for audit, i.e. measurement of this element of work.

Home visits are likely to generate the best environment for the PDSN's work — parents are more relaxed and nurses can gain insight into the other pressures that impinge on family life. The diabetes educational process can, however, be impaired if there is competition from the television, other children and the dog!

PDSNs need local guidelines and protocols for work that can be carried out on the telephone, relating to adjustments of insulin and advice during illness; these should be worked out together with the consultant. PDSNs, along with many other nurses, have concerns relating to the legality of providing information to families over the telephone. There is currently no explicit guidance to nurses regarding this, and the legal position still needs to be effectively clarified[14].

CLINIC ORGANISATION

The role of the PDSN in the organisation of the clinic is fundamental. This is particularly the case when age banding is used, i.e. children of comparable age come to the same clinic. The PDSN is well placed to construct the clinic groups so that friendships between families can develop, especially if they also live near each other. In our clinic each child receives appointments for the whole year, allowing families to plan ahead.

The children routinely have four clinic visits per year, of which:

— two are routine visits
— one is for the annual review
— one is for an education session.

Education of the children and families must be ongoing; research in Newcastle in the 1980s suggested that education was possible using a group format, which improved parent and child knowledge of diabetes and glycaemic control. Watson and Court[12] have described how this has been developed within the clinic process. The PDSN's role as educator is a major ongoing responsibility, which can take place opportunistically at times of change, at camp (see later) or formally in a 'new patient clinic', but mostly will occur during the home visits and by telephone during problem-solving. It is essential that the team has common approaches — one of the PDSN's roles is to feed back to team members any inconsistency in guidance identified by her contacts with families. Similarly it is important to recognise that families and children obtain their information from a wide range of sources, and that these can be contradictory:

• Books, which may be out of date
• Neighbours and relatives with diabetes who may have been educated differently in the past
• The family doctor and practice nurse
• The school doctor and nurse
• The school dinner lady or teacher that has diabetes
• The media (scaremongering)
• Their diabetic peers (teaching 'bad tricks').

The role of the PDSN is to correct misinformation, to promote good practice and to educate the wider constituency where this is possible. Formal strategies for this may include the development by the PDSN of groups or education workshops in order to deal with particular concerns. For example, there may be groups for:

— parents of very young diabetics
— newly diagnosed 'parents'
— weight control in adolescents (held in conjunction with dietitian and psychologist).

Workshops may be held for:

— primary school teachers
— nursing colleagues
— Games/PE teachers.

Other opportunities to educate the wider public arise at times when money has been collected for children with diabetes and is being presented, often with local media present.

In our clinic we do not have a set age at which we transfer young people to the adult clinic, this is decided on an individual basis. This is, however, an important opportunity for the PDSN to review individually a young person's knowledge of diabetes and awareness of potential pitfalls as they approach a time of increasing independence and sometimes isolation. It is clearly important to liaise with adult services carefully in order to minimise the drop-out rate from clinic surveillance that frequently occurs at this time.

The PDSN is well placed to inform families about other agencies such as the British Diabetic Association (BDA) and to encourage young people to join. There are comparable organisations in America, Australia and some European countries, all of which belong to the International Diabetes Federation (see Appendix 2 — Useful Addresses). The BDA has its own checklist of what care should be available to children and supports the St Vincent Declaration guidelines for minimal standards of care[15]. They also reinforce the family's own responsibilities to accept and respond to the diabetes service offered to them.

The Paediatric Diabetes Team should give their advice and assistance to any local initiatives which offer help and support for families; fund-raising and the development of a local parents' group are examples. While supporting such a group, the PDSN should not feel pressurised to be the main instigator or the sole organiser.

HOLIDAYS

Many children with diabetes will attend activity holidays specifically for children with this condition. These may be organised nationally by the

BDA, or locally by individual clinics. This subject is discussed in greater detail in Chapter 18. The PDSN should act as a facilitator for informing families of the varied opportunities available, in getting appropriate paperwork sorted out and ensuring that the child and family have been well prepared. One way of informing families is to have a news board in the clinic to which families and staff can both contribute. It is not unknown for schools to be very reluctant to take children with diabetes away on school trips, or, if they do, to impose unrealistic demands on families. This 'crisis' time is a chance to educate teachers and to set up support for them that allows a child to go on the trip in a normal way; the PDSN can be seen working as an advocate for the child. Similarly, if the family are planning holidays abroad this gives the PDSN a good opportunity to revise aspects of diabetes care with the child and the family. Information and advice may be needed about how to cope with long journeys, flying across different time zones, heat, humidity and different types of food (see Chapter 11).

The PDSN needs to keep up-to-date with changes in the equipment being developed for blood testing and injections (Figures 8.9 and 8.10. See also Chapter 11). This may be achieved by keeping contact with representatives from the major firms supplying such equipment. For a child it is important to be able to choose their own equipment. However, the selection they can choose from must be up-to-date, safe to use and suitable for use by a child.

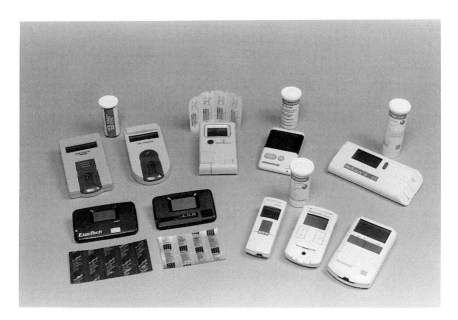

Figure 8.9. A selection of blood glucose meters. (Reproduced by permission of the University of Newcastle upon Tyne)

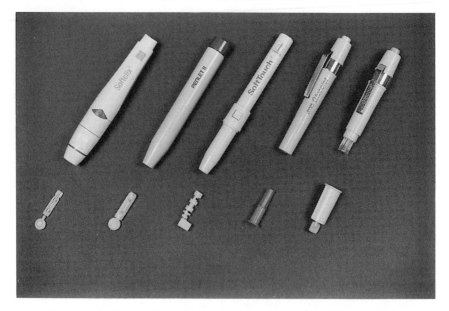

Figure 8.10. A selection of blood-letting devices. (Reproduced by permission of the University of Newcastle upon Tyne)

Whilst the care and education of the children and families is the principal role of the PDSN, there are other aspects which need to be considered that affect the child directly or indirectly. The network of people who are involved in a child's life can be extensive and varied. It is important that activities enjoyed prior to diagnosis are interfered with as little as possible, by keeping the interests of the child central to any arrangements. The PDSN may need to be patient and be prepared to spend a great deal of time with extended family members, teachers, the football team coach, dance instructors and leisure group leaders, amongst others. The child needs to feel confident in the supervision received from an adult carer, and the carer needs the knowledge to provide safe care. When this works well it can promote self-confidence in the child, improve peer group acceptance (rather than rejection) and generate increasing confidence in carers to include children with diabetes in all activities.

SUMMARY AND CONCLUSIONS

The role of the PDSN is varied and at times complex, being an amalgam of carer, advocate, co-ordinator, educationalist, councillor, nurse and liaison officer. The following attempts simply to list the principal elements.

1. Clinical care.
2. Liaison with:
   - School (school meals, trips away, emergency care, school nurse support)
   - Primary Health Care teams (emergency care, prescriptions, changes in clinical management, nurse support)
   - Employers.
3. Teaching:
   - Children and parents
   - General Practitioners' study days
   - Nurses (English National Board course 928, P2000 student nurse and nursery nurse courses)
   - Ward staff update
   - Teachers—away day seminars on chronic conditions of childhood that affect a child's education.

It is important to recognise the individual contributions to the educational process that all members of the 'Team' make and how these emerge as a coherent educational package for children and families. We would argue that the PDSN is fundamental to the success of this process.

4. Advocacy and counselling:
   - Assisting families with applications for social benefits and supporting them during appeals tribunals (Disability living allowance)
   - Support during discussions at the school—health interface
   - With employers
   - With parents and their adolescents when relationships are 'fragile'
   - With young people over drugs, smoking, alcohol, contraception and driving insurance
   - With families that are irrevocably breaking up.
5. Organisational skills:
   - In the running of the clinic (need for computing skills to facilitate audit)
   - In the organisation of outside-clinic activities/camps
   - Parent group support
   - Fund raising.

Children with any chronic condition are being encouraged to enjoy as full and as active a life as possible at school and at home. PDSNs should promote this philosophy by encouraging the child/young person with diabetes to achieve the skills, knowledge and self-confidence to be able to manage diabetes in a safe, well controlled manner. This is likely to be achieved best where a real partnership for care develops, initially between parents and health professionals and then with the young person as they achieve independence. The contribution to be made by the PDSN is considerable. It is their understanding of the physical condition, the monitoring of growth and development and the ability to appreciate the psycho-social needs of families which are so important. In addition the PDSN is well placed to recognise the times when additional support from dietetic, medical and psychological colleagues becomes necessary.

ACKNOWLEDGEMENTS

The authors thank Benedicte Kakou, PDSN, Robert Debre Hospital, Paris and Katja Zuur, Juliana Children's Hospital, Holland for providing their updated information.

REFERENCES

1   BDA. *British Diabetic Association Report 1996: Diabetes in the United Kingdom.* London: BDA, 1996.
2   Royal College of Nursing. *Paediatric Nursing: 1995. A Philosophy of Care. Issues in Nursing and Health.* London: Royal College of Nursing, 1995.
3   Department of Health. *A Vision for the Future.* London: HMSO, 1993.
4   *Directory of Diabetes Specialist Nurses.* London: British Diabetic Association, 1995.
5   *Paediatric Diabetes Special Interest Group Directory, 1995.* London: Royal College of Nursing, 1995.
6   Tattersall, R. B., Gale, E. A. M. (eds). *Diabetes Clinical Management.* Edinburgh, London: Churchill Livingstone, 1990: 132.
7   Forsander, G. Family attitudes to different management regimens in diabetes mellitus. *Practical Diabetes International* 1995; **12:** 80–5.
8   Royal College of Nursing. *Paediatric Diabetes Special Interest Group Working Party Report: The Role and Qualifications of the Nurse Specialising in Paediatric Diabetes.* London: Royal College of Nursing, 1993.
9   Clinical Standards Advisory Group. *Standards of Clinical Care for People with Diabetes.* London: HMSO, 1995.
10 Kubler-Ross, E. *On Children and Death.* New York: Collier Books, 1985.
11 Ewles, L., Simnett, I. *Promoting Health: A Practical Guide to Health Education.* Chichester: John Wiley, 1991.
12 Watson, S., Court, S. Group education in the diabetes clinic using a format. *Practical Diabetes* 1994; **11:** 142–4.
13 Stephenson, A. Learning for life. *Paediatric Nursing* 1992; **3–4:** 6–8.
14 Glasper, A. Telephone triage; A step forward for nursing practice. *British Journal of Nursing* 1993; **2:** 2.
15 World Health Organisation and International Diabetes Federation. The St. Vincent Declaration. *Diabetes Medicine* 1990; **7:** 360.

9

The Concept of Control

DEBBIE MATTHEWS

INTRODUCTION

The noun 'control' is defined as a restraint, a regulation or a check. Complete biochemical control of diabetes is the normalisation of blood glucose concentrations together with other disordered metabolites such as lipids and growth factors. However, because of deficiencies in the therapeutic modalities for diabetes, complete control of the condition is not yet possible. This chapter is not about personal control but describes the objective assessment of diabetic control, the definition of control and the reasons for wanting good diabetic control, and discusses the factors which affect control.

THE ASSESSMENT OF GOOD CONTROL

The assessment of diabetic control may be laboratory-based, as in the case of glycated haemoglobin and fructosamine assays, or home-based, as in the monitoring of blood or urinary glucose.

LABORATORY MEASUREMENTS

Glycated Haemoglobin

The measurement of glycated haemoglobin is widely used in both clinical practice and research to assess glycaemic control, as the blood level of glycated haemoglobin reflects the integrated blood glucose concentration over a period of six to eight weeks. The term 'glycated haemoglobin' refers

Childhood and Adolescent Diabetes. Edited by S. Court and B. Lamb.
© 1997 John Wiley & Sons, Ltd.

to a series of minor haemoglobin components, HbA1a–c, which are stable ketoamine derivatives of adducts formed between glucose and the amino-terminal valine of one or both β chains of normal adult haemoglobin, HbA. They were first isolated by cation exchange chromatography in 1958[1]. Following this, several studies demonstrated a significant decrease in glycated haemoglobin levels about four weeks after improving glycaemic control in patients with diabetes[2].

The most commonly used methods to assay glycated haemoglobin fall into two broad groups: those which depend on charge to separate glycated HbA1 from HbA, which include ion-exchange chromatography, High Pressure Liquid Chromatography (HPLC) and agar-gel electrophoresis, and those which depend on some other property and measure 'total' glycated haemoglobin, such as affinity chromatography. At present, none of the methods available for quantifying glycated haemoglobin is ideal; there is no consensus on either a reference method or glycated haemoglobin standard. The test results from one laboratory cannot be compared directly to those obtained in another laboratory. This means that each laboratory must establish its own normal ranges and standards for glycated haemoglobin. Ideally, separate ranges for children should be derived.

The advantages of glycated haemoglobin as a test of diabetic control are that it is objective, independent of the patient's co-operation and independent of the time of the last meal, and that it reduces diabetic control to a single number which reflects blood glucose concentrations during the previous six to eight weeks. The major disadvantages of glycated haemoglobin are the non-standardisation of the assays and the finding that short periods of poor control, up to two weeks, lead to a disproportionate increase in HbA1 concentration. The measurement gives no information about the lability of blood glucose concentrations.

Fructosamine

Fructosamine is a measure of the non-enzymatic glycation of proteins in blood, the major constituent of which is albumin. Because of the shorter half-lives of serum proteins in comparison to haemoglobin, the measurement of fructosamine reflects integrated glycaemia over a much shorter time period, about two weeks. The fructosamine assay uses the ability of ketoamines to act as reducing agents in alkaline solution. The assay is easily automated, rapid, cheap and highly reproducible[3]. However, there is concern about the specificity of the assay, and factors other than glycated protein may also contribute to the reaction. Another problem is that short-term fluctuations in serum protein levels can lead to variations in measured serum fructosamine of up to 10%.

The advantage of the method is that it may be used to detect a response to a therapeutic manoeuvre earlier than with glycated haemoglobin. On the other hand, since glycaemic control in children can vary significantly over a two-week period due to factors such as intercurrent illness or holidays, fructosamine measurements may not reflect average glycaemic control over the usual three-month period between clinic visits. It has been shown that fructosamine is a poor indicator of HbA1 values, with wide 95% confidence limits, indicating that it is impossible to predict accurately longer term glycaemic control from fructosamine measurements[4]. Since major studies on the prevention of microvascular complications in diabetes have used HbA1 levels to assess glycaemic control, it is suggested that measurement of HbA1c should be used in all children with diabetes in preference to the measurement of fructosamine. Fructosamine measurements may be a useful adjunct for short-term monitoring of changes in insulin therapy.

Advanced Glycation End-Products

As blood glucose increases, glucose rapidly attaches non-enzymatically to the amino groups of proteins. Some early glycated products are degraded but those formed on collagen, DNA or other long-lined macromolecules undergo further rearrangement to form advanced glycation end-products (AGE). Through their effects on protein function and signal transduction, it is likely that AGEs have a central role in the pathogenesis of diabetic complications. It has been suggested recently that the measurement of haemoglobin-AGE may provide a longer term measure of diabetic control, reflecting blood glucose concentration over a greater proportion of the red cells' life, and may reflect more closely the extent and risk of diabetic microangiopathy[5]. Haemoglobin-AGE may be measured by a competitive ELISA technique. However, the method is relatively new and has not yet been evaluated as a measure of glycaemic control in children.

HOME-BASED MONITORING

Blood Glucose

Isolated random blood glucose readings yield little information about overall control because they tend to be performed at the same time of day and may not be representative of overall blood glucose levels. However, blood glucose readings performed frequently and at different times provide useful information about glycaemic control. Capillary blood glucose self-monitoring with reagent strips and/or a reflectance meter has been in use from the 1970s onwards. There are various systems in use, many of which are entirely satisfactory.

Most reagent strips consist of glucose oxidase immobilised with peroxidase and a chromogen. The colour developed is proportional to the glucose concentration and may be compared visually with a reference chart or read in a reflectance meter. The usual test sites are the sides of finger ends, *not the fingertips*, and should be used in rotation. Toes can be used during infancy, and ear lobes are also occasionally used. The development of spring-loaded devices and very fine lancets to obtain capillary blood has made the process less painful and more acceptable.

Blood glucose monitoring is generally acceptable to children and some adolescents. The frequency of testing varies within and between individuals, from several times a day to rarely, but a request for one test a day at varying times is reasonable for a child or adolescent who is in good health. The target should be to keep blood glucose levels at 4–10 mmol/l but this goal may be adjusted according to individual circumstances. Regular monitoring can provide a useful profile allowing adjustment of insulin dosage or diet to be made appropriately as indicated. It allows for confirmation of both hyperglycaemia and hypoglycaemia and therefore gives some indication of the lability of blood glucose concentrations.

The variability of blood glucose concentrations may be expressed in a number of different ways. The M value is a quantitative index of the deviation of several blood glucose measurements from a mean standard. The mean amplitude of glycaemic excursions (MAGE) is a measure of within-day glycaemia stability[6]. These measures reduce detailed data to a single number which is useful for research. However, in the clinic, simple observation of home blood glucose records is probably more useful for assessing the stability of glycaemic control.

The main disadvantage of home blood glucose monitoring is that it is highly 'user-dependent' and requires the patient and their family to be well motivated and educated in order to carry out and derive benefit from it. All methods depend on scrupulous technique to be reliable. Some are very time-sensitive and a deviation of a few seconds in the various sequences of testing can lead to unreliable results. Inadequate sample size gives a falsely low reading. These anomalies are discovered by some children and used to manipulate results. The relatively old method of BM stick testing, which is relatively time-stable and allows for a visual check, may be the most reliable where 'difficulties' in sampling are encountered.

Urinary Glucose

The home monitoring of urinary glucose using disposable strips is still common, although it has been superseded by blood glucose monitoring in many paediatric clinics. The technique is attractive since it is non-invasive although it only gives a crude reflection of the prevailing blood glucose concentration and may be misleading. Glycosuria is the net result of two distinct processes, glomerular filtration and the tubular reabsorption of glucose, both of which may differ among patients. Thus, the interpretation of results may be made difficult by the variability of the renal threshold for glucose in the individual child. The average renal threshold is about 10 mmol/l but a negative urine test may be found with a blood glucose concentration of 2–22 mmol/l and 2% glycosuria may occur with normoglycaemia[7]. Urine testing does give some assessment of blood glucose levels between voiding and can be very helpful as part of an overall assessment. Unfortunately urinalysis does not give information about hypoglycaemia so there is a tendency by some children to aim for some glucose in the urine, which may lead to higher average blood glucose levels.

THE OVERALL ASSESSMENT OF CONTROL IN THE DIABETIC CHILD

In summary, no method of monitoring a child's diabetic control is entirely satisfactory. The measurement of HbA1 is objective but retrospective. It provides a measure of integrated glycaemic levels and, therefore, does not give any indication of where problems in diabetic control arise. It should be noted that HbA1 determination may be the only way of assessing management in the child or adolescent who refuses to carry out any home-based monitoring. Blood glucose monitoring provides instant information for the patient and family, indicates the lability of blood glucose levels and may guide day-to-day management.

A problem may arise when there is a large discrepancy between blood glucose monitoring results and glycated haemoglobin. Children who produce sheets of normal blood glucose concentrations but have elevated levels of HbA1 may be fabricating the results or are only testing when they think their blood sugars are normal. An unexpectedly low HbA1 in a child with high daytime blood glucose concentrations may indicate an abnormal haemoglobin or alert the family and clinician to the presence of prolonged nocturnal hypoglycaemia.

It should be noted at this point that the monitoring of diabetes control will not lead to improved control unless it is backed up by intensive support and education. This point will be discussed further later on. In summary, the practical methods available for assessing control are:

- Capillary blood glucose
- Urine glucose
- Fructosamine
- HbA1c
- AGE
- Growth.

REASONS FOR ACHIEVING GOOD DIABETIC CONTROL

Having discussed the assessment of diabetic control, one must now investigate the reasons why good control is desirable, together with the goals of diabetic therapy. Diabetic control may be considered in terms of the short-, medium- and long-term goals.

SHORT-TERM GOALS

On a day-to-day basis it is desirable to control diabetes adequately to allow the patient to feel well, to prevent the symptoms of hyperglycaemia such as polyuria and polydipsia and to avoid as far as possible hypoglycaemia and recurrent diabetic ketoacidosis. Well managed diabetes should have little or no effect on school attendance, academic performance or sporting and other activities.

MEDIUM-TERM GOALS

In the medium term, the goal of diabetic control is to promote normal growth and physical maturation. Severe growth failure secondary to chronic poor blood glucose control, the Mauriac syndrome, is a rare phenomenon nowadays. However, it has been shown that height velocity is a highly sensitive index of blood glucose control. Studies show that there are significant effects on the growth of children with diabetes, including a reduced pubertal growth spurt in girls and growth retardation in boys[8]. Excessive weight gain is common, particularly in adolescent girls with diabetes. However, the relationship of obesity to glycaemic control is not well defined and may occur in adolescents with both good and poor glycaemic control.

LONG-TERM GOALS

In adults and adolescents there can now be little doubt that improved glycaemic control can positively affect the long-term risk of developing nephropathy, retinopathy and neuropathy. In the Diabetes Control and Complications Trial (DCCT) over 1400 subjects with insulin dependent diabetes aged 13–39 years were followed for up to nine years[9]. There were two groups of patients; those receiving intensive therapy achieved a steady mean HbA1c of 7% and those receiving conventional therapy achieved a mean HbA1c of 9%. The risk of new retinopathy was reduced by 76% in the intensively treated primary prevention cohort and the risk of progression of retinopathy was reduced by 50% in the intensively treated secondary intervention cohort. Similar reductions were seen in patients on intensive therapy for rates of new microalbuminuria, proteinuria and neuropathy.

These results are most encouraging but in clinical practice it would be most helpful to know if it is necessary to achieve an HbA1c level of <7% in order to realise the benefits of intensive therapy, or whether reducing HbA1c from 9% to 8% confers some benefit. Because the DCCT did not randomise patients to different levels of glycaemic control, such questions cannot be answered with certainty. However, secondary analysis of the data suggests a continuous risk gradient for the control–complications relationship which means that any improvement in glycaemic control is likely to be associated with reduced risk of complications[10].

The relative benefits of intensive versus conventional treatment were nearly identical in adults and adolescents in the DCCT. However, the DCCT allows very few conclusions to be drawn about the treatment of children before puberty. It has been suggested that the contribution of the pre-pubertal years of diabetes on long-term microvascular disease is minimal. However, these conclusions have been challenged recently[11]. Certainly proliferative retinopathy may appear during late adolescence in children with long-standing diabetes, suggesting that the pathological process commences in the pre-pubertal years.

The major adverse effect found in the DCCT was a three times increased risk of severe hypoglycaemia in the intensively treated group. There was no evidence that this led to increased mortality or severe morbidity and there was no trend toward deteriorating neuropsychological or cognitive function over the course of the study. However, hypoglycaemia remains the therapeutic hazard most feared by children with diabetes and its impact must not be underestimated. There is some evidence that recurrent hypoglycaemia leads to cumulative damage to cerebral function and impairs intellectual capacity. Behaviour and cognition are certainly disrupted during a hypoglycaemic episode, which may be detrimental to schooling. Thus, an increased incidence of hypoglycaemia may be particularly hazardous in children.

The duration of diabetes and the quality of diabetic control are important determinants of microvascular disease, but because of individual factors do not necessarily predict their development in individual patients. The genetic and environmental factors responsible for individual susceptibility remain unknown. In the DCCT there was an incidence of 25% new cases of microalbuminuria. This clearly suggests that factors other than overall glycaemic control are as important in the aetiology of microvascular complications. It is possible that large variations in blood glucose concentrations over extended periods may contribute to microangiopathy. Although improved overall glycaemic control reduced the appearance of microalbuminuria in the DCCT, much more impressive primary prevention has been achieved in both animal and human studies by the use of ACE 1 inhibitors[12].

In summary, good control of diabetes is desirable to prevent symptoms of hyperglycaemia, to allow normal growth and development, and to prevent long-term microvascular disease. Probably only moderate control is needed to ensure the first two goals, keeping blood glucose concentration around 10 mmol/l. The prevention of long-term microvascular disease requires tighter glycaemic control, which may be appropriate for the post-pubertal child. However, one should pause before striving for near normal glycaemic control in pre-pubertal children since it carries a risk of frequent and serious hypoglycaemic episodes with no proven benefit in terms of long-term complications. Other factors may be just as important in determining long-term microvascular disease, and further research is indicated.

THE PRACTICAL CONTROL OF DIABETES

We must now consider the factors which influence the monitoring of diabetic control, the setting of therapeutic goals and factors which affect the child's control of his diabetes.

THE MONITORING OF DIABETIC CONTROL

The monitoring of blood glucose is invasive but quite convenient and simple to perform. There is a degree of fascination associated with blood letting for many children. Many older children and adolescents find urine testing repugnant and the need for privacy to collect urine samples and perform tests is inconvenient. It has been shown that the simpler and quicker the monitoring test and the less unusual the circumstances in which it is performed, the likelier it is to be done. Thus, except in very young children, blood testing is frequently preferred to urine testing. Devices which give results rapidly are beneficial and newer blood glucose reflectance meters which give results in a few seconds rather than a couple of minutes may be very helpful.

For a parent, child or adolescent to carry out blood glucose monitoring they need to be convinced that this is useful. Monitoring is only really of practical value if it leads to corrective action. It is important that all monitoring tests and tests of HbA1c levels are discussed fully with the child and his family and any necessary changes in therapy made after full discussion. There is no general agreement about the frequency of blood glucose monitoring and it depends on many factors such as the level of control sought, the motivation of the child and his family, and compliance. Children should not be overburdened with too many requests for tests and parents should not be converted into zealots in blood glucose monitoring. Children and adolescents reluctant to test may fabricate records to increase the number of tests apparently done or to improve on results obtained. This may be suggested by discrepancies between blood glucose monitoring records and the HbA1c level and confirmed by recalling values from 'memory' reflectance meters. If fabrication is occurring, it is important that this is managed sensitively in a non-judgmental manner. It may help to discuss with the child the purpose of the monitoring and that the testing is for the benefit of the child and not for the doctor, specialist nurse or dietitian.

SETTING THERAPEUTIC GOALS

Compliance with diabetic therapy over long periods of time presents many difficulties for children, adolescents and families. Realistic goals for diabetic control should be worked out on an individual basis and may differ considerably between children depending on a variety of factors such as personality, duration of diabetes and age. Strategies such as positive reinforcement may help families and adolescents to set long-term care goals and to monitor their own success at achieving and maintaining those goals. Praise is given whenever those aims are achieved. Conversely, criticism by the Diabetic Team will discourage the child and is likely to damage their compliance. It is important that the diabetic clinic is not run solely on biochemical results.

FACTORS AFFECTING THE CHILD'S CONTROL OF HIS DIABETES

Motivation and compliance are two important factors affecting diabetic control. The young child takes little responsibility for his diabetes and it is his parents who manage the condition. On the whole, parents are well motivated and likely to comply with monitoring, insulin therapy and dietary advice. It is important during this stage that the child is educated about diabetes so that he is able to participate appropriately in his care and is prepared for taking over responsibility for his diabetes at a later age. Some parents themselves set unrealistic therapeutic goals for their children and may frustrate the child by depriving him of normal activity, setting him apart from other children, perhaps causing him to become shy and withdrawn or aggressive.

As adolescence is reached teenagers become increasingly responsible for managing their diabetes. Their priorities are likely to be more closely identified with those of their peer group rather than of their parents. Maintaining good control of their diabetes becomes more difficult for adolescents, who may not perceive themselves as threatened by diabetes or its complications. Advice offered should be flexible and considerate reflecting their changing motivations. A teenager is more likely to listen to advice on how to avoid embarrassing episodes of hypoglycaemia or polyuria when out with peers rather than possible complications as a 'boring old adult'. No matter how difficult the circumstances we still have a responsibility to help the adolescent maintain as good a metabolic control as possible.

Diabetic control is affected by teenagers having inadequate under-standing of the condition and its management. Control may deteriorate if teenagers are given responsibility for their diabetes before they have sufficient cognitive abilities. Education presented in a suitable format for adolescents is essential to ensure effective self-management and improved diabetic control. However, there is a difference between what adolescents know and what they actually do. Thus, education is not confined to the provision of information alone but must encompass the much more complicated task of encouraging adolescents to put their knowledge into practice.

Handing over responsibility for diabetic control may be difficult for parents. However, although excessive parental intervention may produce good diabetic control, it may leave adolescents with poor self-esteem or cause an oppositional stance to be taken in the future. It has been shown that a child's assumption of responsibility for management of his diabetes is associated with poor glycaemic control in children under 12 years of age[13]. Thus, it is important that parents do not relinquish responsibility too soon. Conversely, over-anxious parents may be concerned about their child's capacity to cope independently and need support and advice themselves to allow their child to take over his own management.

The deterioration of glycaemic control so frequently observed among adolescents is usually attributed to behavioural changes, poor motivation and compliance. However, it is now clear that this is not the complete explanation and that the endocrine changes of puberty also contribute to poor glycaemic control[14]. Although poor compliance during adolescence is not unexpected, it is most important that when good compliance occurs, it is rewarded by an improvement in glycaemic control. This may be particularly difficult to achieve in view of the pubertal hormonal and metabolic milieu. If adolescents learn that their monitoring and adjustments to therapy have little effect, despondency may occur and result in reduced motivation and compliance. It is, therefore, the responsibility of the diabetic team to respond quickly and appropriately to any problems with diabetic control.

Hypoglycaemia is an important cause of an adolescent losing confidence in their ability to control their diabetes. The fear of hypoglycaemia is likely to be greater than the fear of future complications. Anxiety about hypoglycaemic symptoms and the unwelcome attention which they attract may discourage some children with diabetes from trying to achieve tight glycaemic control.

It would be easy to attribute the improvement in glycaemic control demonstrated in the DCCT to the more intensive insulin regimens used and simply to adopt them for all adolescents. Unfortunately, however, simply intensifying treatment does not seem to affect glycaemic control. A more reasonable conclusion is that the DCCT intensive therapy was effective in providing additional frequent support from the diabetic team in addition to heightened personal involvement and commitment of the patients concerned. The imposition of more demanding insulin regimens and the counterproductive effects this may have on teenage compliance suggest that the question as to the best regimen to be used in a typical teenage group has to be resolved by further trials. Many teenagers may simply be unwilling to follow such demanding treatment programmes, with the attendant risks of increased hypoglycaemic episodes.

CONCLUSION

In conclusion, glycaemic control may be assessed in several ways, both laboratory-based and home-based. Although none of the methods is ideal, a good measure of overall glycaemic control may be obtained. Because of accumulating evidence linking complications with the degree of metabolic control, tight glycaemic control is desirable. However, while each child with diabetes should be managed with the intent to maintain metabolism as near normal as possible, this must be compatible with the psychological and physical well-being of that child and his family. If these constraints are ignored, good biochemical control may be achieved but at the expense of the child's overall development with likely adverse effects on his future adult life.

REFERENCES

1   Allen, D. W., Schroeder, W. A., Balog, J. Observations on the chromatographic heterogeneity of normal adult and foetal haemoglobin. *Journal of the American Chemical Society* 1958; **80:** 1628–34.
2   Koenig, R. J., Peterson, C. M., Jones, R. L., Saudek, C., Lehrman, M., Cerami, A. Correlation of glucose regulation and hemoglobin A1c in diabetes mellitus. *New England Journal of Medicine* 1976; **295:** 417–20.
3   Johnson, R. N., Metcalf, P. A., Baker, J. R. Fructosamine: a new approach to the estimation of serum glycosyl protein. An index of diabetic control. *Clinica Chimica Acta* 1982; **127:** 87–95.
4   Shield, J. P. H., Poyser, K., Hunt, L., Pennock, C. A. Fructosamine and glycated haemoglobin in the assessment of long term glycaemic control in diabetes. *Archives of Disease in Childhood* 1994; **71:** 443–5.
5   Wolffenbuttel, B. H. R., Giordano, D., Founds, H. W., Bucala, R. Long-term assessment of glucose control by haemoglobin-AGE. *Lancet* 1996; **347:** 513–15.

6   Service, F. J., Nelson, R. L. Characteristics of glycemic stability. *Diabetes Care* 1980; **3:** 58–62.
7   Baum, J. D. Home monitoring of diabetic control. *Archives of Disease in Childhood* 1981; **56:** 897–9.
8   Salardi, S., Tonioli, S., Tassoni, P., Tellarini, M., Mazzanti, L., Cacciari, E. Growth and growth factors in diabetes mellitus. *Archives of Disease in Childhood* 1987; **62:** 57–62.
9   DCCT Research Group. The effect of intensive treatment of diabetes on the development and progression of long term complications in insulin-dependent diabetes mellitus. *New England Journal of Medicine* 1993; **329:** 977–86.
10 DCCT Research Group. The relationship of glycemic exposure (HbA1c) to the risk of development and progression of retinopathy in the Diabetes Control and Complications Trial. *Diabetes* 1995; **44:** 968–83.
11 McNally, P. G., Raymond, N. T., Swift, P., Hearnshaw, J. R., Burden, A. C. Does prepubertal duration of diabetes influence the onset of microvascular complications? *Diabetic Medicine* 1993; **19:** 906–8.
12 Cranston, I., Evans, M. Diabetes — trials, tribulations and pay-off of tight control. *Journal of the Royal College of Physicians of London* 1995; **29:** 431–4.
13 Fonagy, P., Moran, G. S., Lindsay, M. K. M., Kurtz, A. B., Brown, R. Psychological adjustment and diabetic control. *Archives of Disease in Childhood* 1987; **62:** 1009–13.
14 Dunger, D. B. Diabetes in puberty. *Archives of Disease in Childhood* 1992; **67:** 569–71.

10

'Food' and its Relationship with Childhood Diabetes

SHIRLEY WATSON

INTRODUCTION

Feeding, especially for mothers, is a fundamental part of the parental relationship with their children. Food, especially sweet food, is used to convey emotions like love, pleasure, reward and approval and is denied when there is disapproval. Snack foods such as biscuits, crisps and confectionery are used to distract and pacify young children, particularly in crowded places, and to replace parental attention. In some cultures the amount of food displayed and consumed is a reflection of the wealth and importance of individuals in their society. Diabetes, with its potential to interfere with parental control, the choice of foods for infants and children and other cultural issues, is likely to cause difficulties of practical management and compliance.

The aims of this chapter are to reflect on 'diet' and its role in the management of diabetes, including concepts which have changed professional perceptions of the relationships between diabetes, the individual and food. The discussion will also highlight particular problems relating to the under-fives, middle years (5–12) and adolescents. Much of the advice given is based on my experiences of helping children with insulin dependent diabetes mellitus (IDDM) and their families in the north-east of England, which has suffered generations of unemployment and associated social and health problems.

Childhood and Adolescent Diabetes. Edited by S. Court and B. Lamb.
© 1997 John Wiley & Sons, Ltd.

Table 10.1. Some landmarks in the history of diet and diabetes

1797	Dr J Rollo	Advocating blood pudding and old rancid meats, e.g. pork; eating as little as possible
1870	Bernard Mauryn	Measured protein and carbohydrate, restricting both
1858	Priory of Paris	Van Holland: 125 g sugar, candy and two meats
		Van Holland: Large portions of rice and cereal

Taken from Ref. 1

HISTORICAL BACKGROUND

The management of 'diet' and diabetes prior to the discovery of insulin in 1921 was perceptive, as can be seen by the examples given in Table 10.1. By the beginning of this century low carbohydrate (CHO) starvation diets were generally used to prolong life. Once insulin therapy began CHO in the diet could be increased, although the tendency was towards restriction. It is now acknowledged that a diet containing more than 50% of its energy from CHO with no more than 10% from sucrose (refined CHO), 15% from protein and 30–35% from fat is the goal for optimum health of the adult population, including people with diabetes (Table 10.2)[2-5]. In adopting these policies the educators have to take into account cultural and social components of food and feeding if advice is to be accepted[6]. The aim of education is when necessary to bring about change in the whole family to ensure success.

For example, areas of deprivation, poverty, unemployment and depression are also areas where there is an increased incidence of heart disease and conditions associated with poor health in relation to food choice[7,8]. Obesity in children is said to be the silent epidemic sweeping America and the Western World. This can be related to dietary habits as well as the general decrease of activity in children[9]. On the other hand,

Table 10.2. Dietary recommendations by various National Diabetes Associations

Percentage of food as energy	ADA, 1987 (American)[a]	BDA, 1989 (British)[b]	FDA, 1988 (Finnish)[c]	ADA, 1994 (American)[a]	EASD, (European)[d]	General popu-lation[e]
Protein (g)	0.8 kg BW	—	15	10–20	—	10–15
Fat (g)	<30	30	30	<30	30	30
CHO (g)	55–60	>50	55	50–60	50–60	>50

[a] American Diabetic Association
[b] British Diabetic Association
[c] Finnish Diabetic Association
[d] European Association of Societies for Diabetes
[e] UK recommendations for the General Population

families who have acknowledged the direction of the media and national advice about changing food habits and increasing awareness of food choice and health need little help to adapt to the advice about diabetes and food.

From the barren desert of knowledge of food and diabetes any research project published was acted on almost without question. For example, the effect of fibre on blood glucose control gave many educators the licence to offer only wholemeal bread as a bread source. Now there is a more realistic view of the effect of fibre, acknowledging that an increase in fibre is our general goal but only soluble fibre has any real effect on glycaemic control[10,11]. The British Dietetic Association's 1989 and 1994 recommendations[12,13] and the 1994 American Dietetic Association's recommendations[14] highlight the philosophy we should now all share about individual assessment and education based on scientific data as opposed to myth.

SPECIFIC FOODS

FIBRE

Dietary fibre is important and intake towards recommended levels should generally be encouraged. The amount of fibre required to achieve improved glycaemic control in young children (i.e. 2 g fibre/100 kcal[15]) would have the effect of decreasing total calorie intake because of the bulking effect of fibre on satiety. It would therefore be difficult to achieve a diet providing 50% of the energy from unrefined CHO with no more than 10% from refined sources. The use of fibrous foods such as fruit, beans and legumes can be encouraged depending upon the age and glycaemic needs of the child. Children under five should be encouraged to eat familiar foods containing unrefined carbohydrate, such as bread, rice, pasta, potato and cereal, without bulking the diet excessively, and an increase of fibre encouraged if necessary as a family issue over the years.

SUCROSE

Research carried out in the north-east of England on schoolchildren in 1980[16] showed that an intake of 50% energy from CHO was the norm but to achieve this 22% came from refined sources. A comparative study repeated 10 years later[16] showed no change in the percentage of energy from different sources, but the main source of sucrose (refined CHO) had changed from table sugar to sugar in drinks (Tables 10.3 and 10.4). The total fat consumption had not changed but milk intake, which has a positive nutritional value, had declined and confectionery appeared in the top 10 sources of protein. This was after 10 years of health education generally

Table 10.3. The proportion and sources of carbohydrate in children's diets — survey of diet in a Northern region dental survey repeated after 10 years of health education[16]

1980	%	1990	%
Confectionery	22	Confectionery	26
Table sugar	16	Soft drinks	20
Soft drink	13	Milk	10
Biscuits & cakes	11	Biscuits & cakes	9
Sweet puddings	11	Sweet puddings	7
Milk	9	Table sugar	7

Reproduced by permission of Ashley Adamson, Nutrition Research Centre, Royal Victoria Infirmary, Newcastle upon Tyne, UK

aimed at an adult population. The habits of young people are determined by fashion, advertising, the media and peer pressure[17].

Sucrose in a mixed diet at levels targeted in the general public has no detrimental effect on glycaemic control[18]. The use of diabetic sweets, chocolate, cakes and biscuits should be actively discouraged because of their expense, calorie content and laxative effect. With evidence that sucrose can be used in a mixed diet, advertising of such products in diabetic publications should be reviewed[19].

FAT

Fat is also a major health issue when dealing with diabetes (Table 10.5). Children with IDDM need to develop good habits with regard to quality and quantity of fat. They are no longer actively encouraged to fill up with protein foods such as cheese and meat but there are still families who use food in this way.

Table 10.4. The proportion and sources of total energy in children's diets — survey of diet in a Northern region dental survey repeated after 10 years of health education[16]

1980	%	1990	%
Meats	13	Meats	16
Bread	10	Confectionery	11
Biscuits and cakes	9	Chips	9
Chips	9	Bread	8
Confectionery	8	Biscuits and cakes	8
Milk	8	Milk	5

Reproduced by permission of Ashley Adamson, Nutrition Research Centre, Royal Victoria Infirmary, Newcastle upon Tyne, UK

Table 10.5. The proportion and sources of fat in children's diets — survey of diet in a Northern region dental survey repeated after 10 years of Health Education[16]

1980	%	1990	%
Meats	20	Meats	23
Butter and margarine	15	Confectionery	11
Milk	10	Butter and margarine	11
Biscuits and cakes	9	Chips	9
Chips	9	Biscuits and cakes	8
Confectionery	6	Milk	6

Reproduced by permission of Ashley Adamson, Nutrition Research Centre, Royal Victoria Infirmary, Newcastle upon Tyne, UK

Foods high in fat and sugar tend to supply cheaper sources of nutrition for families on limited income. Motivation to improve or change family habits may be difficult in areas of high unemployment and poverty.

Children under three need approximately 40% of energy from fat in a healthy diet and failure to thrive which is directly related to health education messages has been reported in this age group[20,21]. Younger children may also be at risk of non-specific diarrhoea when taking a diet of less than 40% of energy from fat[22].

Fat Advice for the Family

- Grill rather than fry food whenever possible
- Only serve chips at home once or twice a week. Remember there are often chips on the menu at school, so try not to have them every day!
- Eat baked or boiled potatoes, pasta or rice more often
- Use beans in meat dishes, thereby cutting down the amount of meat necessary
- Try to choose snacks which are lower in fat instead of crisps all the time. An exchange list will help to choose healthier snacks
- Try to cut the visible fat off meat and bacon
- Use less butter or margarine, or use a lower fat spread. Do not add fat to vegetables before serving
- Try not to use milk too often with snacks or meals. Children over the age of five should use a skimmed or semi-skimmed type. Remember pastry is made with fat so avoid too many pastry foods such as pies and pasties
- If hungry do not eat meat, eggs or cheese between meals. Split the snack into smaller portions and spread it over the afternoon. If more active, then an extra 10 g of CHO will not affect blood glucose
- Nuts, although low in carbohydrate and high in fibre, are very high in fat so try not to include these too often in large amounts.

The overall aim is to reduce the percentage of calories from fat, particularly saturated fat, by giving positive alternative suggestions which reflect sympathy to cultural, economic and environmental issues.

ETHNIC GROUPS

Traditional food habits of ethnic groups, e.g. Asian families, are high in unrefined CHO and fibre; however, the influence of the Western diet features strongly in families who have settled here. The use of traditional family meals should be encouraged, with advice on changing the source of or restricting fat as appropriate. The advice about reduction of sucrose and energy-dense sucrose products applies whether it is halwa, gur, candy or sugared fizzy drinks. Dietary information should reflect the ethnic foods used and a knowledge of their cultural dietary needs is essential.

EDUCATION

The main message of nutritional education will depend on national food habits; for example, extracts from the Fifth Nordic Nutrition Conference[23] show that the staple diet in Iceland consists of fish, milk and meat. The intake of grains and fruit is not high, presumably because few are grown there and vegetable production is limited. As a result the percentage energy from fat varies from 41 to 48% whilst that from carbohydrate varies from 33 to 39%. Extracts from a German study[24] of childhood intakes in relation to heart disease show sucrose intake to be 14% of total energy as opposed to 22% in a study in the north-east of England[16]. In the German study 39% of calories were derived from fat (18% from saturated, 5% from polyunsaturated and 16% from monosaturated) and 48% from carbohydrates. Education is unlikely to be successful unless the whole family is targeted to make reasonable and realistic changes. The messages or lessons learned in the early stages stay the longest, therefore they have to be correct and acceptable.

CARBOHYDRATE EXCHANGE SYSTEMS

Traditional methods of communicating nutritional messages associated with diabetes have involved exchange systems. These included carbohydrate prescriptions with weighed CHO 10 g exchange lists given, or, as in America, an exchange system involving CHO, fat and protein.

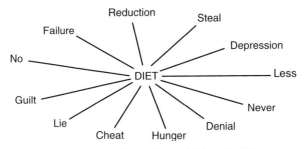

Figure 10.1. Negative connotations of diet for a child with diabetes

A complicated exchange system may satisfy the scientist but there is little evidence that such prescriptions are accurate[25]. However, the health educator deals not just with imparting knowledge but also with monitoring compliance, quality of life, health and the ability to live socially with diabetes within and without the family. All of these factors need to be taken into account when deciding on an educational approach. For example, consider the negative connotations of the word 'diet' (Figure 10.1). The ideal educational messages need to encourage a 'Food Plan' without the use of negative words, such as diet, seen by most adults as a temporary state. Children of overcontrolling parents generally suffer by the use of the 'diet' concept causing emotional and psychological disturbances that may affect compliance. Positive advice should be given to balance any increase of other nutritional components, once sucrose sources are reduced. For example, one young man, on being told he had to cut down on sweets and confectionery but have regular snacks, consumed on average seven packets of crisps daily! Careful thought must be given to advice and more emphasis placed on what they can eat as opposed to what they cannot.

A CHO exchange system could never be an exact science and was never meant to be. It is used as a general guide to families of newly diagnosed children, but the degree of implementation depends on the family's normal food habits. The 10 g exchange system is used to push unrefined CHO intake to the upper limits of what the child can physically manage to eat, not to restrict the child's intake.

A dietary assessment initially identifies the areas of refined CHO which can be reduced, e.g. drinks, confectionery, table sugar, etc., and the unrefined CHO prescription can be tailored to the child's normal eating habits with an emphasis on regular meals and snacks, particularly before bed. If it is necessary to increase unrefined CHO this is easiest just after diagnosis, because of the anabolic effect of insulin and increased appetite. The child is encouraged to eat more CHO, which is adjusted according to appetite once the initial hunger subsides as it is equally harmful to compliance to be forced into eating.

Table 10.6. Examples of CHO exchanges

Foodstuff	CHO (g)
One small potato	10
One medium chappati	25
One large pitta bread	40
One-third large tin beans	20
One-third large tin spaghetti	20
Two fish fingers	10
Two large tablespoons rice	10
One Weetabix	10
Two cream crackers	10

Examples of CHO exchanges are given in Table 10.6. Protein is encouraged in normal portions at main meals but discouraged for snacks or between meals. An idea of normal portions sometimes has to be suggested, depending on family habits. Fat is targeted by giving a list of low-fat snack ideas and advice (Table 10.7).

ILLNESS

During illness when appetite is poor, small but frequent drinks or snacks (10–30 g of CHO) should be consumed regularly, for example:

- Toast and jam (20 g)
- Cereal and milk (20 g)
- Small ice-cream (10 g)
- Cup of milk (10 g)
- Cup of milk and honey (15–20 g)
- Ten grapes (10 g)
- Half a cup of Lucozade (10 g).

Not all families will grasp these messages and some may need advice on alternative ways to manage. One mother, for example, had no short-term memory due to a childhood illness but could follow simple written instructions. She had little self-esteem but was successful in following a large wallchart with digital times, words and drawings of her child's day. We made coloured cards for her; yellow for breakfasts, green for main meals and red for snacks. The chart would read:

Breakfast, yellow card from box . . . .
Snack, red card from box . . . .
Lunch and tea, green card from box . . . .

On each card were examples of meals or snacks normally eaten by the family with appropriate amounts of carbohydrate. It was, on the whole, successful and kept the family together, as well as improving the mother's self-esteem because she was a success.

PRACTICAL ADVICE

On the following pages we will describe the dietary treatment of children at different ages and stages of diagnosis, as well as discussing the problems that children with diabetes commonly face.

UNDER-FIVES

Infants and Toddlers

Milk is the main component of the infant and toddler diet. The infant and parent may become dependent on bottle feeding, especially night feeding, and incur feeding difficulties normally associated with prolonged use of the bottle and restricted use of solids. This is understandable — hypoglycaemia in this age group can be frightening because of the infant's inability to communicate, and particularly if fitting has been experienced with hypoglycaemia.

For babies under six months regular milk feeds, either breast or bottle, are encouraged to maintain normal glycaemia. There should be little change in practice except for avoiding fasts of more than three to four hours. One big risk is the overnight period when the fasting time may have been eight to ten hours. Raw cornflour can be used for very young children in the last feed, as this has been shown to have an effect on glycaemia for approximately six hours. It has been suggested that raw cornflour is not used by infants under two years because of immature amylase production. Our experience has shown that infants under two years do respond well to cornflour. The evening dose for an infant is 2 g per kg body weight; this can be mixed with fruit juice or milk as a drink. The solution needs frequent agitating to keep the raw cornflour in solution. Cornflour can also be mixed with pureed fruit or mashed banana, for while it has no taste the texture can influence acceptance. Raw cornflour can also be useful for infants whose appetites are fluctuating due to illness; 1–2 g of cornflour per kg body weight can be given mixed with feeds once or twice daily as required.

Weaning

Early introduction of weaning at three months may also be necessary to improve glycaemia with the introduction of rice and fruit purées. The advice given for introducing solids should be the same as for non-diabetic infants, as the products used are recommended to be sugar-free. Unrefined carbohydrate should be encouraged at each meal in the form of rice, cereals or potato, and after six months pasta and wheat products can be given.

The target carbohydrate intake for a toddler is 100–150 g daily, and parents need advice on snacks and food portions that can be given. Infants and toddlers vary in the amount of food actually consumed compared with that offered, and appetites vary from day to day. A 10 g or 5 g exchange system may not be necessary for parents of children in this age range but ideas equivalent to their values will reassure parents about their child's blood sugar and safety.

As discussed earlier, food, especially sweet food, is used for a number of emotional reasons. If parents, therefore, feel that they want to give chocolate, small amounts can be given without fuss at the end of a meal containing unrefined CHO. This message should be extended to other members of the family, especially grandparents who may feel that it is their right to spoil their grandchildren and giving sweet food is an easy way to do that. Usually at this age children with their peers are accompanied by adults and so explanations can be given and sweets kept for after meals. Guidelines to help parents use food appropriately, for example not giving sweet foods as a reward or a treat, should help with the health issues associated with sucrose-containing foods and the likelihood of long-term compliance.

Hypoglycaemia is best treated by identified glucose treatments which the child will always associate with this condition. This practice will help to prevent hypos and food manipulation in the future.

Feeding Problems

The use of glucose polymers may be helpful during illness and during the period known as the 'terrible twos', the battle of wills between the toddler and the parent while he/she is establishing their 'self'. Food refusal is a powerful psychological focus for the family of a toddler with diabetes. The child may drink if eating is out of the question, and a 5–10% solution of a glucose polymer in milk, juice or yoghurt, for example, may give time for a cooling off period, reducing parental anxiety. Another trick is to provide a bottle of the toddler's usual fruit drink, but not the sugar-free variety, so that the toddler thinks he has achieved success but if he drinks a normal sugar drink the parent can relax a little. The next step is to use small portions of food not associated with that particular meal, such as segments of satsuma or tangerine, a few crisps, grapes or raisins, which may be useful to avoid anxiety over hypoglycaemia; more food could be incorporated in the next meal or snack if necessary.

Parents appreciate advice given for difficult feeding problems including:

- Making food look interesting: for example, making sandwiches into shapes
- Making faces on plates
- Using finger foods rather than relying on the spoon so that toddlers feel in control
- Using distractions; these can work both ways, either to diffuse a desperate situation so that the parent can feed the child, e.g. video or favourite song, or to make them less interested in food. Sometimes the 'train in the tunnel' approach is too much action and not enough eating
- Making feeding time a social occasion; when everyone is eating the toddler is not the only focus
- Giving the toddler some control, i.e. choice of two or three things to eat, where to sit, which plate to use, etc.

One family with a boy aged two and a half followed advice about introducing chocolate after a meal in the form of one finger of Kit Kat (a thick chocolate-coated biscuit) which was 25% of his mealtime CHO. This worked well until he asserted himself by standing at the cupboard door demanding that he had the same at every opportunity, which the parents found hard to deal with. They were advised to rid the household of all evidence of Kit Kat bars and such items so that when he asked, they could show him the empty tin. This approach had to be consistent until he eventually lost interest. Now Kit Kats are still given but not demanded daily.

Shopping can be difficult for parents with toddlers, especially two- and three-year-olds. Many families allow their children sweets or crisps while shopping, to make the task less stressful for the parent. The child can see this as a wonderful 'power and control' time because a tantrum can have dramatic effects. In the end the parent must decide on how to handle the situation, and if they are consistent with their approach it is possible to reach a compromise. For example, they could stop taking them shopping for a while, offer healthier choices or 'tough it out'.

Parties

Children's parties can be worrying occasions. Parents of a child with diabetes need to educate, and instil confidence in, parents of other children that their child will be safe. Some families may close the door on the child with diabetes out of fear of the unknown. This happened to the family of a two-year-old diagnosed just before Christmas—no party invitations came. It was suggested that the family hold a party themselves for their child inviting as many friends and parents as they could to show that nothing had changed.

There are a number of approaches to the enjoyment of party food, including going to the party and plating appropriate foods in advance. This

Table 10.7. A comparison of foods used as snacks in the UK

Food	CHO (g)	Fat (g)	kcal
Average fruit—apple, orange, pear	10	0	50
Plain biscuit—digestive type	10	3	70
Crisps—average bag	10–15	10	150
Potato puff type snacks, e.g. Quavers	10	5	100
Four dried apricots	10	0	40–50
Kit Kat—two-finger	15	5	110
Custard cream biscuit	10	3	60–70
Garabaldi biscuit × 2	10	2–3	70

is usual and reasonable for the parents of infants and toddlers who know their child's food preferences. It is never easy for a parent to know when to leave the child at a party but it seems sensible to follow the example of the other parents. As children become more independent they are allowed to choose foods. This is still possible if the child has diabetes and a good approach, as long as food has not become an obsession. Children rarely finish party food due to the general excitement of the occasion and they usually need to eat more to cope with the various party games. If the hosts are agreeable sugar-free drinks can be served, which are better for everyone. Ice-cream and cake will usually be used up in soft play, excitement or other activities. It is the practice in this country to give a birthday bag full of sweets which can be used over the next few days in the child's normal routine.

When to give insulin depends on the time of the party, exercise and amount of food. It may be possible to give insulin before the party tea if it is at an appropriate time, e.g. late afternoon, but most young children's parties are held earlier. In this case insulin can be given after the party at the usual time and the amount eaten gauged by the pre-insulin blood sugar and the child's appetite (Tables 10.8 and 10.9). Generally most children would not be able to consume a meal at this time but may be able to have more before bed. The amount can be estimated by the before bed blood sugar. If the blood sugar has not settled the next day any adjustment to insulin can be addressed then. This eliminates the problem of the effect of excitement, exercise and poor post-party appetite on reducing blood sugar excessively and risking nocturnal hypoglycaemia.

As the child matures it may be necessary to reason with them, depending on the individual. For example, given the freedom to choose where there is an excessive amount of sweet foods at a friend's party, the choice will probably lead to excessively high blood sugar, thirst, bed-wetting, etc. In this case parents can categorise food into green and red choices. The child

Table 10.8. Advice on carbohydrate intake on normal and party days

Normal day

INSULIN	Breakfast 30–40 g	Snack 10 g	Lunch 50–60 g	Snack 10 g	INSULIN	Tea/dinner 40–50 g	Snack 20–30 g

Party day (party starts at 3.00 pm)

INSULIN	Breakfast 30–40 g	Snack 10 g	Lunch 30 g	Party food	BLOOD TEST	INSULIN	Tea/dinner 20–30 g	Snack 40 g

can have as many green foods as he/she wants, i.e. crisps, sandwiches, savoury snacks, and the amount of red or sweet food will depend on their age and activity level.

CHILDREN FROM FIVE TO 12 YEARS

The school years see the child progressing from family dependence to adolescence and independence. The influence on young people during this time comes from family and peers, and from advertisements trying to sell

Table 10.9. Some suggestions for managing insulin and food after a party for a younger child

Result of pre-tea blood test	Appetite	Suggested action
High	Hungry	Give 1–2 extra units soluble insulin before snack at tea time, normal supper
High	Not hungry	Give normal insulin, larger supper
Low	Hungry	Normal evening dose of insulin, normal tea, normal supper
Low	Not hungry	Snack tea, 1–2 units less insulin, larger supper

more sugar-coated cereals and fat-loaded confectionery. The scale of the problem of compliance and food is almost directly related to the national and regional consumption of confectionery, e.g. sweets, sweet biscuits, chocolate, cakes, fizzy drinks, as children with diabetes wrestle with their identity and their acceptance by peers.

Having diabetes during these years has the advantage of continued dependence on the family for the bulk of their food. Education is repeatedly focused on the family[26]. If any change in food habits is necessary then it is most successful for the child if the whole family adapt to healthy eating advice. This need not all be done immediately but gradually, so that the family do not feel 'guilt' or overwhelmed by the suggestion of change. The child needs to be helped to adapt their lifestyle when outside the home so that they still feel accepted socially. Most of this acceptance is associated with confectionery issues, such as when and how much chocolate, cakes, sweets, etc. you can eat. Diet is a four-letter word with negative connotations. Food plans and changing habits are best encouraged by giving healthy choices.

The Confectionery Issue

Children of this age are rarely non-compliant with excess unrefined CHO food, but will be exposed to situations when it becomes impossible not to give in to peer pressure. Parents should be encouraged to avoid the words 'cheat' or 'steal' when dealing with non-compliance as this creates guilt in the child; these words are associated with negative feelings about themselves and lead to low self-esteem (Table 10.10). It is normal to want to eat, and the role of the educator is one of negotiation to minimise the effect of bad glycaemic control and possible obesity due to non-compliance.

Try to look at the foods that the children are exposed to and the timing of their biggest pressure, then negotiate a reasonable amount. This gives them a choice of foods, sweets or chocolate which will have less effect on blood glucose than their uncontrolled previous habits. It is best to avoid suggesting half a packet or a third of a bar, which is unlikely to work for psychological reasons. Extra food and insulin when at the cinema or out with friends should be openly negotiated without guilt, although if it happens too often it can lead to obesity.

How to Negotiate Change

It helps parents to be told that all young people with diabetes face these problems. Children need opportunities to communicate with their parents that they are having a difficult time. Using terms like 'normal', and 'friends

Table 10.10. An exercise in perpetuating low self-esteem in a boy with diabetes

Event	Emotions	Consequences
After school: Peer pressure, 4.00 pm visiting local shop, 80 g CHO in sugared sweets	Happy	Being part of the crowd, feeling that you belong
Home	Guilt	Feeling apprehensive as you approach home
Pressure from Mum to do blood test before tea	Unhappy, angry	Argument as you refuse to do blood test
Not hungry at tea, leave half the meal	Anger, frustration, despair	Argument, Mum wants to know why you are not eating Not allowed out to play football as still refusing to do a blood test
Mum finds sweet papers in your pocket	Anger, guilt	Sent to your room
By supper you are starving but you are refused extra food until you do a blood test	Humiliation, unhappy	
Blood test is 22	Sadness, guilt, failure, hopelessness, unloved	Extra soluble given; Mum used words like 'cheat'; argument
		LOW SELF ESTEEM

buying sweets makes it difficult for some young people with diabetes', help when counselling for difficult situations. Worry, stress and unhappiness are associated with eating of sweet foods. The following questions should be asked.

- Is he allowed sweets etc. at any other time?
- Is it that he needs to buy something when with his friends, so that he feels normal?
- If sweets were included at another time would he be happy?

It is not a good idea to withdraw food if blood sugar is high, it will not make the child feel better and children need food to grow. A more flexible approach can be adopted, such as a smaller tea but slightly bigger supper. Explore other possible reasons for high blood sugars: stress, growth, lumpy injection sites. It is best to let the family decide on the issues, for example, 'My child wants to eat with his friends and he does not want to buy diet drinks or sugar-free gum.' Suggest reasonable alternatives—eating with friends; buying food to eat later; blood testing at teatime to look at insulin requirements. Honesty should be encouraged without blame when large amounts of food have been consumed, allowing for corrective measures. Discipline over other issues should not interfere with diabetes-related 'contracts' as this has a detrimental psychological effect on acceptance of their condition. It is better to miss a favourite TV programme if discipline is needed. Family rules changed to help the child with IDDM may make other children in the family feel resentful.

Regular exercise can help to control diabetes, so activity should always be encouraged. Many children, knowing they have overindulged, regularly increase exercise by playing football or running in the evening.

Snacks

Although parents may find including all the children in a regular routine of snacks and suppers more expensive, it does help with compliance of the young child with IDDM. If no other child is eating at a snacktime compliance can become a problem, for example at school, risking hypoglycaemia. School visits by team members are essential to ensure that snacks are handled properly and children not left to hide biscuits, etc. Snacks should ideally be taken in breaktimes. The suggestions for snacks at these times should be as subtle as possible, avoiding noisy suggestions such as apples or crisps. As the child becomes older, parents may be less anxious about hypoglycaemia, although the child may be more terrified of this experience happening whilst in class. While a blood sugar profile may suggest that snacks are not necessary, they may be needed to satisfy the child's anxiety. A flexible approach to timing is required as many families still think it necessary to eat each snack or meal at exact times whilst in class rather than waiting until a natural break occurs. The use of watch alarms suggests a level of precision that is unnecessary, unrealistic and gives the wrong message.

Education

The education of the child about IDDM is very important at these ages as knowledge gained now will be invaluable[26,27]. The aim is to give them information about all aspects of diabetes including food management, so that they can manage safely while on school trips or staying with friends. Confidence can be lost when difficulties arise away from home, but if managed well, this should benefit their self-esteem. This is especially true of children who were diagnosed before five years of age as they will have little practical knowledge of diabetes in general. Aspects of increasing fibre and reducing fat can be tackled by education of the child if parents have previously refused to take suggested changes on board.

Table 10.11. Food frequency chart

Food examples	More than once daily	Once a day	Two to three times a week	Once a week	Never or occasional
Wholemeal bread					
Chapattis					
Rice/pasta					
Potatoes boiled or baked					
Pastry					
Cakes/sweet biscuits					
Added sugar					
Sugared drinks					
Sweets/chocolate after meals					
Fruit					
Yoghurt					
Sweets/chocolate in between meals					

Food frequency charts, like those illustrated (Table 10.11), serve as a better tool for determining changes required in fibre, fat and sugar habits than formal dietary assessment. The children may complete them independently, or with help, and the results discussed. Objectives are then set and the process repeated to establish shifts in food habits. This tool is a non-confrontational aid and gives children an idea of how they can change, or at least of what they should be doing.

Advice for Girls

Girls are particularly prone to post-puberty obesity[28] and so the nutritional adviser needs to be aware of puberty stage and changes. Doses of insulin and amount and type of food required need to be carefully monitored. Problems may have developed due to low self-esteem, guilt and binge eating. Relationships between child and parent may be difficult as the parents are finding it equally difficult to 'give up' parental control and management issues. Sympathetic and practical advice along with psychological input is often necessary during this difficult period.

The following advice about binge eating could be given to a young girl.

1. Use non-energy-dense foods during binge sessions, e.g. vegetables, sugar-free jellies and home-made sugar-free ice lollies (a list should be provided).

2. Take regular exercise, like dancing for 20 minutes a day to your favourite music or skipping in the privacy of your own back garden. Exercising with a friend or family member is more likely to be successful, and may also solve communication problems and break down barriers between family members.
3. Accept that you have a problem — if you lapse back into binge eating do not reproach yourself or deny yourself food to make up for it. Start again straight away.
4. If you can stop at one thing allow yourself some of your favourite food once or twice a week to prevent the starve/binge scenario.
5. Try to plan something else to do at your worst times, for example, visit a friend, do a jigsaw or go out for a walk.
6. If you are offered counselling, accept it; it will help you and your family.

Exercise

If there is a balanced approach to the use of confectionery there is no need to use exercise as a chance for eating chocolate. Exercise should be part of the prescription, and families should be educated as to whether extra food is necessary, particularly when exercise is taken directly after a meal. Exercise at school rarely needs extra CHO. Prolonged or extensive exercise such as competitive training for swimming or running needs extra unrefined CHO in the meal or snack before, as well as monitoring and increasing food afterwards. The fear of hypos will encourage parents to exaggerate the amount of food required on these occasions. The experienced athlete will know what their own routine should be.

If the child is participating in activity away from home, it is understandably safer to encourage extra food or snacks as the general rule.

THE ADOLESCENT

This wonderful time may bring new concerns as adolescents battle to take control of what, when and how much they eat. The multiple insulin injection or basal bolus system was heralded as an ideal solution to the problem of adolescent diabetes control. However, some young people on this regime eat when and what they like with no monitoring or change in insulin dose, some may omit the lunch dose altogether. Control of diabetes is not their main priority.

Food Choices

Girls tend to exercise a lot less than boys, and have a greater potential for obesity and subsequent food problems, such as gross manipulation of insulin therapy to control weight or even anorexia nervosa. All need careful and sympathetic handling[28]. Boys become just as irregular with food choices and timing but generally are still growing fast and remain physically active so require more insulin and energy.

Adolescents with diabetes make similar lunch choices to most of their peers (Table 10.12): a bag of chips or french fries and a packet of sweets, or four savoury pastries and a can of normal coke and a cream bun. These are children that you have seen regularly and educated over the years, but non-compliance is a feature of their age and it is best to set realistic goals and choices; for example, look at what food is available locally and go for a 50/50 healthy/rubbish split.

It could be argued that having a rubbish lunch does not matter, when a healthy breakfast and tea are eaten. If education is the key to informed choice then never miss an opportunity to educate, especially at a time when the young person is wholly in charge of what they eat. Independence can be encouraged by teaching a flexible attitude to adjusting insulin doses or giving extra soluble insulin when going out for a meal. This is made easier with multiple injection regimes. The emphasis should be on freedom of choice made safer by knowledge and the willingness to respond sensibly to changing circumstances.

Alcohol

It seems that alcohol becomes a feature at a younger age each year. We consciously discuss the use of alcohol, its dangers and its effect on diabetes from the age of 14, but it may be necessary to consider this earlier. Realistic goals should be set and the advice offered much depends on the habits of

Table 10.12. Typical adolescent food choices at lunch

Food	CHO (g)
Chocolate bar	20
Doughnut	40
Cream bun	30
Packet of sweets	20
Bag of chips	50
Cake	40
Carton of milk	10
Sandwich	30
Carton pure orange juice	20
Pastie (savoury snack)	30
Fruit	10
Bread bun	20
Carton of mixed salad from local store using pasta, beans or rice	40

young people in your area. A locally produced booklet (Appendix 10.1) discusses safe amounts of alcohol and the pitfalls and effects of spiking and mixing drinks, particularly cocktails. Practical advice is given on eating when alcohol is intended to be a feature, e.g. to eat more if drinking and not to drink on an empty stomach. However, no matter what is said to a young person, it is the nature of their age to challenge and test the advice given by adults.

Education

An effective method of teaching this age group is to give groups of young people with diabetes a theoretical problem and ask them to come up with a solution. The teacher also learns from observation the social problems that these people face[27]. Talking about the future rarely motivates change, but finding out what effect diabetes has on their day-to-day lifestyle may focus the young person on a reason for compliance. Two typical examples of daily problems are thirst and nocturnal enuresis. These make the young person tired and less able to concentrate at school. Consistently high blood sugars may cause mood swings and a general feeling of lethargy and depression. Boys may be less effective in sport and may be motivated to do better. Girls may want to make the best choices for skin care and to prevent obesity. This age of adventure needs careful handling.

Individuals with diabetes and their families need continued support and education. Non-compliance is a normal and understandable reaction to diabetes but can be managed without the young person losing self-esteem. Reasonable and realistic goals should be set and conventional ideas about food and diabetes challenged where appropriate. Children with a lifetime of diabetes ahead of them are at great risk from the complications of diabetes, but with sympathetic support and realistic education from the beginning, and encouraging change where necessary within the family, we would hope to give the best possible start with the least psychological damage.

The aim of nutritional education is to reflect the national nutritional guidelines, but social, family and psychological issues must be considered as high priorities.

REFERENCES

1 Ellenberg, M., Rifkin, H. *Diabetes Mellitus. Theory and Practice.* 4th Edn, Volume II. Garden City: Medical Examination Publishing Company, 1990: 540–1.

2 Food and Agricultural Organisation of the U.N. *WHO/UNU Report: Energy and Protein Requirements.* WHO Technical Report Series 724. Geneva: WHO, 1985: 1–205.

3 *Recommended Daily Amounts of Food, Energy and Nutrients for Groups of People in the United Kingdom.* London: HMSO, 1981: 1–27.

4 Nutrition Sub-Committee of BDA. Dietary recommendations for diabetics for 1980s. *Hum Nutr Appl Nutr* 1982; **36A:** 378–94.

5 Diabetes and Nutrition Study Group of the European Association for the Study of Diabetes. Nutritional recommendations for individuals with D.M. *Diabetes Nutr Metab* 1988; **1:** 145–459.

6 Murcot, A. The cultural significance of food and eating. *Proc Nutr Soc* 1982; **41:** 203–10.

7 French, A. D., Carmichael, C. L., Furness, J. A., Rugg-Gunn, A. J. The relationship between social class and dental health in five year old children in the North and South of England. *Br Dent J* 1984; **156:** 83–6.

8 Cook, J., Altman, D. G., Moore, D. M. C., Topp, S. G., Holland, W. W., Elliott, A. A survey of nutritional status of school children: relation between nutrient intake and socioeconomic factors. *Br J Prev Soc Med* 1973; **27:** 91–9.

9 Gortmaker, S. L., Dietz, W. H., Cheung, L. W. Inactivity, diet and the fattening of America. *J Am Diet Assoc* 1990; **Sept:** 1247–52.

10 Mann, J. I. Dietary fibre and diabetes. In: *Dietary Fibre in the Management of the Diabetic. Proceedings of British Diabetic Symposium, Oxford.* Medical Education Series, 1984: 7–13.

11 Jenkins, D. J. A., Taylor, R. H., Wolever, T. M. S. The diabetic diet, dietary CHO and differences in digestibility. *Diabetologia* 1982; **23:** 477–84.

12 Kilnmouth, A. L. Dietary recommendations for childen and adolescents with diabetes. *Diabet Med* 1989; **6:** 537–47.

13 Magrath, G., Hartland, B. V. Dietary recommendations for childen and adolescents with diabetes. *Diabet Med* 1993; **10:** 874–85.

14 Feistinker, L. Nutrition recommendations for diabetics. *J Am Diet Assoc* 1994; **94:** 507–11.

15 Kinmouth, A. L. *et al.* Whole food and increased dietary fibre improved blood glucose control in diabetic children. *Arch Dis Child* 1982; **57:** 187–94.

16 Adamson, A., Rugg-Gunn, A., Butler, T., Appleton, D., Hackett, A. Nutritional intake, height and weight of 11–12 year olds. Northumbrian childen in 1990 compared with information obtained in 1980. *Br J Nutr* 1992; **68(3):** 543–63.

17 Thomas, B. J. How successful are we at persuading diabetics to follow their diet- and why do we sometimes fail? In: *Nutrition and Diabetes.* (Turner, M., Thomas, B. J., eds.) London: Libbey, 1981: 57–66.

18 Mann, J. I. Simple sugars and diabetes. *Diabet Med* 1987; **4:** 135–9.

19 Nutrition Sub-Committee, British Diabetic Association. Dietary recommendations for children and adolescents with diabetes. *Diabet Med* 1989; **6:** 537–47.

20 Stordy, B. J. Is it appropriate to apply adult healthy eating guidelines to babies and young children? *Proceedings of a Conference: Growing Cycle; Child, Mother and Child, November 1994.* National Dairy Council Publications, 1995.

21 Stordy, B. J. Healthy eating for infants–mothers' actions. *Acta Paediatr* 1995; **84(7):** 733–41.

22 Cohen, S., Hendrick, K., Eastham, E. J. Chronic non-specific diarrhoea. *Am J Dis Child* 1979; **133:** 490–2.

23 Steingrimosttir, L. Nutrition in Iceland. 5th Nordic Nutrition Conference. *Scand J Nutr* 1993; **37:** 10–12.
24 Somogyl, J. C., Elmadfa, I., Walter, P. New aspects of nutritional status. *Bibl Nutr Diet: Diet A* 1994; **5:** 100–4.
25 Hackett, A., Court, S., McLauren, C., Parkin, J. M. Dietary variations in diabetics. *Arch Dis Child* 1988; **63:** 794–8.
26 Hackett, A., Court, S. *et al.* Do education groups help diabetics and their parents? *Arch Dis Child* 1989; **64(7):** 997–1003.
27 Stephenson, A., Watson, S. *Working Hand in Hand for Children with Diabetes.* Booklet on Education Tools used to Teach Children with Diabetes of all Ages. (Available from S. Watson, Paediatric Dietetic Service, Royal Victoria Infirmary, Newcastle upon Tyne, UK)
28 Steel, J. M., Young, R. J. Abnormal eating attitudes in young insulin dependent diabetics. *Br J Psychiatr* 1989; **155:** 515–21.

APPENDIX 10.1

ALCOHOL
AND YOU

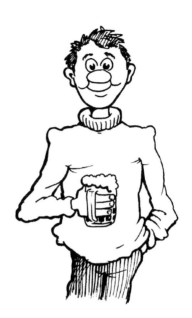

Because of the dangers of alcohol you should avoid the low carbohydrate lagers or high gravity beers such as LCL, Carlsberg Special, Pils, Stella etc. These ferment for longer, so that more sugar can become alcohol. They are therefore not recommended for people with diabetes.

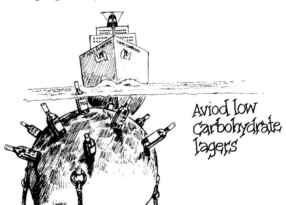

Aviod low carbohydrate lagers

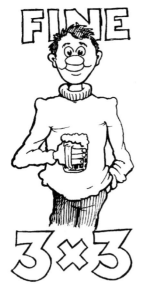

Ordinary beers and lagers can be taken in the recommended amounts for the general public, two or three drinks up to three times a week.

Try not to exceed two or three drinks of cider two or three times a week. There is also a low alcohol cider available.

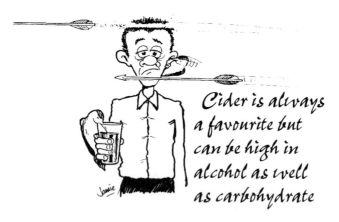

Cider is always a favourite but can be high in alcohol as well as carbohydrate

Medium or dry wine has a low carbohydrate and moderate alcohol level. Alcohol free wine is also now available. Remember that low alcohol wine is also a good idea but does contain some alcohol.

Dry Martini has a low carbohydrate and a low to medium alcohol content. With a slimline or low calorie mixer for example, soda water or slimline tonic, two or three pub measures would have very little carbohydrate and a moderate alcohol content.

Low alcohol and alcohol free beers are available in most pubs and taste OK (honest!)

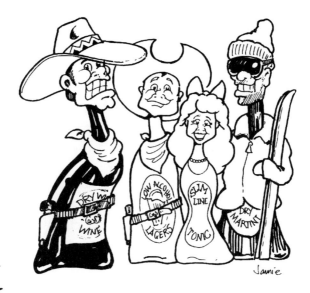

The Good

Too many spirits are probably best avoided as they are high in alcohol. Once again, no more than three pub measures with a slimline mixer are recommended.

Beware the effect of mixing spirits with other alcoholic drinks, especially in cocktails, "3 for the price of 2" or "doubles for £1". Remember "Happy Hours" can lead to an unhappy night.

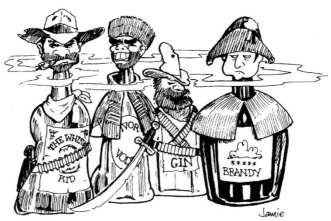

<u>*Never*</u> drink on an empty stomach.

<u>*Never*</u> replace meals or snacks with alcohol especially before bed.

<u>*Always*</u> have a sandwich type snack during or after drinking.

<u>*Adding*</u> alcohol to anyone's drinks without their knowledge is stupid and dangerous, especially if they have diabetes.

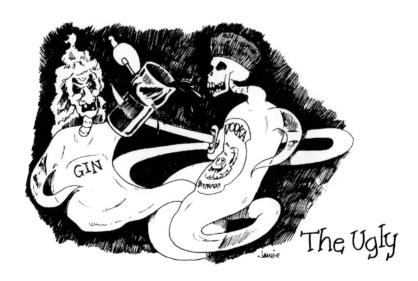

The Ugly

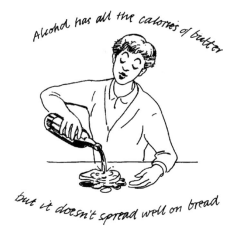

Alcohol has all the calories of butter

but it doesn't spread well on bread

If you are watching your weight remember alcohol is as high in calories as fat.

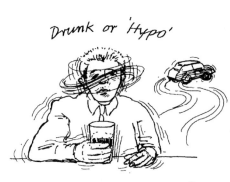

Drunk or 'Hypo'

Do you know the difference?

As a person with diabetes you can hold a driving licence safely. Drinking and driving would not only jeopardise your licence but also your life and the lives of others. A hypo under the influence of alcohol may be very dangerous. Drunk or hypo, could you tell the difference?—Your friends won't!

Alcohol and Hypos

People with diabetes may drink alcohol safely but should be aware of certain facts. Alcohol stops your body releasing glucose into the bloodstream during a hypo. Therefore a hypo under the influence of alcohol may be very dangerous.

Credits

Illustrations by Jamie O'Brien and Jan Munro

Ideas and text by The Newcastle and Gateshead Paediatric Diabetes teams

11

Insulin Strategies

JERRY WALES

INTRODUCTION

There is much more to managing diabetes than insulin therapy, but this is the cornerstone of treatment and the source of much (unjustified) confusion. There are a bewildering number of commercially available insulins that, in the UK alone, could be combined in more than 200 000 possible ways. This chapter will discuss the rationale behind some of the more practical and often used insulin strategies.

CHEMISTRY

Insulin can be extracted from animal sources (beef or pig) but it is usual to employ 'human' insulin in childhood diabetes, although there is no great scientific rationale for this. It is felt that for prolonged therapy the least immunogenic preparations are desirable. As most children will never receive anything other than the human insulin preparations the possible concern about a 'change' in symptoms of hypoglycaemia described in adults is not an issue.

Most currently available human insulin is manufactured by genetic manipulation of yeast (suffixed by *pyr*) or *Escherichia coli* (*crb*), although previously animal insulins were humanised by enzymatic modification of porcine insulin (*emp*). 'Designer', modified insulins with a shorter or longer half-life will be discussed later in the chapter, but one such product, Humalog® (insulin lispro), is currently available, although only licensed for the over-12s.

Childhood and Adolescent Diabetes. Edited by S. Court and B. Lamb.
© 1997 John Wiley & Sons, Ltd.

In vitro insulin forms a hexameric (three double molecules or dimers) crystal that dissociates in the presence of diminishing insulin concentration to dimeric and then monomeric insulin that circulates in the peripheral circulation and is bioactive. (Physiologically, insulin in monomeric form, plus the connecting C-peptide and small amounts of other forms of the molecule, is secreted into the portal circulation.) Because of the time required for this dissociation, the appearance of insulin activity after subcutaneous injection of pure 'soluble' or 'short-acting' preparations is thus delayed by 20–60 minutes, is at its maximum two to four hours later, and continues for up to eight hours after administration.

The commonest strategies to prolong insulin activity are to bind insulin to a simple peptide, protamine, to form the isophane insulins or to crystallise the insulin in the presence of zinc to form the lente insulins (the larger the particles formed, the longer the half-life). Isophane insulin, being bound 1:1 to protamine, can be mixed in various ratios with soluble insulin to derive pre-mixed preparations. The excess of zinc in the lente insulins would combine with soluble insulin to delay its action and so must be mixed shortly before administration, and in a set fashion to prevent contamination of soluble stock-bottle insulin by zinc. This requires a formal technique for the traditional method of mixing insulin, as detailed in Table 11.1.

INJECTION TECHNIQUE, INJECTION SITES AND FACTORS AFFECTING ABSORPTION

The fact of injectable therapy looms large in any initial discussion of diabetes care after diagnosis. Modern 29, 30 or even finer gauge needles allow for relatively pain-free administration into the subcutaneous fat layer. However, this apparently simple procedure can produce huge variations in

Table 11.1. Method for mixing zinc, lente insulin and soluble insulin. The important point is to avoid a needle or syringe contaminated with or containing excess zinc coming into contact with the stock of soluble insulin

1. Place the two insulin bottles on a flat surface.
2. Draw up as much air as the total dose into the syringe.
3. Inject the same quantity of air as lente dose into the bottle containing medium-acting insulin without inverting the bottle or touching the surface of the cloudy liquid with the needles.
4. Invert the soluble insulin bottle, inject remaining air and withdraw the short-acting dose of insulin.
5. Return to the lente bottle, invert and withdraw the dose of medium-acting insulin.
6. Inject immediately.

response to insulin, complications at the injection site and adverse psychological reactions to the whole process.

Children are often thin, especially in the mid-childhood ages, and their subcutaneous fat layer becomes a difficult target. Sites with the thickest layer (avoiding blood vessels and nerves) should be chosen (although there is often reluctance by the child to use the stomach). Pinching up a skinfold doubles the available fat thickness and the needle should be inserted, without any form of preparation other than basic hygiene, at 90[deg] to the pinched skin (which often translates as 45[deg] to a limb). This technique, along with short needles incompletely inserted, is necessary to avoid intramuscular injection which is painful, produces bruising and variations in insulin absorption. The surface area of the sites used should be approximately the size of the patient's hand placed on their limb, but anaesthesia after repeated injection into the same site over time results in coin-sized sites because of preferential usage. Insulin is lipogenic and produces fat hypertrophy at the sites (Figure 11.1). Small, hypertrophic sites, especially if zinc preparations are used, are poorly vascularised and retard the absorption of insulin.

Each child and family develop their own strategy to cope with the pain of the injection itself. Common tricks are the use of a familiar 'routine', distraction, 'gating' the area by rubbing the site for one minute sufficient to produce a sensation of local warmth prior to injection or the use of an ice-cube wrapped in a handkerchief to give local anaesthesia.

Often a small amount of insulin is lost by leakage after injection and this can sometimes represent a significant percentage of the total dose in small children.

To prevent disfiguring lipohypertrophy it is good practice to try to spread out the area of injection as much as possible and to rotate the site of injection from left to right, arm to leg, stomach to buttock, etc. While desirable in terms of 'site management' this practice does introduce yet more variability in insulin absorption. Injection into the four most commonly recommended sites — arm, thigh, abdomen and buttocks — is shown in Figures 11.2–11.5. Self-injecting into a thin arm can be difficult but raising a skinfold against a doorframe is possible. Broadly speaking the rate of absorption is affected by the temperature and blood supply at the injection site. Current evidence suggests that insulin is most rapidly absorbed from abdominal injection sites, next the arm and most slowly from the buttocks. These in turn are affected by ambient temperature and clothing, the compartment into which the injection is given, and any rubbing or exercise that occurs around the time of injection. There will tend to be a more rapid onset of action from more centripetal injections given just before exercise.

Children are often on small doses of insulin and the traditional method of drawing up insulin in a syringe could lead to major errors. Even with 0.3 ml

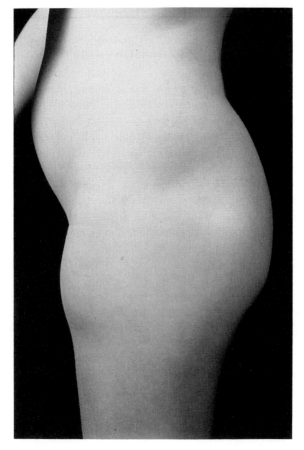

Figure 11.1. Fat hypertrophy of left thigh

syringes and fixed needles the proportion of the dose that can be varied by the introduction of a bubble, or a slight misjudgement of drawing-up, is relatively large. This is one of the advantages of the newer insulin 'pen' injection devices which allow for much greater accuracy even with small doses.

Although some children as young as five can self-inject, their technique, when unsupervised, may be less than optimal. Omission of insulin, manipulation of the dose for psychological or social reasons and to achieve weight loss are common practices which can add to the variability inherent in the absorption of insulin. These issues are discussed in other sections of the book.

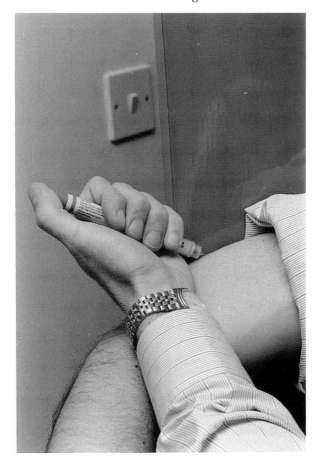

Figure 11.2. Injection into upper arm using door frame to raise a skin fold

FACTORS AFFECTING INSULIN AVAILABILITY

Insulin 'stock' should be stored in a domestic refrigerator and away from sunlight, the latter being the most important degrading factor in normal circumstances. It is acceptable to keep 'pen' (see later) insulin cartridges when in use at room temperature, inside the pen. A child on a small dose of insulin may take weeks or months to empty a 1.5 ml cartridge or the larger 3 ml bottles used for self-mixing insulin, and incorrect storage will lower the insulin activity at the end of this period. While pharmaceutical companies take every effort to ensure uniformity, there are anecdotal reports from

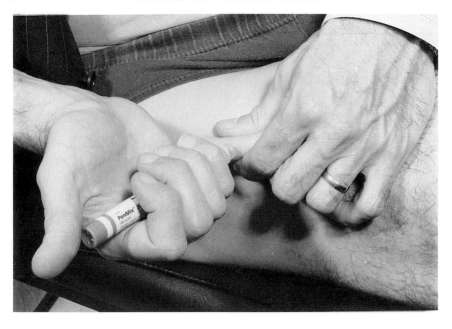

Figure 11.3. Injection into right thigh

patients of inter-batch variation, possibly related to transport and intermediate storage.

The activity of insulin is antagonised by many of the hormones produced in abundance at puberty. Growth hormone (GH) secretion is a pulsatile phenomenon, largely at night and augmented at the time of puberty. The large amounts of circulating GH account for the 'dawn phenomenon' — a rise in sugar levels seen pre-breakfast — that leads to an unavoidable worsening of control at this age, because currently available insulins are particularly poorly active eight hours after injection without producing unacceptable earlier night-time hypoglycaemia. It may be possible in future to use GH antagonists or insulin-like growth factor-1 to overcome this effect, but this is still under investigation.

The action of androgens and oestrogen to increase muscle mass, lower subcutaneous fat and modify behaviour, coupled with extra GH, means that the dose of insulin required to maintain reasonable control increases substantially (rarely up to 2 units per kg per day) through puberty before reducing again in the late teens and twenties. Many girls find that they require more insulin in the three or four days prior to their period, and if the cycle is sufficiently regular this increase can be pre-planned.

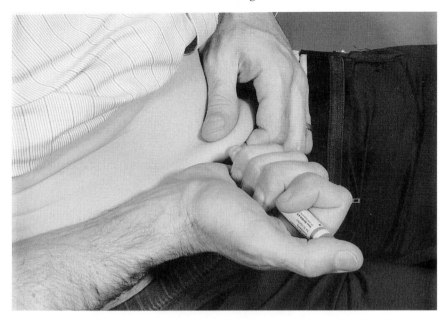

Figure 11.4. Injection into abdomen

Giving insulin at least half an hour before a meal, particularly breakfast, allows insulin to be circulating before the glucose levels start to rise. This simple management strategy can result in a much more normal overall level of blood glucose over several hours. In practice, given the relatively chaotic nature of most households with children, the timing varies, especially at breakfast, from 40 minutes before to well after the meal. The content of the meal ingested (as opposed to offered) is also a variable which is almost impossible to control in childhood. Children are capricious not only in their dietary habits but also their pattern of exercise, which is highly dependent on the season/daylight hours and school holidays. Finally the naive immune system of most young children means that life consists of a succession of upper respiratory and other viral ailments that increase the need for insulin, but at the same time interfere with the appetite.

A list of the main factors affecting the absorption and fate of injected insulin is given in Table 11.2. For these reasons a child injecting 4.5 units of soluble insulin 20 minutes before a breakfast of cereal and milk from an old vial into their hypertrophic thigh site on a sunny day when they are well will produce a very different sugar profile from the same individual the next day, starting a 'cold' on a rainy morning and injecting 3.85 units into their pristine arm 20 minutes after a small breakfast of toast and jam.

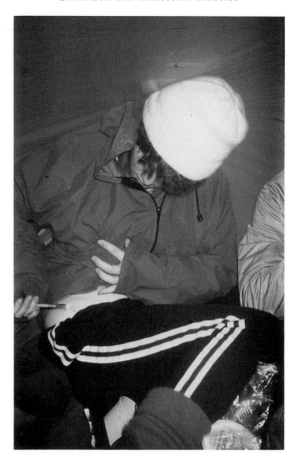

Figure 11.5. Injection into buttock

PRACTICAL INSULIN REGIMES

In the light of the above one should not be too rigorously scientific in the choice of a particular brand of insulin given in a particular manner. Each clinic is likely to gain experience with a limited number of regimes with which they feel comfortable, but should always be willing to try new approaches at the request of the family or in the light of circumstance.

There are three broad forms of insulin (short-, medium- and long-acting) which may be combined in a variety of different regimes ranging through once, twice or multiple injection regimes. Pure, crystalline or soluble human insulin has a theoretical time-action profile of: onset = 0.3–1 h; time to peak 2–4 h; duration 8 h. Medium-acting, isophane or lente insulins vary in onset from

Table 11.2. Factors affecting insulin action on sugar profiles

- Wrong compartment (fat/muscle)
- Loss of insulin
- Site: where?
       state (leakage)?
- Site: abdomen, arm, legs, buttock?
       state (lipo-hypertrophy)?
- Rubbing / temperature / exercise
- Dose errors (including dose manipulation)
- Storage / degradation
- Puberty: growth hormone
              sex steroids
              periods (menstrual cycle)
- Timing of meals
- Variable content of meals
- Variable exercise
- Infection and illness
- Stress

1 to 4 h, peak at 6–10 h and last up to a day. The longest acting insulins start working at 3–8 h, peak at 6–20 h and can effectively last up to 36 h such that daily injections theoretically produce a relatively steady background state.

ONCE- OR TWICE-DAILY REGIMES

As many children at presentation have a residual 20% of pancreatic function that produces insulin, especially after meals (the 'honeymoon' period), there is some logic in starting a twice-daily regime of isolated medium-acting insulin at diagnosis. A usual starting dose is 0.5 units per kg per day given two-thirds in the morning before breakfast and one-third before the main evening meal. In children over five years of age there is rarely a need to use anything other than multiples of 2 as starting doses, or future increments, which allows for more precise drawing up of insulin. This regime provides a period of observation during which an approximate total daily dose can be calculated to achieve a balance between good control and frequent hypoglycaemia. As the honeymoon period closes there will be a deterioration in control apparent especially after meals. At this point soluble insulin can gradually be added to the regime, 2 units at a time in those older than five years, until an approximate distribution of two-thirds medium to one-third soluble is achieved at both ends of the day. A typical dose would be in the order of 0.75–1 unit per kg per day in a pre-pubertal child (see above). Pre-mixed insulin can be used at any point, with fixed proportions (available as 10/90; 20/80; 30/70; 40/60 and 50/50) of short- to medium-acting insulin. Different mixtures can be used morning and evening or as needs dictate. These fixed mixture regimes have the benefit of simplicity, though there is a perceived loss of flexibility. The amount of soluble insulin can be adjusted to affect mainly the blood sugar levels mid-morning to early afternoon and before bed, and the medium-acting insulin adjusted to control the levels before the evening meal and pre-breakfast respectively.

Some newly diagnosed children, usually in the first five years of life, can achieve reasonable control on a single morning dose of medium-acting insulin. This state can persist for a surprisingly long period of time and is usually preferable to more frequent injections provided overall control remains good. While anxiety exists that these children will be resistant to more frequent injections when required for improving control, in practice common sense prevails and inevitable change is accepted.

MULTIPLE INJECTION REGIMES

Sometimes it can prove very difficult to achieve good control with only two injections a day. Also the older child with diabetes is disadvantaged by the relatively restricted nature of the timing and amount of their meals and insulin dose. An approach that allows some liberalisation of this regime, as well as the theoretical advantage of more 'physiological' insulin profiles, is to inject a medium- or long-acting insulin once a day (basal) in combination with soluble (bolus) insulin before meals. For example, better control and more flexibility can be obtained with three injections a day, giving soluble insulin before breakfast and lunch with a mixture of short- and medium-acting insulins before the main evening meal.

The more typical basal bolus regime extends this further by giving soluble insulin before the main meals and a medium- or long-acting insulin at bedtime. The timing of the administration of the longest acting basal insulins is less crucial.

The bolus insulins should be given at least 20 minutes (but see above) before the three main meals and allow for flexibility in both the timing of the meals and the amount eaten by varying the time and dose administered. It is possible to have a more normal 'existence' of three meals of varied amount, no snacks and more spontaneous social eating with this regime but it does require more frequent injections, an injection at school and the need for forethought and planning, which limits its usefulness in practical terms to the committed pre-teenager or adolescent. The regime is designed to be flexible, but as a guide half to two-thirds of the previously calculated total daily dose (if newly diagnosed then start at 0.5 units per kg per day) should be given as a night-time basal insulin and the remainder equally divided in the first instance between the three main meals. The bolus insulin dose is then modified to take into account sugar levels after meals (dependent on quantity and composition) and the basal insulin adjusted to maintain near normal sugars on waking.

INJECTION DEVICES

Numerous injection devices exist, the simplest of which is a plastic syringe with a prefixed needle. Increasingly the ease of use, accuracy and convenience of insulin pen injectors (Figure 11.6) means that they are becoming the preferred device for patients. Many different pen injectors are available (Figure 11.7), using disposable cartridges of soluble, long-acting or pre-mixed insulin, capable of giving from 30 to 40 units of insulin in 1- or 2-unit increments. For the older patient, needing more than 40 units of insulin per injection, disposable pre-filled pen injectors giving up to 80 units at a time are also available, avoiding the need for double injections. All these units are effectively big syringes with a dial-up dosage facility. Unexpectedly high (less frequently low) sugar levels should prompt inspection of the device for mechanical problems and retained bubbles and questioning about storage in direct sunlight, on radiators, etc. If there is any doubt then the device should be exchanged for a new one. Many users of the above syringes and pens find that they can re-use the same needle for more than one injection, but this should be at the discretion of the patient.

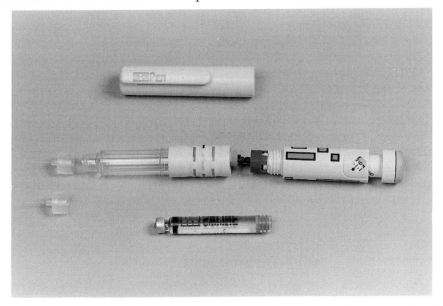

Figure 11.6. Components of an insulin pen injector. (Reproduced by permission of the University of Newcastle upon Tyne)

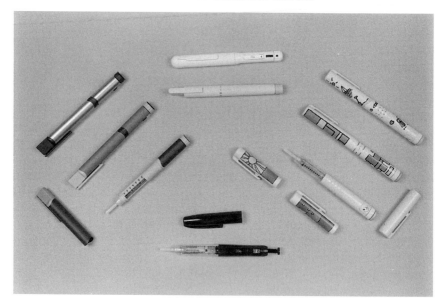

Figure 11.7. A selection of pen injector devices. (Reproduced by permission of the University of Newcastle upon Tyne)

Various types of spring-loaded automatic injection devices can be used that hide some or all of a patient-loaded syringe in a spring-loaded tube that will inject the insulin on activation. Some are bulky, noisy and cumbersome to use whilst pinching a skin fold, but may be preferred by some patients. There is also a spring-loaded pen injector available, the Diapen® (Figure 11.8). There are several marketed gas-driven or self-pressurised devices that blow insulin through the skin in a 'painless' manner if correctly adjusted and used. They are all expensive and, for the majority of patients, offer little advantage as a means of administering treatment.

Users of multiple injection regimes can be offered a subcutaneous cannula that, once inserted, can stay in place for a day or more — subsequent injections being into the cannula. These cannula may be uncomfortable, can become infected and allow for too much variation of delivered dosage to be of anything but limited application.

LESS COMMON INSULIN REGIMES AND NEW APPROACHES TO THERAPY

The most 'pseudo-physiological' means of administering insulin is to infuse insulin continuously into an indwelling subcutaneous, intraperitoneal or intravenous catheter. The rate is adjusted to a basal daytime rate according

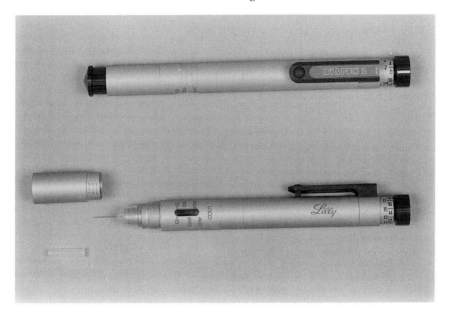

Figure 11.8. Diapen pen injector. (Reproduced by permission of the University of Newcastle upon Tyne)

to need (and approximately one-third of this rate at night), a button can be used to give increments of bolus insulin at mealtimes. The subcutaneous route is the most convenient but still may cause discomfort and infection at the site. Problems may occur with blockage of the tubing leading to the cannula or electromechanical problems with the pump. These methods are now largely confined to exceptional circumstances where tight control is imperative, such as periconceptionally in some high-risk women and in rare 'brittle' diabetics with incipient major complications or painful neuropathy. Intravenous insulin is the treatment of choice for diabetic ketoacidosis and is discussed in Chapter 13.

Alternative routes of insulin administration are being investigated, but as yet are not recommended for routine use. Insulin may be administered mixed with a 'carrying agent' intranasally, given transdermally by iontophoresis, given orally in various slow-release formulations or by suppository, by buccal absorption or even as a nebulised aerosol. None of these methods has yet been developed to the stage where they are likely to have impact on the care of children in the near future.

Insulin may be modified to alter its structure in such a way as to reduce or prevent hexamerisation and thus have a faster time–action profile or to retard its action and produce longer 'basal' profiles without the need for the use of zinc or protamine.

The major need in paediatric practice is for a rapidly acting insulin that will work soon after injection when administered before a meal. Early attempts at insulin modification resulted in some promising time–action profiles but with enhanced mitogenicity in animal models. However, stage 3 trials are underway in children using a rapidly acting monomeric analogue, Humalog® or insulin lispro with a good animal safety profile, and it is possible that they will have an important place in therapy in the near future. Currently Humalog is only licensed for children over 12 years of age. It has a rapid onset of action of around 15 minutes and a shorter duration of action of only two to five hours. Most clinical experience has been gained in the USA where it is used with medium-acting insulins. It is not yet available pre-mixed with longer-acting insulins.

Implantable or trans-surface delivery devices, either semi-mechanical with feedback control from bio-sensors or using gel-encapsulated porcine islet cells, are being investigated and hold the potential promise of near-physiological insulin delivery. The ultimate physiological replacement, human islet cell or pancreatic transplants, are unlikely to have a major impact on management in the near future because of problems with donor supply and the toxicity of even modern immunosuppressive regimes.

ADJUSTING DOSE—ILL HEALTH, OPERATIONS, EXERCISE AND TRAVEL

At times of intercurrent illness the patient should test for ketones in the urine and increase the frequency of blood sugar testing. Under no circumstances should insulin be omitted. If the child is not too unwell and the blood sugar is between 10 and 20 mmol/l with only a trace or small amount of ketones present then an extra 2 (<5 years) or 4 (>5 years) units of soluble insulin may be given. If the child is, or becomes, more unwell and/or the sugar exceeds 20 mmol/l, especially in the presence of increasing, moderate or large amounts of ketonuria, then the family should contact their usual emergency support number for advice and possible hospital admission without delay. An intravenous diabetic ketoacidosis regime will be instituted as described in Chapter 13.

A comprehensive perioperative regime for major and minor surgery is given in Table 11.3.

Spontaneous exercise is best dealt with by an increase in short-acting carbohydrate input. Regular, planned exercise, as may occur with a training regime for team or moderately high-level sporting activity, is more logically coped with by adjustments of insulin dose. Strenuous exercise has both a short-term effect (for which emergency sugar supplies should be carried), and an effect lasting up to 18 hours, largely mediated

Table 11.3. Perioperative insulin regimes

1. EMERGENCY SURGERY

Inform Diabetes Team on admission.
Weight, U & E+glucose, bicarbonate, osmolality.
(Blood gas if bicarbonate less than 10 mmol/l).

Follow diabetic ketoacidosis protocol.

Operate when rehydrated and blood pressure stable, sodium and potassium in normal range and blood sugar less than 20 mmol.

POST-OPERATIVELY: Follow diabetic ketoacidosis protocol.

2. MAJOR ELECTIVE SURGERY (MORNING LIST)

Liaison with Diabetes Team well before date
Diabetes clinic visit two to three weeks ahead to discuss control and pre- and postoperative management with child and parents.

Admit day before surgery.
Pre-meal and pre-bedtime BM sticks on the ward.

PRE-OPERATIVELY: Weight, U & E, FBC, true blood glucose, urine for ketones. Normal tea/supper, with normal insulin dose subcutaneously. Starve from midnight, water only to 3.00 a.m. in discussion with anaesthetists.
**First on list.

Intravenous fluid infusions from 8.00 a.m.+insulin infusion (see section 6).
Measure BM sticks pre-theatre and half-hourly during surgery.

POST-OPERATIVELY: Measure BM sticks half-hourly for first two hours, hourly for four hours and then two-hourly until next morning, then discuss with Diabetes Team.
Continue IV infusion and insulin infusion until taking **adequate** oral fluids and snacks.

If gradual return to full diet is planned, consider move to soluble subcutaneous insulin three times/day before meals.

If eating and drinking **normally** by teatime on day of operation, give usual subcutaneous insulin plus meal but continue to check BM sticks as above. Stop insulin infusion half hour after giving teatime subcutaneous insulin. (**For child on once daily insulin continue IV therapy till half an hour after next morning dose of insulin followed by breakfast**).

3. MAJOR ELECTIVE SURGERY (AFTERNOON LIST)
Liaison with Diabetes Team well before date
Diabetes clinic visit two to three weeks ahead to discuss control and pre- and postoperative management with child and parents.

continued

Table 11.3. *continued*

PRE-OPERATIVELY: Admit day before surgery pre-meal and pre-bedtime BM stick on the ward pre-operatively. Normal tea/supper, with normal insulin dose subcutaneously. Pre-operative weight and on morning of surgery, U & E, FBC, glucose, urine for ketones. Allow normal breakfast no later than 7.30 a.m., then starve, but check with anaesthetists for exact timing.
**First on afternoon list.

Insulin:
If on twice a day mixed insulin give 60% of usual dose of soluble insulin subcutaneously before breakfast, but no medium-acting insulin.

Basal bolus ('pen') regimes — usual soluble subcutaneous insulin therapy before breakfast.

(**For children on one injection medium-acting insulin per day give 25% of normal morning dose as soluble subcutaneous insulin before breakfast**).

Intravenous fluid infusions from 12 noon+insulin infusion (see section 6).
Measure BM sticks pre-theatre and half-hourly during surgery.

POST-OPERATIVELY: Measure BM sticks half-hourly for first two hours, hourly for four hours and then two-hourly until next morning, then discuss with Diabetes Team.
Continue IV fluids and insulin infusion until taking **adequate** oral fluids and snacks.

If gradual return to full diet is planned, consider move to soluble subcutaneous insulin three times/day before meals.

If eating and drinking **normally** by breakfast on first post-operative day, give usual insulin plus meals. Check BM sticks pre-meals. Stop insulin infusion half hour after giving morning subcutaneous insulin. If in doubt please discuss with Diabetes Team.

4. MINOR SURGERY (MORNING LIST)

Notify Diabetes Team well before event.
**Plan for child to be first on the list.

PRE-OPERATIVELY: Admit afternoon before or early morning of day of planned surgery; pre-meal and pre-bedtime BM sticks.
Normal subcutaneous insulin with tea, day before (all regimes).
Starve from midnight (water to 3.00 a.m. or as ordered by anaesthetist).
No breakfast; subcutaneous insulin.
Check blood glucose/BM stick pre-operatively.

IV fluid infusion from 8.00 a.m. + insulin infusion (see section 6).

POST-OPERATIVELY: Measure BM sticks hourly for four hours then in discussion with Diabetes Team.
Fluids+snacks when conscious.
If not tolerating fluids then stay overnight and continue infusion till next morning. Otherwise give normal subcutaneous teatime insulin**, then meal. Stop insulin infusion half an hour after teatime subcutaneous insulin.

---

continued

Table 11.3. *continued*

Discharge home after tea if eaten **normally**. (Instruct parents to phone Diabetes Team for advice if worried in night.)

Normal subcutaneous insulin from next day.

(**For children on a single daily morning dose of medium-acting insulin, give one-third of the daily dose before tea**.)

5. MINOR SURGERY (AFTERNOON LIST)

Liaise with Diabetes Team well before event. Allow normal breakfast no later than 7.30 a.m.

N.B. Breakfast and morning subcutaneous insulin can be given at home. Insulin dose, see below. Parents should be instructed to seek advice on dose from Diabetes Team well before the planned surgery.

PRE-OPERATIVELY. **Plan for child to be first on the afternoon list**. Measure BM stick on arrival.

Oral fluids until three hours pre-operatively (check with anaesthetists) and monitor BM stick while starved pre-operatively on an hourly basis.

IV fluid infusion from 12.00 noon with insulin infusion (see section 6).

POST-OPERATIVELY: Measure BM sticks hourly for four hours, then in discussion with Diabetes Team.
Fluids+snacks when conscious.
If not tolerating fluids and food **normally** then stay overnight and continue infusion till next morning.
Otherwise could go home after usual subcutaneous insulin and late tea. Stop IV infusion half an hour after subcutaneous dose. (Instruct parents to phone Diabetes Team for advice if worried in night.) Normal subcutaneous insulin next day.

Insulin
If on twice-a-day mixed insulin give 60% of usual dose of soluble breakfast insulin subcutaneously, but no medium-acting insulin. Usual dose before tea and then home.

Basal bolus ('pen') regimes — usual breakfast soluble subcutaneous and afternoon soluble+long-acting subcutaneous insulin therapy.

(**For children on one injection medium-acting insulin per day**
(a) Give 25% of normal morning dose as *soluble* subcutaneous insulin before breakfast.

(b) Give one-third dose of patient's normal **medium**-acting subcutaneous insulin before tea, then home.)

IV fluid infusion guide

1/5 (0.18%) normal saline and 4% dextrose *plus* potassium 10 mmol/500 ml.

---

continued

Table 11.3. *continued*

Weight (kg)	1/5 normal dextrose saline (ml/hour)
10	40
20	60
30	70
40	80
50	90
60 plus	100

6. INSULIN INFUSION GUIDE
50 u soluble insulin (0.5 ml) added to 49.5 ml normal (0.9%) saline in syringe pump (1 ml solution=1 unit soluble insulin).
Infuse at standard rate of 0.05 u/kg/hour. Measure BM stick hourly.
Then:
Adjust insulin infusion rate (discuss if unsure):
Blood glucose above 15 mmol/l—increase by 25%.
Blood glucose below 7 mmol/l—decrease by 50%.

through depletion of muscle glycogen. Thus for planned training the short-acting insulin immediately before the exercise should be reduced (or omitted entirely for the most strenuous exercise) to a level that, with experience, allows for freedom from hypoglycaemia during the event. The medium- or long-acting insulin immediately after the exercise should also be reduced by up to 25%, again the exact amount being dictated by practice and experience.

Travel necessitates forethought regarding storage of insulin in warm climates, a letter for customs regarding the need to carry insulin and needles and syringes (the British Diabetic Association produce an ID card which serves the same purpose), emergency contact numbers and insurance for the destination and also an adjustment of insulin dose to cope with travel across time zones. For trips involving a change of less than four hours, adjustments of dose are rarely necessary. For longer journeys an easy and practical solution is to give 15–20% of the total daily dose of insulin as soluble before main meals on the plane and to revert to the usual regime on arrival in the new time zone. Glucose-testing strips, insulin, emergency sugar and glucagon should be carried on the plane. Hot climates bring disturbed nights to the unacclimatised and this, coupled with holiday activities, means that it is wise to consider an overall reduction in dose to avoid spoiling a family holiday by severe hypoglycaemic attacks.

CONCLUSIONS

The chemistry of currently available insulins plus the variability inherent in the life of a child or adolescent make over-rigorous approaches to insulin treatment futile. A team member should be prepared to be sympathetic and flexible to try to achieve the optimum control for any particular individual or family by experimenting with different types and modes of administration of insulin as dictated by experience.

FURTHER READING

Betz, J. L. Fast-acting human insulin analogs: a promising innovation in diabetes care. *Diabetes Education* 1995; **21:** 195–200.

Buysschaert, M., Minette, P., Ketelslegers, J. M., Pairet, J. V., Vogels, M., Lambert, A. E. Comparison of blood glucose profiles and glycaemic control in type 1 diabetic patients treated with Actrapid-Monotard® or Actrapid-Protophane® (NPH) insulins. *Diabetes Research* 1987; **4:** 31–3.

Gibb, D. M., Foot, A. B. M., May, B., Parish, H., Strang, S., Grant, D. B., Dunger, D. B. Human isophane or lente insulin? A double blind crossover trial in insulin dependent diabetes mellitus. *Archives of Disease in Childhood* 1990; **65:** 1334–7.

Holly, J. M., Dunger, D. B., Edge, J. A., Smith, C. P., Chard, T., Wass, J. A. Insulin-like growth factor binding protein-1 levels in diabetic adolescents and their relationship to metabolic control. *Diabetic Medicine* 1990; **7:** 618–23.

Howey, D. C., Bowsher, R. R., Brunelle, R. L., Woodworth, J. [Lys(B28), Pro(B29)]-human insulin. A rapidly absorbed analogue of human insulin. *Diabetes* 1994; **43:** 396–402.

Kaufman, F. R., Devgan, S., Roe, T. F., Costin, G. Perioperative management with prolonged intravenous insulin infusion versus subcutaneous insulin in children with type I diabetes mellitus. *Journal of Diabetes Complications* 1996; **10:** 6–11.

MacPherson, J. N., Feely, J. Insulin. *British Medical Journal* 1990; **300:** 731–6.

O'Hagan, M., Greene, S. A. Pre-mixed insulin delivered by disposable pen in the management of children with diabetes. *Diabetic Medicine* 1993; **10:** 972–5.

Sane, T., Koivisto, V. A., Nikkanen, P., Pelkonnen, R. Adjustment of insulin doses of diabetic patients during long distance flights. *British Medical Journal* 1990; **301:** 421–2.

Thow, J., Home, P. Insulin injection technique. *British Medical Journal* 1990; **301:** 3–4.

Tunbridge, F. K. E., Newens, A., Home, P. D., Davis, S. N., Murphy, M., Burrin, J. M., Alberti, K. G. M. M., Jensen, I. Double-blind crossover trial of Isophane (NPH) and Lente based insulins. *Diabetes Care* 1989; **12:** 115–19.

12

Setting Standards of Care, Audit, Data-Handling and Registers

KEN ROBERTSON AND GEOFF R. LAWSON

SETTING STANDARDS

So many documents come to us nowadays containing the phrase 'Standard setting' that we could be forgiven for forgetting that medicine is founded on the traditions of introspection and improvement. However, it is fair to say that the recent official emphasis on audit has hardened up the approach to the delivery of health care in as effective a way as possible. Nor should we neglect efficiency in times of diminishing resources to cover increasing demands.

In diabetes, as in many other branches of medicine, there has been a profusion of documents professing 'gold standards' of care. The majority however, have been based on adult practice and thus are inapplicable to childhood diabetes. Adult diabetology is heavily, and rightly, skewed towards the early detection and management of complications. In childhood, evident complications are rare—although they must be sought—so standards must be broader, taking account of the changing needs of a growing child while, at the same time, recognising the accumulating evidence that good control must begin pre-pubertally for maximum protection.

LOCAL TAILORING OF NATIONAL GUIDELINES

This is no place to open a debate about the relative merits of and differences between Protocols and Guidelines. Suffice it to say that, for those not at the

Childhood and Adolescent Diabetes. Edited by S. Court and B. Lamb.
© 1997 John Wiley & Sons, Ltd.

forefront of a speciality or subspecialty, they can provide a very useful starting point for the planning and provision of a service. Furthermore, with growing emphasis on Health Care Purchasing, such documents are increasingly being read by those responsible for the allocation of resources, so it is important that providers (i.e. clinicians) have a clear idea of their contents.

Reinvention of the wheel is usually a fruitless policy. For this reason it is helpful, when preparing documents for local use, to start with the recommendations of a National Body such as the St Vincent Task Force in the UK. For precisely the reason that such bodies do not wish to be prescriptive in their advice, the statements will be general and often flexible. Such documents are meant only as a framework for local tailoring and the latter process should take account of all the peculiar factors that influence care delivery in a real clinic in their individual settings. The mistake too often made is to produce a document so bland that it sets no standards at all — 'Patients with diabetes will be reviewed regularly and will receive education' does not provide an objective that will attract meaningful commitment. Statements such as this have appeared in the guidance for at least one region in the UK and a moment's thought implies that the standard could be satisfied by someone setting up a stall at the school gates. However, there is a natural apprehension that any goals will be viewed by purchasers as thresholds upon which may depend payment. This blinkered approach to standard setting must be resisted by the demonstration of good systems of care moving towards achievable targets. Any centre's performance must be considered in the context of how others are faring.

ST VINCENT DECLARATION AND CHILDREN

Children receive little attention in the St Vincent Declaration[1] (Appendix 1) but the following sentence emphasises the importance of co-ordinated care:

> Ensure that care for children with diabetes is provided by individuals and teams specialised both in the management of diabetes and of children and that families with a diabetic child get the necessary social, economic and emotional support.

Regional and local task forces have the role of turning this into an action plan.

AUDIT

POINT AND PURPOSE

There have been many attempts to define audit but the following five 'Es' encompass the concepts:

- Expectations: of patients, medical and nursing staff
- Enquiry: driven by the desire to learn more about specific areas of practice
- Evaluation: without objective evaluation, enquiry is meaningless
- Education: the previous three stages educate and provide opportunities for the last
- Enhancement: the purpose of the whole exercise is to enhance care[2].

To these may be added a sixth 'E', for Essential because in order to manage any clinic for a chronic disease successfully it is vital to step back regularly to take a look at what is being achieved — or not.

INTRA-CLINIC AUDIT

One of the stumbling blocks in diabetes audit is the tendency to dwell upon glycosylation indices such as HbA1c, total HbA1 and fructosamine. This is understandable insofar as these are objective measurements which correlate with disease outcome. However, the plethora of methodologies make interpretation very difficult. Most laboratories do not offer a paediatric reference range and some use the manufacturer's range from the side of the box rather than establishing a local range. These details matter — in Glasgow the reference mean was lowered by 0.5% when a reference range was compiled from 100 children in hospital for reasons other than diabetes. Regular analysis of the spread of glycosylation values across the clinic can give an indication of general performance. Identification of those individuals doing badly is useful for targeting of care.

There are, of course many other objective measures that can, and should be, audited. Growth monitoring is mandatory, with early recognition of individuals who are falling on the centile charts. Completeness of annual review type data such as retinal examination, blood pressure, dietary review and skills checking should be surveyed. The rate of readmission to hospital after initial diagnosis is a rough indicator of efficacy of diabetes education. A dramatic increase in the incidence of severe hypoglycaemia or referrals to the clinical psychologist may indicate the need for a team policy rethink. A periodic review of default patterns is vital if individuals are not to slip through the net, as may occur if clinic staff simply send multiple repeat appointments.

If a system involves only one doctor who sees all the patients at every clinic then consistency of approach is more likely but if, as in many clinics, there are several doctors involved, some only on a short-term basis, it is even more important to take a regular overview. In any case, trends are rarely apparent when concentrating upon an individual and if, as suggested above, local guidelines are in place then performance must regularly be gauged against these.

INTER-CLINIC AUDIT

We all want to know how we are faring in relation to our peers, and now we have to satisfy purchasers of health care that we are performing well. Regular meetings of professionals involved in the care of children with diabetes constitute the first step towards improving the care for all. This can be enhanced further with objective peer assessment. It is first necessary to ensure adequate provision of professionals so that all children can receive appropriate medical and dietetic advice. Rural areas have more problems, but where there is no paediatric dietitian or diabetes nurse specialist it may be possible to set up shared care with a larger centre.

Allowing for differences in clinic populations (age, duration of diabetes) assessment can be made of overall performance in terms of eye screening, blood pressure checks, microalbuminuria screening, etc. Deficiencies act as a spur to those clinics not coming up to the predefined mark. Highlighting of such deficiencies in a regional context is a valuable step towards securing more resources.

Comparison on the grounds of blood sugar control is fraught with problems. It is estimated that there are around 21 different methodologies for assaying HbA1c and HbA1. In an audit of diabetes care in Scottish centres (DIABAUD) 10 methods were in use. Only 23 of 51 clinics were using a local reference range and two of 20 paediatric clinics used a paediatric reference range. There is now widespread recognition that values from different assays, or even values obtained from the same method in different centres, cannot be compared directly. Several suggestions have been offered on how comparisons can be made and, of course, the main reason that this is desirable is to gain some indication of comparison with the Diabetes Control and Complications Trial[3] (DCCT) which showed dramatic reductions in the rate of progression to microvascular complications in an intensively treated group.

European guidelines suggested classification into good, borderline and poor control, with the last category five or more standard deviations from the mean of the normal range. Kilpatrick *et al.*[4] have shown this is completely unreliable, leading to different classification of patients dependent upon analysis method. Similar arguments apply to comparisons on the basis of multiples of the mean of the normal range. Quite simply, the only way to compare centres is for samples to be sent to a single laboratory. If the local and central laboratory assays are linear then sending samples from a proportion of patients to the central laboratory (perhaps 100 samples) will allow construction of a regression line, the equation of which can be used to 'convert' local values to central values. Such an exercise has been completed recently by 22 centres in 18 countries throughout the world who sent samples to the Steno Laboratory in Copenhagen[5]. There were differences between centre mean values for HbA1c of up to 2% but the diversity of management complicated interpretation — with issues such as how a clinic comes by its patients (e.g. selection of patients versus population-based clinics) being relevant.

No international (or even national) standards exist for calibrating methods, thus it is likely that the only way of ensuring consistency is by pegging local laboratories to a national or international centre as above. Although this may appear to be an argument for the clinical biochemists, glycosylation analysis is so vital to patient management in diabetes that clinicians must participate in the debate. That clinicians have an interest in biochemical methodology may be both novel and surprising to colleagues in Clinical Pathology but, none the less, it is essential.

DATA HANDLING

OPTIMISED PAPER SYSTEM

No regular audit or analysis will be possible unless careful thought is given to data collection. The traditional medical clinic is a fairly haphazard affair with doctors renowned for their idiosyncratic notekeeping methods. Any single-disease clinic lends itself to structured notekeeping. As a minimum, a clinic record sheet should be prepared which will act as a focus for the consultation and an *aide mémoire* for those seeing the patient. There may be sections for the individual professionals or a single form but the essence should be a concise document with little opportunity for ambiguity. Tick boxes are useful and every effort should be made to minimise the amount of free text required. The latter is difficult to analyse and, worse, is frequently illegible. An example of such a chart is given in Appendix 12.1.

PAPERLESS SYSTEM

It is a truism that a computerised database should not be designed around a paper form. However, the existence of a structured approach to notekeeping is an essential prerequisite to computerisation. The Holy Grail of 'techies' is to dispense with paper altogether and have the computer as the only repository of patient information. While this has a certain appeal it has not been accomplished anywhere, nor will it be for some time, not least because current software cannot yet emulate the immediacy of well kept paper records.

WHAT TO RECORD

Running a diabetes service requires more than just recording clinic visits. There must be a fail-safe mechanism for recording visits by team members to homes, schools and nurseries, as well as a logging system for telephone contact since this is a valuable guide to the level of support required by individual families and for resource allocation. Paper records will already contain details of hospital admissions but a summary sheet giving dates and reason (diabetes-related or not) may be a useful aid to audit.

DATASET

Consideration should be given to published datasets such as the UK Diabetes Dataset[6] but this is not paediatrically orientated. Everyone will have their own ideas about data that require collection in the children's diabetes clinic. Those without neurosthesiometers will probably regard vibration thresholds as too esoteric but there are obviously certain items that require recording. They can be broadly divided into routine and annual review items.

Routine Items

1. Growth parameters — height and weight should be recorded and plotted on the appropriate centile charts.
2. Urinalysis for glucose and ketones — it is worth considering whether this is valuable, although commonly done.
3. Glycosylation index (HbA1c etc.).
4. Blood sugar (if assayed) — see 'urinalysis'.
5. Insulin regimen including insulin type and doses.
6. Injection device.
7. State and position of injection sites: (H)ealthy, (U)nhealthy.
8. Hypoglycaemia — notoriously difficult to quantify and to grade, especially retrospectively. It may be helpful to record the worst hypoglycaemic episode since the last visit on the following scale:

> 0 None at all
> 1 Biochemical or mild and self treated
> 2 Mild and required help
> 3 Required HypoStop and/or Glucagon
> 4 Required admission to hospital.

Clearly, there are overlaps and local agreement is required over grading in young children who will always require help, but this approach at least gives a guide to prevalence.

It is also useful to record who saw the patient, for audit and medicolegal reasons.

Annual Review

This will vary widely but the following items will be commonly found (Appendix 12.2).

1. Eye examination — acuity and retinal examination.
2. State of feet — e.g. presence of verrucae.
3. Pubertal status — endocrinologists like to measure categories precisely but it may be reasonable to divide pubertal status into Pre-pubertal (Tanner I), Pubertal (II, III, IV) and Post-pubertal (V). This avoids the need to be continually peering down trousers and inside blouses — something which does little for the doctor–patient relationship! The age of menarche should be recorded.
4. Urinary albumin excretion.
5. Thyroid function.
6. Autoantibodies — specifically, anti-thyroid, anti-gliadin, anti-endomysial and anti-reticulin antibodies. Some may add anti-adrenal.
7. Lipids — the value of this is debatable but it may be valuable to check fasting lipids in any child who has a family history of ischaemic heart disease.

A record of diabetes education topics covered may also prove helpful for audit of the service.

Finally, any other concurrent illness should be recorded, e.g. asthma, epilepsy, enuresis, etc.

COMPUTERS

Computers are no longer viewed as optional adjuncts to clinical management. The demands upon all of us to produce information on workload as well as clinical and outcome measures have resulted in more and more clinicians coming to rely upon databases for their day-to-day work. They are no longer the preserve of a few eccentric pioneers. A good system should be intuitive so that an absolute minimum of expertise is required to enter and retrieve data.

COMMERCIAL VERSUS BESPOKE SYSTEMS

There are now a considerable number of commercial vendors offering comprehensive diabetes management systems. Unfortunately, however, these tend to be expensive, sometimes require hardware modification and are generally designed for adult populations with heavy emphasis on microvascular complications. If children have not been considered then there may be no fields for pubertal status and growth. If modifications to the forms and fields are simple then this is not a problem, but some suppliers charge for such changes thus limiting flexibility. Bespoke (locally tailored) systems will avoid such problems but the difficulties here are most often related to lack of support if the designer (often a keen junior staff member) moves on. If you opt for a local system then you should ensure that it is fully documented and is built using a well recognised database engine so that someone else could, if necessary, make modifications in the future. Systems implemented in a DOS environment are less attractive than those designed to run under Microsoft Windows℠, but the latter are slower and require more sophisticated, and expensive, hardware. The other critical question is whether you intend to have a stand-alone, single-user system or require a networked version so that several practitioners can have simultaneous access to the database. You should seek expert advice before procuring any system.

DIABETES AND THE HOSPITAL INFORMATION SUPPORT SYSTEM

Many hospitals now have comprehensive Hospital Information Support Systems (HISS). These can be thought of as stock control systems for patients — capturing biographical details at the point of entry of the patient to the hospital and thereafter building up an 'account' by accreting information about all that happens to that individual during their stay or association. Thus details of X-rays, laboratory tests, diagnoses and treatments are gathered by separate 'modules' within different departments, but all are tied to the patient by a unique identifier which will usually be a system-generated number but later may be a national number such as the new NHS number in the UK. The identifier is retained by the system so that further episodes can be logged for this individual. The heart of any HISS is the Patient Administration System (PAS). This is the repository for biographical details, including name, address, date of birth, and general practitioner. The PAS is the hub around which all other modules revolve.

Some HISS systems are sophisticated enough to allow generation of 'user-specific screens' which can be tailored to capture information pertinent to a disease such as diabetes. This may provide enough functionality for most purposes, but not many systems are so flexible. Some systems do not even allow patient data to be linked to a clinical diagnosis and will be unable even to list the number of diabetics being seen at a centre.

The other option is to 'interface' the HISS with a separate diabetes system such as described above. The principal questions to be asked are, 'what does the diabetes system need from the HISS and what does the HISS require from the disease specific system?' The answers will be locally determined but, in general, a PAS link is desirable so that the biographical details held in the diabetes system are current and do not require to be re-keyed. Interfacing is a complex issue and further discussion is beyond the scope of this book. However, this is a vital area for consideration if you are planning to implement a new system.

DATA ENTRY IN THE CLINIC

There are several diabetes management systems which are designed for use in the clinic but paper output is still required so that other hospital staff have access to the information. Some adults may find it off-putting to see their doctor interacting with a computer during a consultation, but children are much more comfortable with the technology and enjoy seeing their name appear on the screen.

OUTPUT

Strange though it may seem, many elderly computer systems had simple methods for entering data but had the unfortunate design feature that extraction was excruciatingly difficult. The essence of a flexible system is the ability to produce standard and *ad hoc* reports with ease. As a minimum, printed output will be required for communication with the general practitioner; this may take the form of clinic letters and annual reports. Audit procedures such as calculation of mean HbA1c for the clinic population can be stored and run many times. Consideration should be given to how to calculate the latter — the simple approach is to take the mean of all the latest values for each patient. This is clearly better than averaging all the values during a given time because some patients may be over- or under-represented. A more laborious way, ideally suited to the computer, is to calculate the mean for each individual over a year then to take the mean of these. The age/duration profile of the clinic will also have to be considered. Print-outs of visits by the team and telephone logs may be valuable and, unless there is 24-hour access to the system, it is wise to print out summaries periodically for retention in the patients' case-files.

Any good system will allow on-the-fly or *ad hoc* report generation so that specific questions can be answered — e.g. how many children under the age of five have had grade 3 or 4 hypoglycaemic attacks in the past six months? how many of these required admission to hospital? If you are contemplating a system that requires programming to produce the answer to such a question — forget it!

REGISTERS

The key to achieving the goals of the St Vincent Declaration will be the solid bedrock of diabetes registers. Quite obviously, it is impossible to show a 30% reduction in diabetic blindness in a region where there is no knowledge of the current scale of the problem. This example shows that more is needed than a simple register of diabetes: morbidity databases built around validated registers are required. This is a tall order.

Registers are more complete if they are compiled by multiple ascertainment using capture–recapture methods[7]. The latter may be biased, however, if the sources of data are not truly independent. The Scottish Study Group (SSG) for the Care of Young People with Diabetes started a register in 1981 of children under 15 years of age developing insulin dependent diabetes. Paediatricians caring for these children register details via a card system. Validation is carried out by comparison with Scottish Medical Record returns of hospital in-patients and a few are added by scrutiny of death certificates. Now that so many newly diagnosed patients are not being admitted to hospital, validation is more difficult but Scotland is geographically well defined and very few children are cared for by doctors who are not members of the SSG. Larger regions have larger problems. Another method of validation is by analysis of pharmacy prescriptions as described in a study from Verona in Italy[8]. Regional, whole-population registers will necessarily include many adult patients (the vast majority) with NIDDM and as an absolute minimum the two groups (IDDM and NIDDM) should be distinguished.

With the coming of St Vincent, many areas are now setting up mechanisms to gather information from diverse sources—general practitioners, hospital doctors, chiropodists and ophthalmologists—in an attempt to gauge morbidity. Clear definitions of data items are essential if inter-regional comparisons such as were recently piloted in England and Wales[9] are not to be worthless.

Any register is a living entity which must be fed if it is not to become wildly inaccurate. Use of a unique identifier such as the NHS number with a currency outwith any given region, coupled with dynamic means of updating the data are essential. For example, development must occur to allow anonymised transfer of morbidity data from existing hospital and GP systems as well as simple methods such as are adopted by companies wishing to update mailing lists—current data are returned to the 'owner' periodically for updating.

All of this may seem a long way from the clinic where we look after individual children with diabetes and their families, but it is only by disciplining ourselves to collect and share audit and morbidity data that we can influence service provision and, ultimately, disease outcome.

REFERENCES

1 World Health Organisation (Europe) and International Diabetes Federation (Europe). Diabetes care and research in Europe: the St Vincent Declaration. *Diabet Med* 1990; **7:** 360.

2 *Moving to Audit — An Education Package for Hospital Doctors and General Practitioners* (ISBN 1 871749 24 7). The Postgraduate Office, Ninewells Hospital and Medical School, Dundee DD1 9SY, 1992.

3 The Diabetes Control and Complications Trial Research Group (DCCT). The effect of intensive treatment of diabetes on the development and progression of long term complications in insulin dependent diabetes mellitus. *N Engl J Med* 1993; **329:** 977–86.

4 Kilpatrick, E. S., Rumley, A. G., Dominiczak, M. H., Small, M. Glycated haemoglobin values: problems in assessing blood glucose control in diabetes mellitus. *BMJ* 1994; **309:** 983–6.

5 Mortensen, H., Hougard, P. on behalf of the Hvidøre Study. Group comparison of metabolic control in a cross-sectional study of 2873 children and adolescents with insulin dependent diabetes from 18 nations. *Diabet Care* 1997; **20:** (in press).

6 Vaughan, N. J. A., Home, P. D. The UK Diabetes Dataset: a standard for information exchange. *Diabet Med* 1995; **12:** 717–22.

7 Bruno, G., LaPorte, E., Merletti, F. *et al.* Application of capture–recapture to count diabetes? *Diabet Care* 1994; **17(6):** 548–56.

8 Muggeo, M., Verlato, G., Bonora, E. *et al.* The Verona Diabetes Study: a population based survey on known diabetes mellitus prevalence and 5-year all-cause mortality. *Diabetologia* 1995; **38(3):** 318–25.

9 McColl, A. J., Gulliford, M. C. *Population Health Outcome Indicators for the NHS.* London: Royal College of Physicians, 1993.

Appendix 12.1

Diabetes Clinic Flow Chart   GP:

Name:.   Hospital number   D.O.B.   /   /   Diagnosed   /   /

Date:								
General Condition								
Illness								
School missed								
Hypoglycaemia * 1,2,3								
Insulin type: dose:	am	pm	am	pm	am	pm	am	pm
Blood sugar profile								
Weight								
Height								
HbA$_{1c}$								
Skin/ injection sites								
Dietary Comments								
Concerns								
Plan of action								
Seen by :-								
Change of insulin type: dose:	YES/NO am	pm	YES/NO am	pm	YES/NO am	pm	YES/NO am	pm
Next appointment								

* HYPOGLYCAEMIA: 1 = mild, self help   2 = moderate, needed some help
   3=severe, needing i.m./i.v. treatment or with seizure or other unusual manifestation
(hemiplegia etc)

Appendix 12.2

Diabetes Care Chart: ANNUAL REVIEW

Date of review: Years since diagnosis**: **0 1** 2 3 4 **5 6** 7 8 9 **10**

Reviewed by: Special comments:

Growth centiles Ht Wt	**Laboratory investigations***	
Current HbA1c Average HbA1c	Serum creatinine	
Insulin dose/kg body weight	Cholesterol	Triglycerides
Hands	TSH	FT4
Skin condition	Auto-antibodies	
Feet	Thyroid	
Blood pressure	Anti-gliaden G A endomysial	
Reflexes	Urine microalbumin***	
Vibration	Other	
Fundoscopy		
Other examination findings		
Puberty	Optician	
School	Dentist	
Chiropodist	Retinal photos**	

* Venous blood for lab investigations to be taken at diagnosis, and then after 1,5 and 10 years if no abnormal results, annually if positive auto-antibodies or other indication.
** Retinal photography to be carried out after the age of 10 after 5 years from diagnosis and every year once puberty established, i.e. menarche in girls, growth spurt in boys.
*** Urine screen for microalbuminuria after 5 and 10 years and annually with established puberty.

DIABETES NURSE SPECIALIST	Telephone number:	Working hours
		Answer phone
		Radio-pager number
CHILDREN'S DIETICIAN	Telephone number:	Working hours
CONSULTANT PAEDIATRICIAN	Telephone number:	Working hours

24 HOUR MEDICAL COVER   Ring xxxxxxxxxxxxx and ask operator to radio-page Children's Diabetes Consultant on Call.

13

Acute Complications of Diabetes

JULIE A. EDGE AND KRYSTYNA MATYKA

INTRODUCTION

The two most common acute complications of insulin dependent diabetes mellitus (IDDM) are hypoglycaemia and ketoacidosis. The former is a major cause of anxiety and alarm to children, their parents and carers, while the latter may be life-threatening and difficult to treat. Ketoacidosis should be avoidable but one of the costs of improving blood glucose control is a rising incidence of hypoglycaemia. This chapter will cover the definitions, causes, presentation and practical management of both conditions.

HYPOGLYCAEMIA

DEFINITION

Hypoglycaemia is the most feared acute complication following treatment of IDDM and is a common problem, especially when aiming for tight blood glucose control.

The brain relies almost exclusively on glucose as its source of energy. In health, blood glucose levels do not fall below 3.5 mmol/l, because as blood glucose levels fall a neurohumeral response is initiated which acts to restore blood glucose levels to normal. Counter-regulatory hormones such as glucagon, adrenaline, cortisol and growth hormone are secreted and there is stimulation of the sympathetic nervous system. This has the net effect of improving cerebral glucose supply as a result of increased hepatic glucose output, decreased peripheral glucose uptake and increased cardiac output. It

Childhood and Adolescent Diabetes. Edited by S. Court and B. Lamb.
© 1997 John Wiley & Sons, Ltd.

Table 13.1. Grading of hypoglycaemia

Mild	Biochemical hypoglycaemia with no symptoms
	Mild symptoms easily treated with glucose/food
Moderate	Required unusual assistance to treat in very young
	External help required in older children
Severe	Parenteral glucagon or IV glucose required
	Seizure, coma, hemiplegia, hospital admission

also leads to the production of a symptom complex (sweating, shaking, palpitations) which alerts the individual to their state and prompts them to eat. If despite these efforts, glucose levels fall further (<3.0 mmol/l) then neuroglycopaenia follows (confusion, incoordination, odd behaviour) with cognitive dysfunction. However, in people with IDDM suffering recurrent episodes of hypoglycaemia (or 'hypos'), even mild episodes, these responses can be blunted and neuroglycopenia can occur without warning. It has been suggested that after a hypo awareness can be impaired for days. Because of concerns about the long-term effects of recurrent severe hypoglycaemia in IDDM it is felt that the blood glucose should not fall below 4 mmol/l — 'four is the floor' — even though in health blood glucose may fall to 3.5 mmol/l.

Hypos are commonly classified as mild, moderate or severe (Table 13.1). Mild refers to self-administration of food or glucose, moderate to requiring some form of external assistance such as help to eat, and severe where parenteral glucagon or glucose is given or severe symptoms such as coma and seizures result. Other definitions referring to adults classify severe hypos as requiring external assistance. As many young children rely on adults to provide them with food even when they have mild symptoms this definition is not appropriate for this age group. Some children will have low capillary blood glucose results without symptoms, so called biochemical 'hypoglycaemia'. Many parents (and some doctors) do not regard these as hypos because of the lack of symptoms. This is wrong. All documented blood glucose values of less than 4.0 mmol/l can be considered a hypoglycaemic event and should not be tolerated on a regular basis.

The true prevalence of hypoglycaemia is not known as minor episodes are not usually reported. Studies looking at the prevalence of severe hypoglycaemia in children and adolescents quote ranges from four to 86 episodes per 100 patient years[1,2].

CLINICAL PICTURE

The symptoms of hypoglycaemia can be very individualised and both child and family will come to recognise their own symptoms in time. From a clinical aspect the symptoms can be divided into three main groups: those due to the neurohumeral response (sweating, palpitations, shaking), those due to neuroglycopenia (confusion, odd behaviour, speech difficulty, incoordination and later coma and convulsions) and non-specific malaise (nausea, headache). Some individuals develop transient hemiplegia (often migraine sufferers) whilst neuroglycopenic, and recovery from this may lag behind restoration of blood glucose levels.

In a recent study of children with diabetes aged 1.5–16 years the most frequent symptoms reported by the children were weakness, dizziness and trembling[3] (often referred to as 'the wobblies'). The commonest parental observations were pallor, sweating, tearfulness and irritability. The authors commented on the frequency with which both parents and children reported behavioural changes during a hypo, something not often mentioned in the adult population with diabetes. Children with newly diagnosed IDDM and their carers need to be educated in the symptoms and signs of hypoglycaemia so that they can recognise them and take appropriate action. It is also wise to warn them that seizures can occur and reassure them that this is not epilepsy.

CAUSES OF HYPOGLYCAEMIA

PRECIPITANTS

Isolated Episodes

One of the greatest challenges in the management of the child with diabetes is the extreme variability in their day-to-day level of activity. Although their lives can be reasonably structured, with a strict routine being set at school, the amount of unplanned exercise, usually in the form of games, will vary greatly from day to day. Although adjustments to insulin dose, diet or both can be made with a planned period of exercise such as a PE lesson or after-school class, this will obviously not be possible with impromptu games of football. Therefore one of the commonest reasons for isolated episodes of hypoglycaemia is unplanned exercise. The other common reason is missed meals due to forgetfulness or lack of time, or occasionally deliberately. Older children in particular hate to be different and may avoid eating if their friends and peers are not, particularly in the classroom. Many would rather miss a meal than be left out of a game in the playground.

Gastro-enteritis

Another important but less well documented cause of isolated episodes of hypoglycaemia is gastro-enteritis. Often, infections lead to hyperglycaemia due to the stimulation of 'stress' hormones (such as adrenaline and cortisol) which lead to mobilisation of glucose stores, and patients are advised to be prepared to increase doses of insulin during infections even if the appetite is poor. During an episode of gastro-enteritis, however, there can be little systemic upset with no anti-insulin hormones being produced. Loss of the intestinal brush border then leads to poor glucose absorption and hypoglycaemia can ensue which can be extremely difficult to treat with oral glucose. In these situations patients may need to reduce the dose of insulin given. Subsequently a period of increasing insulin requirement may ensue if the initial period of diarrhoea and vomiting is followed by systemic symptoms; however, it is more likely to be followed by a more prolonged period of low blood sugars, presumably as the intestinal brush border recovers from the insult.

Recurrent Hypoglycaemia

This occurs when there is a persistent imbalance in the dose of insulin and quantity of food consumed, with the addition of exercise as a further variable. Particular attention needs to be paid to the diet and insulin regimen if there are recurrent episodes. Children who take up a sport on a regular basis may need adjustment to their insulin regimen as well as advice on carbohydrate consumption. It is also important to remember that delayed hypoglycaemia can occur, sometimes up to 24 hours after strenuous exercise, as the body replenishes its stores of glycogen. If this is a recurring problem, it may be important to advise extra carbohydrate both before and after heavy bouts of exercise. Children should not feel that they cannot participate in sport or that their performance will be compromised because of their diabetes.

Nocturnal Hypoglycaemia

Hypoglycaemia at night-time is a terrifying prospect for the carers of children with IDDM. It is a common problem, with studies quoting prevalence rates during single overnight blood profiles from 34–80%[4,5], with the great majority of episodes being asymptomatic (usually slept through). The risk of nocturnal hypoglycaemia is related to the kinetics of the long-acting insulins which lead to overinsulinisation in the early part of the night with levels waning towards morning. Thus hypoglycaemia commonly occurs around 2–4 a.m. and is then followed by a dawn rise in glucose levels. Young children are more at risk as they go to bed much earlier in the evening and have a longer period of fasting overnight. There are few reliable predictors of nocturnal hypoglycaemia but it has been suggested that a glucose level greater than 7 mmol/l at 10 p.m. will avoid the great majority of hypoglycaemia at 2 a.m. A reasonable guideline to give parents is to give extra carbohydrate before bedtime if the blood glucose is less than 7 mmol/l[4].

There has been concern that sudden unexpected death in young people with IDDM who are otherwise well (so-called 'dead in bed' syndrome) may be due to unrecognised severe nocturnal hypoglycaemia. It is possible that hypoglycaemia could lead to arrythmias in an individual with subclinical autonomic dysfunction but there is no evidence for this hypothesis at the current time and further research is awaited.

MANAGEMENT

Everyone with IDDM should carry some form of fast-acting glucose with them at all times. In the case of a very young child this would need to be carried by the main carer, be it parent, nanny, teacher, or so on. It needs to be both palatable for the individual involved (dextrosol tablets are of no use if that person would never eat them) and practical to carry (a bar of chocolate is likely to melt). The practical management of an episode of hypoglycaemia will depend on the severity of the episode, the temporal relationship to meals and what is available in the form of treatment.

The initial step in the management of any episode of hypoglycaemia whenever possible is to check the blood glucose, remembering the importance of ensuring that the fingers are completely clean on testing. Following confirmation of the diagnosis a step-by-step approach should be used which will depend on the level of consciousness of the patient as well as on the degree of co-operation (Figure 13.1). Hypoglycaemia occurring just before a meal still needs to be corrected with fast-acting carbohydrate prior to ingestion of the meal as the long-acting carbohydrate in most meals will take time to act — an effect which is compounded by the delayed gastric emptying which can occur during hypoglycaemia. Nausea is common both during and after an episode of hypoglycaemia and may affect management, but it will subside as the glucose level improves. The treatment of hypoglycaemia at night-time is the same as that during the day but can be complicated by a very sleepy child who is not in the least interested in eating, and so high-sugar drinks and Hypostop® may be more useful at this time.

Mild Hypoglycaemia

Following confirmation of the diagnosis, around 10–20 g of fast-acting carbohydrate should be offered. A sugary drink such as Lucozade®, concentrated fruit juice or high-sugar squash is probably easiest to administer but what is given will depend on what is available. Some children may be reluctant to comply initially but with encouragement will

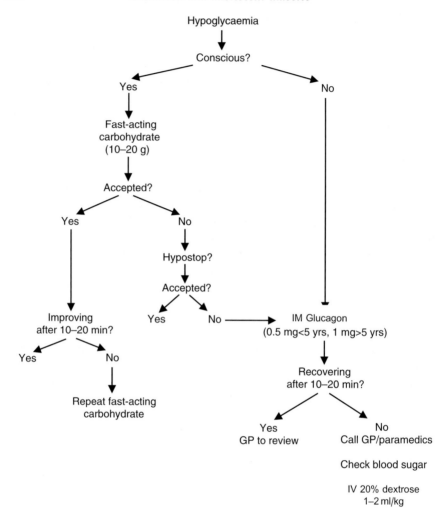

Figure 13.1. Step-by-step approach to the management of hypoglycaemia. For further clarification, see text

eventually co-operate. If the symptoms have not settled within 10–20 minutes it is worth checking the blood glucose (to ensure it is still low) before giving a further 10–20 g of fast-acting carbohydrate. Following recovery, the child should have 10–20 g of long-acting carbohydrate such as toast or wholemeal biscuits, to avoid rebound hypoglycaemia.

Severe Hypoglycaemia

If the child refuses to take any food or drink, Hypostop® (a glucose gel) can be squeezed into the side of the mouth and is absorbed directly from the buccal mucosa. If this is successful it should be followed by long-acting carbohydrate as already mentioned.

With an unconscious or fitting child (or one who just will not co-operate), no attempt should be made to force glucose into the mouth, as aspiration is a serious possibility. Instead, the child should be removed from any place of danger and placed in the recovery position, if possible. Glucagon (0.5 mg for children under five years or 1 mg for the over-fives) is then injected intramuscularly or subcutaneously. This should work within 15–20 minutes. If the episode occurs at home with the parents it would be sensible for the general practitioner or paramedics to be called at the time of administering glucagon as, should glucagon not be effective, glucose should be given intravenously (1 ml/kg of 20% or 2 ml/kg of 10% dextrose). It is important to re-check the blood glucose before giving further intravenous dextrose as some children may remain comatose despite a return to normal blood sugar levels and harm can be done by making them hyperglycaemic. Children do not need to be admitted to hospital following an episode of severe hypoglycaemia unless the child is felt to be at risk of further episodes or is unwell. However, it is advisable that children should be reviewed by a medical practitioner to ensure that no other treatment is necessary. Subsequently, nausea and vomiting can occur following administration of glucagon and may hamper recovery. Rebound hyperglycaemia can also occur following hypoglycaemia (often due to over-treatment) and glycaemic control can be upset for the rest of the day.

It is important to remember that children who arrive in Casualty following an episode of severe hypoglycaemia involving a convulsion may have a blood sugar level in the normal range, leading to uncertainty as to whether the episode was caused by hypoglycaemia. The blood glucose level may well be normal in the post-ictal phase as counter-regulatory hormones would have been stimulated in response to hypoglycaemia and extensive investigations to look for another cause for the convulsion should not be instituted unless clinically indicated.

Following recovery, an explanation for the episode should be sought, if possible, so that further episodes can be avoided. This may include advice regarding exercise or diet or possibly an adjustment in insulin regimen (for recurrent hypoglycaemia).

CONSEQUENCES OF HYPOGLYCAEMIA

The immediate consequences of hypoglycaemia can be quite mild but can also include coma and convulsions. The latter not only compromise the safety of the child but will frighten both the carers and the child involved. This may then affect glycaemic control, with the family preferring higher blood sugars rather than facing the possibility of another serious episode of hypoglycaemia. The delayed consequences of recurrent hypoglycaemia may include blunted counter-regulatory responses to hypoglycaemia (as mentioned above); these will expose the child to further episodes of hypoglycaemia which can be severe. Finally, there has been recent concern about the long-term implications of recurrent hypoglycaemia on cerebral function, especially in children diagnosed under the age of five years[6] (when the brain is still developing). Although there are no firm data at the present time there is enough anxiety to encourage the complete avoidance of hypoglycaemia if at all possible.

DIABETIC KETOACIDOSIS

Diabetic ketoacidosis (DKA) remains a serious and life-threatening condition. The incidence and mortality of DKA have not changed despite increased awareness among primary health care teams that diabetes can occur even in the very young. At diagnosis 25% of children still present in DKA, and in those children under the age of four years this proportion is 40%[7]. Readmission rates with DKA during childhood are around 0.2 per patient year[8]. Cerebral oedema complicates approximately 1% of episodes of DKA, and largely accounts for the fact that DKA is still the major cause of death in children with diabetes.

There is no agreed definition of DKA, but in practice the term refers to decompensated diabetes resulting in hyperglycaemia, acidosis and the presence of ketones. Blood glucose is generally raised, but in some 8% of cases it may be less than 15 mmol/l. The factors which precipitate DKA in children and adolescents are slightly different from those in adults, and are summarised in Table 13.2.

The basic pathophysiology of DKA has been covered in Chapter 2, but it may be worth reviewing the fundamental abnormalities. Blood glucose rises owing to increased hepatic production of glucose secondary to an increase in glucagon/insulin ratio in the portal circulation, and reduced peripheral glucose uptake due to insulin deficiency and insulin resistance. Levels of all the counter-regulatory hormones (catecholamines, cortisol and growth hormone) rise, contributing to the hepatic overproduction of glucose. The hyperglycaemia then results in an osmotic diuresis and dehydration. Elevated levels of the ketone bodies, acetoacetate and beta-hydroxybutyrate, result from insulin deficiency, which causes mobilisation of free fatty acids from adipose tissue, and the rise of the glucagon/insulin ratio in the portal blood which leads to their preferential oxidation to ketone

Table 13.2. Precipating factors in diabetic ketoacidosis

Young children	Adolescents
Newly diagnosed diabetes, particularly in toddlers	Under-dosage with insulin, injections either missed entirely or dose reduced to prevent hypoglycaemia
Emotions and stress	Binges, particularly girls
Infections, viral and bacterial	Excessive alcohol in addition to above
Occasionally missed injections	

bodies instead of re-esterification to form triglycerides for transport out of the liver[8]. Most of the acidosis in DKA is accounted for by the production and dissociation of these organic ketoacids, but lactic acidosis from hypoperfusion, and the high levels of free fatty acids also contribute.

DKA is associated with severe fluid losses. The water deficit is made up of varying combinations from the osmotic diuresis, vomiting, hyperventilation, and occasionally pyrexia. The sodium losses may also be variable, depending on the predominating fluid type lost, and also on the adequacy of renal perfusion. There is always total body depletion of potassium and phosphate ions, even though plasma levels may be low, normal or high. There will also usually have been some attempt by the child or parent to correct the fluid losses with increased oral consumption of fluids of different compositions. Generally, more water is lost than sodium, prompting many authors to suggest that rehydration with hypotonic solutions would be appropriate[9]. However, there are several reasons why this may not be appropriate in children, particularly in the light of recent ideas about the aetiology of cerebral oedema, which are discussed below.

Hyperosmolar coma is rare in children, but does occasionally occur; serum osmolality usually exceeds 300 mOsmol/l, and ketosis is absent. The management is very similar to that of DKA, except that it has been recommended that insulin is given more slowly to prevent too rapid a fall in blood glucose and plasma osmolality[10].

CLINICAL ASSESSMENT

The clinical features of DKA are shown in Table 13.3. In young children, the acidotic breathing pattern and the smell of ketones on the breath may suggest a respiratory infection. The very young in particular may be diagnosed as having status asthmaticus or severe pneumonia, but DKA must be considered in any sick child, and a capillary blood glucose measurement carried out, as the consequences of missing the diagnosis can be devastating.

Table 13.3. Clinical features of diabetic ketoacidosis

Symptoms	Signs
Polyuria	Lethargy
Thirst, polydipsia	Dehydration
Weight loss	Blood pressure normal, rarely low
Abdominal pain	Kussmaul respiration, or later depressed
Weakness	Smell of ketones on breath
Vomiting	Temperature normal
Air hunger	Disordered consciousness in 20% of cases
Confusion	Unconscious in 10% of cases

A rapid assessment should be made of the conscious level (preferably using the Glasgow Coma Score (GCS)), the degree of dehydration and presence of shock. A full clinical assessment can be made once resuscitation is underway. The child should be weighed. This may be difficult at times but if a weigh bed is available not only can it be used to weigh a very ill child but is extremely useful in subsequent fluid management. Only the larger children and adolescents will be too heavy to weigh with an adult holding them and subtracting the adult weight. If an actual weight is not possible because of the clinical condition, the most recent clinic weight or an estimated weight from centile charts should be used as a guideline. It has recently been recognised that the degree of dehydration in children is often overestimated by clinical methods, and that clinical signs of dehydration, in particular loss of skin turgor or elasticity, occur at around 3% dehydration, and not at 5% as is often quoted. Capillary refill times may be a useful technique for the assessment of dehydration in small children[11].

Abdominal pain is a common feature, but a period of rehydration and insulin and electrolyte replacement should be allowed before a surgical emergency is assumed. If the conscious level is impaired, or neurological status changes during treatment, the GCS should be serially recorded, and deteriorating conscious levels investigated as an emergency. A cardiac monitor should be set up to monitor T waves.

LABORATORY ASSESSMENT

The diagnosis of DKA can be confirmed by capillary blood glucose measurements provided that reagent strips are fresh, that meters are well maintained and that staff are trained in their use. Treatment can then be started while the results of further tests such as plasma electrolytes are awaited. Suggested laboratory investigations are listed in Table 13.4. Arterial or capillary blood should ideally be used for acid–base assessment, but venous pH/bicarbonate may be a reasonable substitute, and

Table 13.4. Suggested laboratory investigations in diabetic ketoacidosis

Investigation	Notes
Blood glucose	To confirm capillary result
Sodium, potassium, chloride, phosphate, calcium	Sodium may still be artefactually lowered due to hyperlipidaemia
Urea, creatinine	
Blood gases, pH, bicarbonate	Should initially be from **arterial** sample
Urinary ketones	
FBC, PCV	Leucocytosis extremely common in DKA and does not necessarily imply infection
Urine culture	
Blood culture, CXR, throat swab	Only if clinically indicated, e.g. raised temperature
Amylase	If abdominal pain severe and continues after initial treatment

FBC=full blood count; PCV=packed cell volume; CXR=chest X-ray

subsequent acid–base status can be monitored using venous or non-arterialised capillary blood gases.

MANAGEMENT OF DKA

DKA can be a frightening condition to treat, particularly in small children. The first essential in any management 'protocol' should be that junior medical staff should be supervised adequately whenever they admit any child they suspect to be in DKA. Also guidelines which are easy to understand are essential. The basic principles of management are to correct fluid losses, institute insulin therapy and to prevent complications such as aspiration of gastric contents, hypokalaemia and cerebral oedema. The *Guidelines for Management of DKA* upon which the following section is based summarise the consensus reached by a number of members of the British Society for Paediatric Endocrinology (see Appendix 13.1), and cannot be considered perfect as complications still arise and the pathophysiology of cerebral oedema is not completely understood.

RESUSCITATION

The first priority is to protect and maintain the airway. If the child's consciousness is impaired, or if abdominal pain is a major feature, a nasogastric tube should be inserted immediately, aspirated and left on free drainage. An oral airway may also be necessary. If respiration is depressed or there is accompanying respiratory pathology, intubation and ventilation may be required. Tissue perfusion may be poor and at least until the first arterial blood gas results are known, oxygen is generally administered by face-mask.

The next priority is to treat shock, which must be corrected rapidly. There is a strong rationale for using colloid rather than crystalloid in this initial resuscitation[12] — 10 ml/kg of a colloid solution such as 4.5% albumin should be infused as rapidly as possible, and this dose repeated until the circulation is restored. The total quantity needed can be titrated against changes in tissue perfusion, or in the most severe cases, against central venous pressure. Urinary catheterisation may be helpful in the comatose larger child but it is not generally recommended.

A decision should be made at an early stage as to where the child should be nursed. If the child is very young, comatose or shocked, or if ward staff are very stretched or inexperienced, then admission to an intensive care unit would be appropriate. Ensure that full instructions are given to the *senior* nursing staff emphasising the need for the observations listed in Table 13.5.

FLUIDS

After restoration of the circulating volume, the main fluid deficit is from the intracellular compartment. Isotonic saline should probably be used at this point, since a failure of plasma sodium concentration to rise during treatment has been associated with a risk of development of cerebral oedema[13]. The volume of fluid to be replaced is based on the clinical assessment of the deficit plus maintenance fluid requirements, with the proviso that ongoing losses are also replaced if significant. The rate at which the fluids are given is an area of contention. It has been standard practice to give fluid rapidly at first, and then slow down the rate[14]. However, since the rapid infusion of large volumes of fluid has been proposed as one risk factor for the development of cerebral oedema (see below), once the circulating blood volume has been restored with colloid, the remaining fluid deficit can be corrected slowly and evenly over the next 24 or even 36 hours. Furthermore, slow rehydration has been used successfully in adults with

Table 13.5. Observations to be carried out during early stages of treatment of DKA

1. Strict fluid balance and urine testing of **every** sample
2. Hourly capillary blood glucose measurements
3. Twice-daily weights
4. Hourly or more frequent neuro observations initially
5. Reporting **immediately** to the medical staff, even at night, symptoms of headache or any change in either conscious level or behaviour
6. Reporting any changes in the ECG trace, especially T wave changes

DKA and, paradoxically, it may lead to more rapid restoration of acid–base balance[15].

Once the blood glucose has fallen to 12 mmol/l, a glucose-containing fluid such as 0.45% saline/5% dextrose, or 0.18% saline/4% dextrose should be started. It has been suggested that cerebral oedema may be related to a plasma sodium concentration which falls or does not show the expected rise as glucose levels fall, so that 0.45% saline may be preferable to 0.18%, although at present this has not been established definitely. However, if the plasma sodium is falling, or if it rises above 155 mmol/l, then a 0.45% saline solution should be used.

INSULIN

Although insulin resistance has been shown to be a feature of DKA, in practice large doses of insulin are not required. A continuous low-dose intravenous infusion of 0.1 units/kg/h soluble insulin is now established as an effective and simple method for reversing the metabolic acidosis, and is associated with a lower incidence of hypoglycaemia and hypokalaemia than higher doses. Lower doses have been suggested but may not be as effective at reversing the metabolic abnormalities. Insulin should be infused using a separate syringe pump, so that adjustments to insulin and fluids can be made independently. A bolus of insulin is not necessary as large doses may cause a rapid reduction in blood glucose which may be undesirable. If the blood glucose falls by more than 5 mmol/l/h, the insulin infusion rate should be halved. Once the blood glucose has fallen steadily to around 12 mmol/l, the blood glucose concentration should subsequently be maintained by altering the glucose concentration rather than the insulin infusion rate, since both insulin and glucose are required for the reversal of ketogenesis and glycogenolysis.

POTASSIUM

There is always total body depletion of potassium even though plasma levels may be low, normal or even high. In order to prevent rapid hypokalaemia from the entry of potassium back into the cells once insulin treatment is started, potassium should generally be added to the first bag of fluid, and the concentration altered according to subsequent plasma electrolyte results. If there is any doubt about renal function, an ECG should be checked for peaked T waves before potassium is given.

BICARBONATE

Although acidosis may be severe, recent randomised prospective studies have failed to show any benefit from the administration of bicarbonate to adults with severe DKA, and two of the studies showed paradoxically delayed improvement after bicarbonate[16,17]. Profound acidosis can theoretically be a cause of poor myocardial contractility, although there is no evidence to support this in children. The commonest reason for the failure of acidosis to resolve is inadequate restoration of the circulating blood volume or late institution of insulin therapy which therefore fails to suppress ketogenesis. It has been our recent practice only to use bicarbonate at a blood pH of less than 6.9, or if there is evidence of poor circulation after adequate administration of colloid. Its use should always be discussed with the senior doctor in charge, and the maximum volume of 8.4% sodium bicarbonate used should be calculated to half-correct the acidosis (i.e. $[1/3 \times \text{body weight} \times \text{base deficit}] / 2 = \text{bicarbonate (mmol) required}$, or (ml) 8.4% sodium bicarbonate).

PHOSPHATE

DKA is associated with severe phosphate depletion due to excessive urinary losses, and like potassium, phosphate levels will fall once insulin treatment is started. However, no complications of phosphate deficiency have been reported in children, and furthermore, several randomised studies of the effects of adding phosphate to the regimen for DKA have shown no clinical benefits[18].

CONTINUING MONITORING

It is essential to monitor fluid balance accurately. The correct use of a weigh bed if available highlights excessive fluid loss and dehydration, which can occur with continuing large fluid losses due to gastric aspirate, and continued polyuria and which require prompt, separate replacement. Blood glucose should be monitored hourly, and plasma electrolytes and acid–base status at least four-hourly, in order to ensure a reversal of the acidosis and hyperglycaemia. If either appears to be worsening, re-evaluation should be carried out by a senior member of staff, and it may be necessary to resuscitate further, or increase insulin doses. Neurological monitoring is essential, and should include serial assessments of the Glasgow Coma Score if there is any disordered consciousness.

CHANGING OVER FROM DKA REGIMEN TO SUBCUTANEOUS INSULIN

Once the child is rehydrated, and is tolerating food and fluids, subcutaneous insulin can be started. The dose should be given half an hour before stopping the intravenous insulin infusion. Urinary ketones may persist for one or two days, owing to the conversion of beta-hydroxy

Table 13.6. Complications of diabetic ketoacidosis

Under-treatment	
Unresolved acidosis	Try further fluid resuscitation
Blood glucose not falling	Increase insulin dose
Recurrence of ketoacidosis	Restart protocol from beginning
Over-treatment	
Unrecognised hypokalaemia	Regular electrolytes, and ECG monitoring
Overtreatment with bicarbonate	
Hypoglycaemia	Reduce but **do not stop** insulin, increase dextrose
Others	
Aspiration of gastric contents	**Always** use NG tube if semi-conscious
Cerebral oedema	
Pulmonary oedema/ARDS	

ARDS, acute respiratory distress syndrome

butyrate (which is not measured by conventional urine sticks) to acetoacetate (which is), as ketoacidosis subsides. However, there may still be a degree of insulin resistance, so that larger doses of insulin than usual may be required to switch off ketogenesis.

COMPLICATIONS OF DKA

These are listed in Table 13.6. With meticulous management and observations, hypokalaemia and aspiration pneumonia are now uncommon, and the greatest risk is from cerebral oedema.

CEREBRAL OEDEMA

Although mortality from DKA in the USA fell between 1978 and 1988, mortality from cerebral oedema has remained the same at around 30%[19]. This is almost exclusively a condition of childhood; over 95% of cases in the largest reported series occurred under the age of 20 years, with one-third under the age of five[20]. It appears to be more common in newly diagnosed diabetes[19,21]. Subclinical brain swelling appears to be common during the treatment of DKA, and may be present even before intravenous rehydration is commenced[22,23]. Whether the severe sudden clinical cerebral oedema is an extension of this process, or whether the two are distinct entities remains to be determined.

Clinical Signs

The clinical signs of cerebral oedema are variable. Most cases occur between four and 12 hours from the start of treatment. There may be either a gradual worsening of coma from admission, or, more commonly, a gradual improvement in the child's general condition, followed by a sudden deterioration, with loss of consciousness, appearance of fixed dilated pupils or respiratory arrest. Occasionally a period of change in behaviour or headache may be noted initially.

Aetiology

Possible contributing factors suggested have included cerebral anoxia from the reduced blood volume and haemoconcentration[24], a high initial plasma glucose concentration[22], excessive rates of intravenous fluid administration[25], and a fall in plasma sodium concentration[12,26]. Animal studies have suggested that insulin itself is required for cerebral oedema to occur, and hypoxia resulting from rapid bicarbonate infusion has also been implicated[27]. However, none of these theories explains all the cases described, and most have also been contradicted in case-series[19]. There have only been three small case–control series reported in the literature, and these have all been retrospective analyses[12,20,28]. There have been no prospective case–control studies in this important area of research.

Management

As soon as cerebral oedema is suspected, hypoglycaemia should be ruled out, then mannitol (in a dose of 0.5 g/kg) given within five or 10 minutes of the initial deterioration in neurological function. The child should be transferred to the intensive therapy unit, and a neurosurgical opinion sought. A computed tomography scan should be carried out as soon as possible to rule out other neurological emergencies. Intracranial pressure monitoring and hyperventilation have been shown to improve outcome. However, only half of patients have a period of neurological deterioration during which intervention might be effective before respiratory arrest. Therefore, prevention of this complication remains one of the most important goals of the management of DKA.

REFERENCES

1   Goldstein, D., England, J., Hess, R., Rawlings, S., Walker, B. A prospective study of symptomatic hypoglycaemia in young diabetic patients. *Diabetes Care* 1981; **4**: 601–5.

2 Diabetes Control and Complications Trial Research Group. Effect of intensive diabetes treatment on the development and progression of long-term complications in adolescents with insulin-dependent diabetes mellitus: Diabetes Control and Complications Trial. *Journal of Paediatrics* 1994; **125:** 177–88.
3 McCrimmon, R. J., Gold, A. E., Deary, I. J., Kelnar, C. J. H., Frier, B. M. Symptoms of hypoglycaemia in children with IDDM. *Diabetes Care* 1995; **18:** 858–61.
4 Whincup, G., Milner, R. D. G. Prediction and management of nocturnal hypoglycaemia in diabetes. *Archives of Disease in Childhood* 1987; **62:** 333–7.
5 Matyka, K. A., Watts, A. P., Stores, G., Dunger, D. B. High prevalence of nocturnal hypoglycaemia in young children with insulin dependent diabetes mellitus studied overnight at home. *Diabetic Medicine* 1996; **13(suppl 3):** A39; 513.
6 Rovet, J. E., Ehrlich, R. M., Hoppe, M. Intellectual deficits associated with early onset of insulin dependent diabetes mellitus in children. *Diabetes Care* 1987; **10:** 510–15.
7 Pinkney, J. H., Bingley, P. J., Sawtell, P. A., Dunger, D. B., Gale, E. A. M. Presentation and progress of childhood diabetes mellitus: a prospective population-based study. *Diabetologia* 1994; **37:** 70–4.
8 Foster, D. W., McGarry, J. D. The metabolic derangements and treatment of diabetic ketoacidosis. *New England Journal of Medicine* 1983; **309:** 159–9.
9 Waldhausl, W., Kleinberger, G., Korn, A., Dudczak, R., Bratusch-Marrain, P., Nowotny, P. Severe hyperglycaemia: effects of rehydration on endocrine derangements and blood glucose concentration. *Diabetes* 1979; **28:** 577–84.
10 Sperling, M. A. Diabetic ketoacidosis. *Pediatric Clinics of North America* 1984; **31:** 591–610.
11 Saavedra, J. M., Harris, G. D., Song, L., Finberg, L. Capillary refilling (skin turgor) in the assessment of dehydration. *American Journal of Disease in Childhood* 1991; **145:** 296–8.
12 Hillman, K. Fluid resuscitation in diabetic emergencies—a reappraisal. *Intensive Care Medicine* 1987; **13:** 4–8.
13 Harris, G. A., Fiordalisi, I., Harris, W. L., Mosovich, L. L., Finberg, L. Minimizing the risk of brain herniation during treatment of diabetic ketoacidaemia: a retrospective and prospective study. *Journal of Pediatrics* 1990; **117:** 22–31.
14 Rayner, P. H. W. Diabetes mellitus; treatment of diabetic ketoacidosis. In: *A Paediatric Vade-Mecum*, 12th edn. (Insley J, ed.). London: Edward Arnold, 1990.
15 Adrogue, H. J., Barrero, J., Eknoyan, G. Salutary effects of modest fluid replacement in the treatment of adults with diabetic ketoacidosis. Use in patients without extreme volume deficit. *Journal of the American Medical Association* 1989; **262:** 2108–13.
16 Hale, P. J., Crase, H., Nattrass, M. Metabolic effects of bicarbonate in the treatment of diabetic ketoacidosis. *British Medical Journal* 1984; **289:** 1035–8.
17 Gamba, G., Oseguera, J., Castrejon, M., Gomez-Perez, F. J. Bicarbonate therapy in severe diabetic ketoacidosis: a double-blind, randomized, placebo controlled trial. *Revista de Investigacion Clinica* 1991; **43:** 234–48.
18 Lebovitz, H. E. Diabetic ketoacidosis. *Lancet* 1995; **345:** 767–72.
19 Levitsky, L., Ekwo, E., Goselink, C. A., Solomon, I. L., Aceto, T. Death from diabetes (DM) in hospitalised children (1970–1988). *Pediatric Research* 1991; **29:** 195A.
20 Rosenbloom, A. L. Intracerebral crises during treatment of diabetic ketoacidosis. *Diabetes Care* 1990; **13:** 22–33.

21   Bello, F. A., Sotos, J. F. Cerebral oedema in diabetic ketoacidosis in children. *Lancet* 1990; **336:** 64.
22   Krane, E. J., Rockoff, M. A., Wallman, J. K., Wolfsdorf, J. I. Subclinical brain swelling in children during treatment of diabetic ketoacidosis. *New England Journal of Medicine* 1985; **312:** 1147–51.
23   Durr, J. A., Hoffman, W. H., Sklar, A. H., El Gammal, T., Steinhart, C. M. Correlates of brain oedema in uncontrolled IDDM. *Diabetes* 1992; **41:** 627–32.
24   Dillon, E. S., Riggs, H. E., Dyer, W. W. Cerebral lesions in uncomplicated fatal diabetic acidosis. *American Journal of Medical Science* 1936; **192:** 360–5.
25   Duck, S. C., Wyatt, D. T. Factors associated with brain herniation in the treatment of diabetic ketoacidosis. *Journal of Pediatrics* 1988; **113:** 10–14.
26   Harris, G. A., Fiordalisi, I. Physiologic management of diabetic ketoacidemia. A 5-year prospective pediatric experience in 231 episodes. *Archives of Pediatric and Adolescent Medicine* 1994; **148:** 1046–52.
27   Bureau, M. A., Begin, R., Berthiaume, Y., Shapcott, D., Khoury, K., Gagnon, N. Cerebral hypoxia from bicarbonate infusion in diabetic acidosis. *Journal of Pediatrics* 1980; **96:** 968–73.
28   Vlcek, B. W. Risk factors for cerebral edema associated with diabetic ketoacidosis. *Annals of Neurology* 1986; **20:** 407.

APPENDIX 13.1

Guidelines for the Management of Diabetic Ketoacidosis Recommended by the British Society for Paediatric Endocrinology

These guidelines summarise the consensus reached by a number of members of the British Society for Paediatric Endocrinology (BSPE) concerning the management of DKA. They cannot be considered perfect as complications still arise and the pathophysiology of cerebral oedema is not completely understood.

EMERGENCY MANAGEMENT

RESUSCITATION

- Ensure that the airway is patent and, if the child is comatose, insert an artificial airway.
- If comatose or recurrent vomiting, insert NG tube, aspirate and leave on open drainage.
- Give oxygen via face mask or airway.
- Insert intravenous cannula and take blood samples (see below).
- If *shocked* (tachycardia, poor capillary filling, hypotension) give 10 ml/kg 4.5% albumin solution as quickly as possible, and repeat as necessary.

Confirm the Diagnosis

This is done on the basis of high blood glucose on capillary blood sampling and a clinical picture of acidotic respiration and dehydration.

Initial Investigations

Investigations of blood glucose, urea and electrolytes, arterial blood gases, packed cell volume (PCV) and full blood count, urinalysis, culture and sensitivity, with or without other investigations if indicated by presence of pyrexia, for example blood culture, chest X-ray, cerebrospinal fluid examination, throat swab, etc., should be carried out.

Weigh the Child

If this is not possible because of the clinical condition, use the most recent clinic weight as a guideline, or an estimated weight from centile charts.

Cardiac Monitoring

Set up cardiac monitor to observe T waves (hypokalaemia can cause cardiac dysrhythmias).

FULL CLINICAL ASSESSMENT AND OBSERVATIONS

Assess and record in the notes, so that comparisons can be made by others later, the degree of dehydration: mild (3%) — dehydration is clinically detectable by dry mucous membranes, reduced skin turgor; moderate (5–10%) — by above plus sunken eyes, poor capillary return; severe (10% with shock) — poor perfusion, thready rapid pulse, reduced blood pressure.

If alert or drowsy institute hourly neurological observations. If in coma on admission, or there is any subsequent deterioration, record Glasgow Coma Score, transfer to ICU, consider instituting cerebral oedema management.

Observations

Ensure that full instructions are given to the senior nursing staff, emphasising the need for the following.

- Strict fluid balance and urine testing of every sample
- Hourly capillary blood glucose measurements
- Hourly or more frequent neuro-observations initially
- Reporting immediately to the medical staff, even at night, symptoms of headache or any change in either conscious level or behaviour
- Reporting any changes in the ECG trace, especially T wave changes
- Twice daily weights.

FLUID MANAGEMENT

Volume of Fluid

By this stage, shock should have been corrected. If not, give a further 10 ml/kg 4.5% albumin over 30 minutes. Then calculate fluid requirements as follows:

requirement = maintenance + deficit, where deficit (litres) = dehydration (%) × body weight (kg). To avoid overzealous fluid replacement, which may be a risk factor for cerebral oedema, calculate deficit as if the patient is no more than 10% dehydrated. Ignore volume of albumin that may have been given to resuscitate. Recommended maintenance fluid values are given in Table A13.1. Add maintenance to deficit and divide total by 24 to obtain the steady rate for the next 24 hours. This amount must be given over 60 minutes.

Table A13.1 Recommended maintenance fluid volumes

Age (years)	Fluid volume (ml/kg/24 h)
0–2	100
3–5	90
6–9	75
>10	50

Type of Fluid

Initially use 0.9% saline. Once the blood glucose has fallen to 12 mmol/l change the fluid to 0.45% saline—5% dextrose.

BICARBONATE

This is rarely, if ever, necessary. Continuing acidosis usually means insufficient resuscitation. Bicarbonate should only be considered in children who are profoundly acidotic (pH < 6.9) and shocked with circulatory failure.

The maximum volume in millilitres of 8.4% sodium bicarbonate for half-correction of the acidosis is calculated according to: [1/3 × body weight (kg) × base deficit]/2, and this amount given over 60 minutes.

POTASSIUM

Potassium should be commenced immediately unless anuria is suspected or there are peaked T waves on the ECG. Add 20 mmol KCl to every 500 ml bag of fluid. Check plasma electrolytes three hours after resuscitation is begun and then at least four-hourly, and alter potassium replacements accordingly. Use a cardiac monitor and observe frequently for T wave changes.

INSULIN

Make up a solution of 1 unit/ml of human soluble insulin (e.g. Actrapid. Novo-Nordisk, Basingstoke, UK) by adding 50 units (0.5 ml) insulin to 50 ml 0.9% saline in a syringe pump. Attach this using a Y-connector to the intravenous fluids already running. Do not add insulin directly to the fluid bags. The solution should then run at 0.1 (units/kg)/hour (0.1 (ml/kg)/hour).

- If the rate of blood glucose fall exceeds 5 mmol/l per hour, reduce the insulin infusion rate to 0.05 (units/kg)/hour.
- Once the blood glucose is down to 12 mmol/l, and a dextrose-containing fluid has been started, consider reducing the insulin infusion rate if blood glucose levels indicate.
- Do not stop the insulin infusion while dextrose is being infused, as insulin is required to switch off ketone production. If the blood glucose falls below 7 mmol/l, add extra glucose to the infusion rather than stopping the insulin.

CONTINUING MANAGEMENT

- Urinary catheterisation should be avoided but is useful in the child with impaired consciousness.
- Documentation of fluid balance is of paramount importance. All urine must be measured accurately and tested. All fluid input must be recorded (even oral fluids). If a massive diuresis continues fluid input may need to be increased to take account of this. If large volumes of gastric aspirate continue, these will need to be replaced with 0.45% saline plus 10 mmol/l KCl.
- Check biochemistry, blood pH, and laboratory blood glucose two hours after the start of resuscitation, and then at least four-hourly. Review the fluid composition and rate according to each set of electrolyte results (see fluid section).
- If acidosis is not correcting, resuscitation may have been inadequate, therefore consider giving more albumin.
- If the blood glucose falls by more than 5 mmol/hour despite reducing the rate of insulin infusion, slow down the rate of intravenous fluid replacement, so that rehydration takes place over 48 rather than 24 hours.

If the blood glucose begins to rise again out of control once dextrose-containing fluids have been started, do not continue with large volumes of hypotonic saline solutions. Re-evaluate the child (? sepsis or other condition), consult senior medical staff and consider starting the whole protocol again.

CHANGING TO SUBCUTANEOUS INSULIN

Continue with intravenous fluids and insulin until the child is fully hydrated. If nausea and vomiting have stopped, there is no reason for the child to be prevented from drinking and eating even while intravenous fluids continue. Once the child is well hydrated and able to tolerate a normal diet, subcutaneous insulin can be started. Do not expect ketones to have disappeared completely before changing to subcutaneous insulin.

Give the first subcutaneous injection 30 minutes before discontinuing the intravenous insulin infusion to avoid rebound hyperglycaemia. A child newly diagnosed as having diabetes should be started on 0.5 units per kilogram body weight per day.

CEREBRAL OEDEMA

The signs and symptoms of cerebral oedema include headache, confusion, irritability, reduced conscious level, small pupils, increasing BP, slowing pulse, papilloedema (not always present acutely) and respiratory impairment.

Management

- Exclude hypoglycaemia.
- If cerebral oedema is suspected inform senior staff immediately.
- Give mannitol 0.5 g/kg stat (2.5 ml/kg mannitol 20% over 15 minutes). This needs to be given within 10 minutes.
- Restrict intravenous fluids to 2/3 maintenance and replace deficit over 72 rather than 24 hours.
- The child will need to be moved to ICU (if not there already).
- Arrange for the child to be intubated and, if necessary, hyperventilated to reduce blood PCO_2.
- Inform neurosurgeons.
- Exclude other diagnoses by CT scan: other intracerebral events may occur (thrombosis, haemorrhage or infarction) and present in the same way.
- Intracerebral pressure monitoring may be required.
- Repeated doses of mannitol (above dose every six hours) should be used to control intracranial pressure.

ACKNOWLEDGEMENTS

We should like to thank all the members of the BSPE, particularly Dr Claire Smith and Dr Jeremy Wales, who have participated in the production of these guidelines.

14

Long-Term Complications — Prevalence and Management

SIMON COURT

INTRODUCTION

For paediatricians as well as families the subject of complications associated with diabetes is highly emotive. In this chapter it is hoped to provide strategies with which to manage the common acute complications as well as providing some insight into the causes and incidence of the chronic complications. More particularly, however, the issue of screening for complications in childhood will be reviewed and a suggestion for an annual action plan presented.

Once the diagnosis of diabetes is made parents will often of their own volition go to the library to read up the subject and will immediately be confronted by the issue of complications. Thus at a time of some sadness they can be further cast down by accounts of the morbidity and mortality associated with diabetes. However, this information is commonly out-of-date and does not reflect modern management. For their child it is the medical advances of the next 50 years rather than the past 50 that are important. It is best to try to pre-empt such a visit by giving appropriate general information at the time of diagnosis, and by answering questions if they arise as honestly as possible. There are a number of general points that can be made, which may help to lessen concern.

1. It is clear that there is variation in susceptibility to complications, i.e. a biological robustness in some patients. (I sometimes use the analogy of

Childhood and Adolescent Diabetes. Edited by S. Court and B. Lamb.
© 1997 John Wiley & Sons, Ltd.

the smoker who escapes cancer.) Unfortunately we cannot at present distinguish this group from others.

2. The current incidence of complications reflects past practice, and the organisation of care has improved very significantly, particularly the development of specialist nurses to support families in the community.
3. Children and families are now given the information and equipment to monitor blood glucose so that they can help themselves attain good control.
4. It is now clear that good metabolic control makes a real difference, and that there are now effective ways of measuring diabetic control.
5. The goal of management is to ensure as far as possible that the young person is well placed to be the beneficiary of any new research, and a great deal of research is in progress.
6. Detection of early subclinical manifestations is increasingly possible and treatment programmes can be started that have a positive effect.
7. Paediatricians now take these issues very seriously.

The British Paediatric Association (BPA) (now The Royal College of Paediatrics and Child Health (CPCH)) and the British Diabetic Association (BDA) have together raised the profile of childhood diabetes. The BDA developed 'The Children and Young People's' section and the BPA published the results of a comparative survey of clinics across the country showing considerable variation in available resources and patterns of care[1]. Diabetes has been identified as one of the national audit conditions.

PAEDIATRICIANS AND THEIR PATIENTS

In 1984 Marteau and Baum wrote a paper entitled 'Doctors' views on diabetes' in which they compared the views of paediatricians and adult physicians who looked after diabetic children[2]. The adult physicians' estimate of morbidity and mortality from juvenile diabetes after 30 years was significantly higher and closer to the published data of the time than estimates made by paediatricians. The two groups also differed in the target blood glucose concentrations they considered optimal for diabetic children, paediatricians tending to accept higher values as satisfactory. They argued that this was likely to be due to the different clinical experiences of the two groups, where paediatricians uncommonly have to confront complications in their patients. In addition they argued that paediatric clinics have a 'culture of optimism' which could influence the perceptions of the clinician. They also added that adult physicians specialising in diabetes might simply be more knowledgeable about complications in general than paediatricians. In this way the gauntlet was thrown down for paediatricians to get their house in order. This has become even more relevant as children are developing diabetes at an earlier age, and as a consequence at any one time a clinic will have around 40% of patients where diabetes was developed under the age of five years. Many patients will have had diabetes for between 10 and 15 years before care is transferred on to adult colleagues, the commonly quoted time-frame for the initial detection of complications. It has, however, been suggested that the years before puberty are not as significant as those after the onset of puberty[3]. Even so, microvascular changes can be identified within a few years of onset and some associated conditions (necrobiosis and cataract) may precede the typical presentation of polyuria and polydipsia.

SCREENING AND PREVENTION

In some respects the whole purpose of diabetic management is the prevention of complications; this applies particularly if educational and psychological, as well as metabolic and structural, changes are included. Primary prevention is discussed briefly in Chapter 1. Secondary prevention requires the identification of a pre-symptomatic phase in the condition, thus allowing a window of time in which to intervene in order to stop or slow down the progression of the condition. Until recently screening for complications and associated conditions has not traditionally been under-taken in paediatric clinics. Despite the paucity of direct evidence from studies in children there are now a number of reasons why screening for certain well recognised complications should be seriously considered. The following basic principles of screening procedures should still apply.

1. The condition has to be serious (visual disability/renal failure).
2. The natural history of the condition should be known.
3. The screening procedure has to be acceptable to the patient, reliable and cost-effective.
4. There should be few false positives and false negatives.
5. There should be accepted treatment for patients with recognised disease.
6. There should be an agreed policy on whom to treat as patients.
7. The cost of detection and consequent treatment needs to be set against the possible expenditure on medical care of the primary condition as a whole.
8. The screening activity should be a continuing process and not a 'once for all' project.

However, from evidence of paediatric practice some of these criteria are not completely satisfied. The St Vincent Declaration (Appendix 1) and the Diabetes Control and Complications Trial[4] (DCCT) have lent a legitimacy to the process of looking seriously at certain screening elements within the annual review process. Clearly there should be a certain caution in extrapolating from adult studies. The DCCT was discontinued because it became clear that the intensive treatment group were significantly advantaged over the conventional treatment group, because intensive treatment effectively delays the onset and slows the progression of diabetic retinopathy, nephropathy and neuropathy in all patients with insulin dependent diabetes irrespective of age, age of onset, baseline glycosylated haemoglobin values and gender. There are a number of more general points that are worth considering. Although the DCCT included adolescents, the numbers were relatively small at 14% and there were no children younger than 13 years. Furthermore, only adolescents who were considered able to comply with the strict regime were enrolled. The regime described as intensive included patterns of surveillance and monitoring that were continued over years, e.g. four blood glucose tests per day, weekly contact with health professionals, insulin administration three or four times per day and glycosylated haemoglobin assay every four weeks. However, what is practical for the motivated adult is impractical for an infant or young child using currently available methods of monitoring. It should also be recognised that levels of glycosylated haemoglobin in the intensive group were rarely in the non-diabetic range, and when they were this was not sustained. In addition there was a cost, in that this group gained significantly more weight, with potential negative effects on exercise, blood pressure and self-esteem. More particularly there was a three-fold increase in significant hypoglycaemic episodes, which in adults was not shown to have long-term cognitive effects — other studies in young children have raised this as a real concern.

The pathogenesis of complications is complex, and a complete description is beyond the scope of this text. There is now no doubt following the DCCT that glycaemic control is of major significance and yet there are patients with very poor control that escape significant complications and others who, by current monitoring standards, are well controlled but have their lives invaded by severe complications. Clearly there are other factors.

1. Genetic susceptibility (clustering in families).
2. Lifestyle factors (exercise, smoking).
3. Gender differences (mortality risks, nephropathy).
4. Pre-pubertal years seem to be of less significance in predicting complications.
5. Points 3 and 4 above point to a role for sex hormones/growth hormone/IGF1, particularly in the development of microvascular complications.

6. Hypertension is now regarded as one of the major risk factors in the development of diabetic complications and mortality and may be as significant as glycaemic control in predicting complications.
7. Hyperinsulinism microvascular disease.
8. High-risk lipid profiles — may be a consequence of poor glycaemic control or may be induced by factors unrelated to diabetes (genetic/dietary).

SPECIFIC COMPLICATIONS

RETINOPATHY

The prevalence of retinopathy is highest in young onset insulin-treated patients but is rarely found under the age of 12 years, and background retinopathy is uncommon before five years duration of diabetes. Prevalence rates vary widely from different countries, but long-term follow-up studies show that retinopathy is an almost invariable finding in conventionally managed childhood onset diabetes. In a recently published study from Finland[5] the prevalence of retinopathy was 28% in a population aged 7.0–19.8 (median 14) years who had had diabetes for 1.8–16.2 (median 6.5) years. They argued that the prevalence of retinopathy has an almost linear relationship with duration of diabetes and that over the subsequent 10 years would reach a level of 80%. Proliferative retinopathy (PR) is a post-pubertal event and causes blindness through vitreous haemorrhage, fibrosis and retinal detachment. PR is rarely seen before 10 years duration, but gives a risk of visual impairment in up to 50% after 20 years duration (retrospective/historical data). It is always preceded by a period of background/minimal retinopathy which does not threaten vision and which can remain stable/harmless indefinitely. Many studies have confirmed the association between poor glycaemic control and the onset/progression of retinopathy. The DCCT confirms that interventions that improve glycaemic control delay the onset and slow the progression of this condition. Although the evidence is less clear in pre-pubertal children, it makes sense to optimise glycaemic control at all ages. There should, however, be different glycaemic goals at different ages (toddlers; middle childhood; adolescents), the avoidance of severe hypoglycaemia being particularly important in the child under five years.

NEPHROPATHY

Diabetic nephropathy is an important cause of morbidity and mortality, and those at greatest risk are childhood onset IDDM patients, with a cumulative incidence of nephropathy after 40 years of disease of at least 40–50%. Some would argue that most patients after prolonged diabetes, that is, for more than 40 years, have evidence of microvascular renal damage but not all develop renal failure. Interestingly, two major diabetes centres (Joslin Clinic, Steno Hospital), on the basis of changing patterns of proteinuria, are predicting a fall in the development of renal failure. Even so, renal failure is currently 17 times more common in patients with diabetes than in those without. In 1982 urinary albumin excretion was identified as a marker of nephropathy (microalbuminuria). The appearance of microalbuminuria is recognised currently as the most reliable marker of subsequent adverse renal and cardiovascular disease in diabetics, but its significance in childhood remains to be completely elucidated. At the present time a multi-centre trial is under way in the United Kingdom, looking at the most appropriate screening methodology in order to address the following issues.

1. To examine the distribution of albumin excretion rates among a childhood diabetic population and their sustainability.
2. To generate a definition of microalbuminuria in children.
3. To determine the albumin : creatinine ratio that will be both sensitive and specific for defining those children with microalbuminuria.

Although poor glycaemic control has consistently been identified as a risk factor for diabetic nephropathy, it appears that not all patients are equally at risk, as some with clearly poor glycaemic control escape serious nephropathy. This suggests the presence of potential protective factors or other destructive factors being involved in the pathological process. Those that have been identified include: age at onset, duration of diabetes, relative insulin resistance, smoking and a family history of nephropathy and hypertension. It has, however, been suggested that hypertension may be a product of nephropathy rather than a cause.

In adults microalbuminuria is defined as an albumin excretion rate (AER) of 30–300 mg/24 hours (or 20–200 μg/min) in two out of three timed collections. These are difficult to undertake accurately in children, but the concentration of albumin in the first morning specimen passed correlated well with the AER over 24 hours. The predictive value of the early morning specimen could be further improved by measuring urinary creatinine in the same sample, thus correcting for the flow rate, giving a ratio of albumin (mg/litre) : creatinine (mmol/litre) (ACR).

The ACR in the early morning sample has been shown to have a correlation coefficient of 0.91 with a timed overnight AER. Using an ACR value of 3.5 mg/mmol in the first morning sample an AER of 30 μg/min was predicted with a sensitivity of 88–100% and a specificity of 90–95%. This is now currently regarded as the screening test of choice. As indicated above, the situation for children is less clear. Karachaliou and colleagues[6] have published ACR values in normal and diabetic children. The mean ACR in normal children was 0.47 (95% tolerance limits 0.14–1.57) but 12/ 129 diabetic children had values above 1.57 (9%). Depending on the definition of microalbuminuria used other workers have described prevalence rates between 7 and 20%. Repeated testing of ACR shows many to be abnormal intermittently, but when values fall between 1.5 and 3.5 mg/mmol these individuals should have their ACR checked annually; if consistently above 3.5 mg/mmol it is this group that could benefit from specific treatment. The DCCT demonstrated the benefits of intensive treatment in the avoidance of nephropathy, with 39% fewer patients developing microalbuminuria and 54% fewer overt nephropathy compared to the conventionally treated group.

Where children have been identified as having persistent and significantly raised microalbuminuria all attempts at improving glycaemic control should be tried. Captopril [an angiotensin converting enzyme (ACE) inhibitor] has been shown to decrease albumin excretion in children with confirmed microalbuminuria. ACE inhibitors are felt likely to be the treatment of choice, but in the current state of knowledge cannot be recommended for routine use in children with proven elevated ACRs. While protein restriction has been shown to be of benefit in adults with overt renal disease, this is unlikely to occur in paediatric diabetic practice and the unpleasant nature of the diet would significantly add to compliance problems.

NEUROPATHY

Although abnormalities of the different modalities of nerve function (motor, sensory, visually evoked responses (VER), auditory evoked responses (AER) and autonomic) have all been demonstrated in children with IDDM, they have not been subjected to the same level of enquiry as nephropathy or retinopathy. The pathogenesis is unclear but is thought to involve two mechanisms:

— diffuse metabolic changes in axons consequent on hyperglycaemia
— microvascular changes involving the endoneuronal capillaries.

Motor nerve conduction has been shown to be abnormal soon after the onset of diabetes with prevalence rates of up to 72%, perhaps suggesting a functional metabolic abnormality. Distal asymmetric polyneuropathy thought to be consequent on both metabolic and microvascular changes was found in 3% of a small group of children less than 18 years of age, but over the following 10 years the prevalence increased to 18% by the age of 29 years. VER abnormalities have been found in 30% of children and the prevalence of autonomic cardiovascular tests is abnormal in 15–30% of children. A scheme for bedside cardiovascular testing has been described[7].

1. Mean resting heart rate (RHR) (60 s).
2. Heart rate variation to deep breathing (DBHR).
3. Response of heart rate to change of position (HR), standing : lying ratio.
4. Fall in systolic blood pressure on standing.
5. Rise in diastolic blood pressure during sustained hand grip.

In this study diabetic children had a significantly higher RHR, decreased DBHR variation, and lower standing : lying HR ratio than non-diabetic controls. Changes of blood pressure (tests 4 and 5 above) were not significantly different in the two groups. A single abnormal result was seen in 42% of diabetic children, 5% in the controls. Two or more abnormal results were found in 24% of the diabetic group but in none of the controls. Cardiovascular autonomic abnormality was associated with longer duration and worse long-term metabolic control. Others have identified male gender and advancing puberty as being associated with peripheral neuropathy. In adult diabetic patients impaired autonomic function has been associated with arythmias, sudden death and an increased mortality rate compared to the general diabetic population. In children and adolescents there is some evidence to suggest an association between altered blood pressure and abnormal autonomic function. However, it is not clear whether early autonomic dysfunction will prove an accurate predictor of later symptomatic autonomic neuropathy, with its poor prognosis. Once again from the DCCT there was evidence of benefit in the intensive treatment group, where clinical neuropathy was reduced.

CATARACTS

The production and metabolism of polyols seems to have an important role in the development of the more chronic complications associated with diabetes. Accumulation of osmotically active sorbitol within the cells may generate cellular swelling contributing to disordered nerve conduction and the development of cataracts. These, however, are an uncommon complication, but children may present to an ophthalmologist with visual symptoms before the diagnosis of diabetes is fully recognised. Cataracts may also develop during the first few years after diagnosis and can be difficult to treat.

SKIN AND JOINT PROBLEMS

Infection

With poor glycaemic control skin infection is not uncommon, bacterial (staphylococcal), candida and fungal infections are all seen in childhood diabetes and may be associated with poor foot care (ingrowing toenails, paronychia). It is worth considering if the family are 'staph' carriers and if the child is a nasal or perineal carrier. Systemic as well as topical antibiotics should be considered.

Necrobiosis Lipoidica

There are a number of very specific dermatological conditions associated with diabetes. Although not common in childhood, the best recognised is necrobiosis lipoidica diabeticorum (NLD). In our clinic, out of 170 children over 15 years we have seen NLD in five children/young people, four of whom were girls. The prevalence in adults is said to be 0.3%, but it is also seen in non-diabetics and in one of our cases NLD antedated the diagnosis of diabetes by many months. The main pathological feature is dermal collagen damage, with surrounding granulomatous inflammation and ulceration. This is commonly secondarily infected but responds to appropriate antibiotics. The underlying condition, however, is very difficult to treat. Topical and systemic steroids have been tried with varying success. When the lesions are quiescent they can be masked by appropriate 'make up' of the kind used by plastic surgical departments. The psychological consequences of these lesions, which characteristically occur on the front of the shins, should not be underestimated in young woman as they commonly have to resort to wearing trousers.

Limited Joint Mobility

Limited joint mobility (LJM) with waxy skin is a well recognised sign in diabetic children. It usually develops between the ages of 10 and 20 years and is related to age rather than duration of diabetes. Reports of prevalence vary between 9% and 31%, suggesting problems of definition within this syndrome. Where this is limited to the little fingers the significance of LJM is in question as a genetic element may explain the presence of LJM in a similar proportion of siblings of diabetic children. LJM was described in 66 children from a group of 357 (prevalence 26%)[8]. They were at least 14 years old and had had diabetes for more than five years. The presence of contractures was significantly associated with glycaemic control (HbA1 concentration), duration of diabetes, age of onset, mean longitudinal cholesterol levels and blood pressure. In addition it was also associated with early retinopathy and albumin excretion. Others have argued that after 16 years of diabetes if LJM is absent patients have a 25% risk of microvascular complications, whereas in those with LJM the risk is 83%[9].

THE SCREENING PROCESS

As discussed earlier in this chapter screening is now being seen as an appropriate activity for children's clinics to undertake. This has become particularly pertinent as increasing numbers of children have had the condition for 10–15 years before handover to the adult service, notwithstanding the discussions about the significance of the years before the onset of puberty towards the development of complications. Screening for complications should be carried out at diagnosis, primarily to provide a baseline. Certain conditions such as NLD and cataracts may be present at the start, and antibody studies will identify those at risk of developing thyroid disease. Appendices 12.1 and 12.2 illustrate the recording sheet used in this clinic and describe the strategy which is incorporated into the annual review. This has evolved over time and has a number of functions. The sheet serves as an *aide mémoire* which is useful if junior doctors are coming into the clinic, and the patient's four visits are presented on a single side of A4 paper. This in turn can be photocopied and sent to the family doctor and family as a record of the visit. The pattern of our clinic visits is described elsewhere, but it includes an annual review, an easy way of undertaking screening and simple to audit. The next section simply and briefly describes those elements that have not been addressed specifically above.

GROWTH

This needs no justification in a children's diabetic clinic. Growth rate and weight gain are both measures that reflect patterns of glycaemic control. It is also important to document insulin dosage per kilogram body weight. Prepubertal dosage in the C-peptide-negative child is close to 0.8 units/kg; during puberty this will rise and should be flagged if rising above 1.5 units/ kg. Once puberty is over the dose should fall towards pre-pubertal levels, otherwise inappropriate weight gain ensues. It is important to recognise the need for privacy when measuring children; weight can be a very sensitive issue and adolescent girls in particular may not wish to be weighed in public. Height should be recorded in the context of parental heights and it is important to document the onset of puberty. We do not feel that a detailed pubertal assessment is required annually.

HANDS, SKIN AND FEET

The first two have been discussed in some detail previously. Looking at feet is important. Significant foot pathology is more common in children with diabetes than in aged-matched controls[10].

- Biomechanical (juvenile pes planovalgus; hindfoot calcaneo varus; digital deformities; hypermobility)
- Onychocryptosis
- Hallux limitus
- Heel bump
- Callus
- Tinea pedis.

Hyperhidrosis was also described, which, alongside poor diabetic control, might account in part for the increased prevalence of fungal infection. Barnett *et al.*[10] suggested regular review of footwear as well as feet, because they placed some of the blame for the increased biomechanical problems on ill-fitting shoes. Those children with LJM also showed digital deformity of the feet.

Shoes and socks are also good indicators of social patterns of care and also family finance. Unfortunately they are also subject to fashion, so that suggestions from doctors may fall on deaf ears. Regular review in the clinic with guidance on toenail cutting would seem sensible, with referral to a chiropodist for more complicated problems.

BLOOD PRESSURE

When measured in out-patients, blood pressure is commonly raised either as a function of the process or because the next element of the annual review is a venous blood sample, even if local anaesthetic cream is used. The importance of hypertension and its relationship to microalbuminuria have been discussed previously. The measurement should be taken after two minutes rest. We use the sitting position and the value is charted against age-appropriate standards. If the blood pressure is raised it should clearly be rechecked at the next visit, but it may be more profitable to have this done at home or in the local surgery. Gompels[11] showed that it was both useful and practical for families to record blood pressure at home using an electronic sphygmomanometer and argued that a representative home series of measurements should be available before any diagnostic or therapeutic decisions could be made. In addition, as familial hypertension may be a risk factor for nephropathy, the blood pressure of parents and siblings could be assessed by this means. It has been suggested that 24-hour ambulatory measurements reflect the relationship between urine albumin excretion and blood pressure more precisely than clinical measurements. In the uncommon clinical situation of a diabetic child with significant microalbuminuria and hypertension, ACE inhibitors are being considered for use but it would clearly be appropriate to discuss management with a paediatric nephrologist.

URINE MICROALBUMIN

Each child is asked to bring a first void urine, in a previously supplied container, at the time of the annual review five and 10 years after diagnosis, and annually for those in established puberty for measurement of urinary microalbumin/creatinine ratios. Those with an ACR greater than 3.5 mg/mmol will then be asked to provide a series of timed overnight urine collections for measurement of AER.

NEUROPATHY

We record knee and ankle reflexes as present, diminished or absent. Vibration perception and proprioception are also included and reflect large nerve function . Vibration can be graded on a scale 0–8 using a Rydel Seiffer graduated tuning fork. We do not currently undertake screening for autonomic dysfunction. Polaroid pupillometry (giving a measure of dark adaptation) has been used to demonstrate subclinical autonomic neuropathy in diabetic children and adolescents, where this was related to duration and glycaemic control. Pupillary variables were not, however, shown to correlate well with the cardiovascular measures referred to previously[12]. Even so, Karavanaki et al. argued that screening for autonomic dysfunction could be justified in paediatric clinical practice.

EYES

We undertake fundoscopy annually through an undilated pupil simply using a darkened room, and also ask for retinal photography (RP) after five years duration and then after 10 years duration if the child is pre-pubertal. RPs are taken at the onset of puberty, then every two years till 16 years of age, then annually. We also encourage the families to have regular vision checks performed by local opticians. Eye tests are free to all people with diabetes.

LIPIDS

Lipid screening is undertaken on a non-fasted sample. Lipid risk factors include the following.

- Elevated total cholesterol
- Elevated low-density lipoprotein (LDL)
- Lowered high-density lipoprotein (HDL)
- Raised triglycerides.

Total cholesterol and HDL-cholesterol remain fairly stable over the day and fasting has little effect; triglyceride levels, however, rise after meals. Azad[13] described a prevalence of dyslipidaemia of 39% in diabetic children compared to 17% in the control group, using a fasted total cholesterol of

Table 14.1. The spectrum of blood lipid concentrations: values of blood lipids (St Vincent Declaration, 1992)

	Concentration (mmol/l)		
	Good	Acceptable	Poor
Total cholesterol	<5.2	5.2–6.5	>6.5
HDL cholesterol	>1.1	0.9–1.1	<0.9
Fasting triglycerides	<1.7	1.7–2.2	>2.2

5.2 mmol/l as the cut-off point, as suggested by the St Vincent working group (Table 14.1). Some have argued for a lower cut-off in children as cholesterol levels rise with age (4.1 mmol/l is the World Health Organisation standard). HDL-cholesterol levels were not shown to be significantly different in the two groups, although in the presence of good glycaemic control IDDM patients can have higher levels of this antiatherogenic lipoprotein.

Lipid screening should be undertaken routinely in the clinic as part of the annual review. When dyslipidaemia is identified, even greater attempts to improve glycaemic control should be made as there is a clear relationship. In addition, advice from a dietitian becomes of particular importance.

AUTO-ANTIBODIES

As can be seen in the chart described in Chapter 12, we undertake this test at diagnosis and then for the next two years as part of the annual review. These studies are then repeated at five and 10 years duration of diabetes. Associated endocrinopathies and coeliac disease are discussed in detail elsewhere in this volume.

SUMMARY

In conclusion, there is increasing evidence that screening in the children's diabetic clinic is appropriate and in this section an attempt has been made to define the different elements that go some way to describe those patients at particular risk of vascular complications. It seems likely that attention to improvement in glycaemic control, abnormal lipid profiles, raised blood pressure and avoidance of smoking together with good foot care will reduce risk of invasive complications.

REFERENCES

1 Swift, P. G. F., Court, S., Crowley, P. M. *et al. The organisation of services for children with diabetes in the United Kingdom: Report of the BPA working party.* London: BPA, 1989 (obtainable from: The British Paediatric Association, 5 St Andrews Place, Regents Park, London NW4, UK).

2 Marteau, T. M., Baum, J. D. Doctors' views on diabetes. *Arch Dis Child* 1984; **59:** 566–70.

3 Kostraba, J. N., Dorman, J. S., Orchard, T. J. *et al.* Contribution of diabetes duration before puberty to the development of microvascular complications in IDDM subjects. *Diabet Care* 1989; **12:** 686–93.

4 The DCCT Research Group. The effect of intensive treatment of diabetes on the development and progression of long term complications in IDDM. *N Engl J Med* 1993; **329:** 977–86.

5 Falck, A., Kaar, M. L., Laatikainen, L. A prospective, longitudinal study examining the development of retinopathy in children with diabetes. *Acta Paediatr* 1996; **85:** 313–19.

6 Karachaliou, F. H., Karavanaki, K., Greenwood, R., Morgan, H., Baum, J. D. Consistency of microvascular and autonomic abnormalities in diabetes. *Arch Dis Child* 1996; **75:** 124–8.

7 Barkai, L., Madacsy, L. Cardiovascular autonomic dysfunction in diabetes mellitus. *Arch Dis Child* 1995; **73:** 515–18.

8 Garg, S. K., Chase, P. H., Marshall, G. *et al.* Limited joint mobility in subjects with IDDM: relationship with eye and kidney complications. *Arch Dis Child* 1992; **67:** 96–7.

9 Editorial. Stiffness of the hands in diabetes. *Lancet* 1981; **ii:** 1027–8.

10 Barnett S. J., Shield J. P. H., Potter M. J. *et al.* Foot pathology in IDDM. *Arch Dis Child* 1995; **73:** 151–3.

11 Gompels, C., Savage, D. Home blood pressure monitoring in diabetes. *Arch Dis Child* 1992; **67:** 636–9.

12 Karavanaki, K., Davies, A. G., Hunt L. P. *et al.* Pupil size in diabetes. *Arch Dis Child* 1994; **71:** 511–15.

13 Azad, K., Parkin, J. M., Court, S. *et al.* Circulating lipids and glycaemic control in insulin dependent diabetic children. *Arch Dis Child* 1994; **71:** 108–13.

ADDITIONAL READING

Cambell, F. M. Microalbuminuria and nephropathy in insulin dependent diabetes mellitus. *Arch Dis Child* 1995; **1:** 4–7.

Kelnar, C. J. H (ed.). *Childhood and Adolescent Diabetes.* London: Chapman and Hall Medical, 1995.

15

Growth in Diabetes and Other Associated Auto-immune Conditions

IAN JEFFERSON

LINEAR GROWTH

The monitoring of sequential changes in linear growth provides the paediatrician with responsibility for looking after children with diabetes with a measure of health and well-being that is not available to our adult diabetologist colleagues. It is of course essential that the measurements are made and recorded accurately and related to the child's age and stage of pubertal development. The accurate measurement of height and weight is one of the most important procedures undertaken in a Paediatric Diabetes Clinic. When interpreted correctly in conjunction with appropriate standards, this can provide important clinical clues to problems in diabetes control and management and/or point to the diagnosis of associated disorders.

When insulin became available for the treatment of insulin dependent diabetes mellitus, medium- and long-term survival became possible but severe growth failure in children remained common, as typified in its severest form by the 'Mauriac syndrome' (hepatomegaly, dwarfism, delayed puberty, recurrent diabetic ketoacidosis, moon-shaped face, protuberant abdomen and fat deposition around the shoulders and abdomen). In a milder form growth failure/delayed puberty is well documented in twin studies and in clinic studies using either control groups or mid-parental target heights.

Childhood and Adolescent Diabetes. Edited by S. Court and B. Lamb.
© 1997 John Wiley & Sons, Ltd.

There is also evidence of an effect on linear growth of the pre-diabetic state although, despite numerous studies, the precise causation remains controversial, largely because of confusion over the control groups chosen. It is felt that any pre-diagnosis effect on 'height at diagnosis' is due to disordered insulin secretion in the initial phase of the auto-immune process, analogous to the hyperthyroid phase that precedes hypothyroidism in Hashimoto's auto-immune thyroiditis. Recent data from Oxford[1] suggest that the effect on height at diagnosis is most marked in the group diagnosed between the ages of five and 10 years, especially in males who were significantly taller than a local control population. Despite the controversy over height at diagnosis there is general agreement that after diagnosis diabetes has an adverse effect on height velocity, with loss of final height standard deviation score (SDS) dependent on age at diagnosis and duration of diabetes. The effect is both pre-pubertal, with an estimated loss of 0.06 SDS per year between diagnosis and puberty, and also pubertal. The precise effect of diabetes on puberty is controversial. Some studies have suggested a general delay in timing of puberty and others suggest that timing is normal; all studies, however, suggest that the recognised reduction in peak height velocity is most marked in girls. The effect on puberty also seems to relate to age at diagnosis, although some studies have suggested it is maximal if diabetes presents clinically just prior to puberty. Recent data, however, suggest the effect is worst in the group diagnosed under the age of five years.

Although the data on the timing of puberty are variable, there is strong anecdotal evidence of delay in some children and, in the female adolescent, an increase in menstrual irregularities, prolonged amenorrhoea (54%, compared with 21% in controls) and in the adult an increase in secondary amenorrhoea and decreased fertility. The ultimate effect of altered height at diagnosis, and changes in pre-pubertal height velocity, pubertal timing and peak height velocity, is an alteration of final adult height. Again the picture is confused, with data suggesting that it may be unaltered or decreased. Recent data suggest that it is related to age at diagnosis, with those children diagnosed under the age of five years having normal height at diagnosis but greatest effect from pre-pubertal and pubertal loss of height velocity and a reduced final height. Children aged five to 10 years have an increased height at diagnosis but pre-pubertal and pubertal loss, resulting in a normal final height, and those diagnosed aged 10 years and over have a normal height at diagnosis and a reduced pubertal peak height velocity but not sufficient to reduce significantly final adult height.

Although with current diabetes management regimens growth is clearly better than it was, it is still adversely affected by the disease state, and in the child who is growing poorly in association with poor blood glucose control linear growth can be accelerated by improvement in blood glucose control.

Generally linear growth does not correlate with control as measured by HbA1c. Any clinic will have children with 'poor control' who are growing and developing normally and some with 'good control' whose height velocity and/or pubertal development is poor. The effect of diabetes and insulin treatment on growth is only partially understood, the growth hormone/IGF1 axis is dependent on insulin, with insulin promoting production of IGF1. In diabetes there is an increase in growth hormone levels (increased secretion and decreased clearance) with increased pulse amplitude and baseline levels, especially in puberty. Despite this, however, levels of IGF1 remain low. It is felt that this is secondary to a decreased portal delivery of insulin that is not addressed by conventional insulin administration. Thus we have a situation of low IGF1 (and poor growth) and high growth hormone which because of its antagonistic effects to insulin increases insulin resistance and worsens control, the effect being most marked in puberty, increasing the normal physiological insulin resistance seen at this time. One of the beneficial roles of C-peptide may be through maintenance of a supply of portal insulin, minimising these effects.

In puberty in males no consistent hormonal abnormalities have been found. There is perhaps more often a dissociation of adrenarche and pubarche, with possible reductions in adrenal androgens and sex hormone binding globulin (SHBG). In females with diabetes and menstrual irregularities reductions in SHBG and IGF1, increases in androstenedione and Insulin Growth Factor Binding Protein (IGFBP1), with an increased luteinising hormone/follicle stimulating hormone (LH/FSH) ratio have been found compared to those with regular periods. There is also an increased incidence of polycystic ovary which is associated with weight gain, poor control and possible greater risks of microangiopathy, although whether this is directly related to the poor control or increased growth hormone levels remains unclear.

Despite these complex issues surrounding linear growth in diabetes, accurate, sequential plotting and monitoring for height and weight progress (on an accurate stadiometer used correctly and on a calibrated set of scales, with clothing adjusted to a constant) provide a most useful clinical monitor of health, well-being and control. Most children, after an initial period of catch-up growth in weight (and possibly height), grow along a centile line for height and weight and any consistent deviation must be investigated in terms of diabetes regimen and/or associated disorder.

Weight particularly gives some very important clues as to overall insulin dosage and dietary compliance. Although it is an oversimplification, weight loss equals poor control associated with insufficient insulin and/or insufficient food and excessive weight gain equals too much insulin and/ or food. The combination of poor control and excessive weight gain must equate to excessive/inappropriate dietary intake and excessive insulin. This

Table 15.1. Theoretical relationship between insulin dose/carbohydrate intake and effects on body weight and glycaemic control

Variables		Effects	
Insulin dose	Carbohydrate intake	Body weight	HbA1c
=	=	=	N
=	↑	=(↑)	↑
=	↓	↓	↓
↑	=	=	↓
↑	↑	↑	↑ (N)
↑	↓	= (↓)	↓↓
↓	=	↓	↑
↓	↑	↓	↑↑
↓	↓	↓	N

Key: N—within normal range; =—correct or appropriate levels; ↑—above appropriate levels; ↓—below appropriate levels; ( )—possible alternative state

is one of the most difficult clinical problems to face, especially in the adolescent/post-adolescent female when physiological insulin requirements are reducing at a time of poor dietary compliance.

The effect of the various combinations of insulin dose and carbohydrate intake on weight gain and glycaemic control can be predicted as shown in Table 15.1 and can provide important clinical clues to recommended adjustments in regimen.

AUTO-IMMUNE ASSOCIATIONS

The clinical association of IDDM with other endocrine disorders has been well established for over a century, but it was the concept of auto-immunity, proven in some of these other endocrine disorders, that provided a possible common thread of causation.

Many papers documented an increased frequency of circulating organ-specific antibodies in patients with IDDM and their first-degree relatives. Genetic evidence came originally from the studies of linkage with the histocompatibility antigen HLA-8 found in IDDM, thyrotoxicosis and Addison's disease. Initial direct evidence of an auto-immune basis for IDDM came from histological studies of the pancreas, showing lymphocytic infiltration of the islets of Langerhans, the term 'insulinitis' was coined by

Von Myenburg[2] and these changes were documented by Gepts[3] in 15 of 22 young patients dying of what was mostly untreated IDDM.

This was supported by later studies of lymphocyte function with the leucocyte migration test showing that lymphocytes of patients with IDDM were sensitised to antigens from the endocrine pancreas. The final piece of evidence came with the demonstration of antibodies to the cytoplasmic component of pancreatic islet cells in 1974 from the laboratories in London[4] and Edinburgh[5] and so established the concept of IDDM as an auto-immune disease. Since that time the observation has been studied and refined to a high degree, immunologically and genetically, although we are still missing a few small pieces of the jigsaw that describes the failure of normal immunomodulation that occurs in individuals who develop the disease.

It is known that there are many auto-immune associations with IDDM. Gastric parietal cell antibody (GPC) is found with a prevalence of 10–15% in childhood IDDM. Rarely, however, does this lead on to the clinical correlate of pernicious anaemia, probably less than 3% per annum of GPC-positive individuals will progress to Vitamin B12 deficiency, although the finding of intrinsic factor antibody may refine this risk. It is argued that monitoring of serum B12 in these individuals need only be every five years, although achlorhydria may be more common, causing iron malabsorption and it may be relevant to monitor serum ferritin more frequently.

Adrenal auto-antibodies (AA) are demonstrable in only 2% of children with IDDM. Addison's disease is rare in the general population (1:50000) but is five times more common in the insulin-dependent population and is often part of one of the polyendocrine syndromes. It must be suspected in the young patient with IDDM with coexistent thyroid disease where there is a strong family history of auto-immune endocrinopathy. Adrenal medullary antibodies are found in 7–16% of children with IDDM but seem to be of no clinical significance.

Other endocrine auto-antibodies are occasionally found to cell types of the anterior pituitary and this can be shown in around 17% of recent onset IDDM and may rarely lead to pituitary failure.

Auto-immune associations are particularly relevant in two chromosomal disorders, Down's syndrome and Turner's syndrome, where the incidence is increased of not only IDDM but also of the other auto-immune endocrinopathies, especially thyroid disease.

Auto-immune thyroid disease is the most common auto-immune endocrinopathy occurring in families with IDDM. The literature on the association is fairly extensive and is well represented by the series from 1981 and 1983 by Riley et al.[6,7] who screened around 1500 young IDDM patients in North America for thyroid microsomal, gastric parietal cell and adrenal antibodies. Thyroid microsomal antibody (TMA) was positive in

23%, with a 2:1 female preponderance. Gastric parietal cell antibody was positive in 11% with a similar female:male ratio, and adrenal antibody was positive in 2% with no sex difference. Evidence of adrenocortical failure was said to develop in one in four of adrenal antibody positive individuals, equating to 1:250 of the IDDM population.

Thyroglobulin antibodies (TGA) were found in 1.6%, which was identical to a non-diabetic control group. Hopwood[8], however, demonstrated an increased rate of TGA in the diabetic population and found a relationship with the development of hyperthyroid thyroid disease.

Riley, in a subset of 771 patients with IDDM (mean age at diagnosis <10 years), found 18% (*n*=136) were TMA-positive with a 4:1 ratio Caucasian: Negro. They were able to continue studying 117 of the TMA-positive IDDM children; eight (7%) were hyperthyroid and 45 (38%) were hypothyroid. They were followed initially for two and a half years and subsequently for five years with tests of thyroid function. Sixty-four (55%) remained euthyroid, although in this group the mean TSH was significantly higher and the mean fT4 significantly lower than in the TMA-negative group. Of the eight who were hyperthyroid, seven were diagnosed already at or before the diagnosis of IDDM and one was diagnosed during the follow-up period. Of the 45 (38%) who were hypothyroid, four were diagnosed pre-IDDM, 10 within one year of diagnosis of IDDM and 31 after the first year of IDDM. The sera were collected and analysed retrospectively and revealed that two children were biochemically hypothyroid at the start of the study but were only diagnosed at the end of the two and a half year follow-up. These patients had had problems with hypoglycaemia and poor school performance, which had been blamed on poor diabetes control but resolved when on thyroxine replacement. In the larger study, the group estimated that of the TMA-positive IDDM group, 1–2% per annum would become hypothyroid. Among the eight hyperthyroid patients, none showed GPC antibodies but three (37.5%) showed the presence of AA, showing this to be a high risk sub-group for the development of adrenal failure and reflecting the common HLA linkage of Addison's disease and hyperthyroidism. The hypothyroid and euthyroid group showed similar rates of GPC (20%) and AA (4.5%).

The frequency of the antibodies did not seem to alter with duration of diabetes, suggesting that the onset of the auto-immune process to multiple target tissues is simultaneous in a subset of about a quarter of individuals who develop IDDM and that monitoring at, or soon after, diagnosis will identify the high-risk group.

Family history and TMA status was checked in 100 patients with IDDM who were TMA-positive. Seventy of the immediate family members showed either a positive history of thyroid disease or were TMA-positive. As part of that study three parents were newly diagnosed as hypothyroid and one was shown to have pernicious anaemia (Figure 15.1).

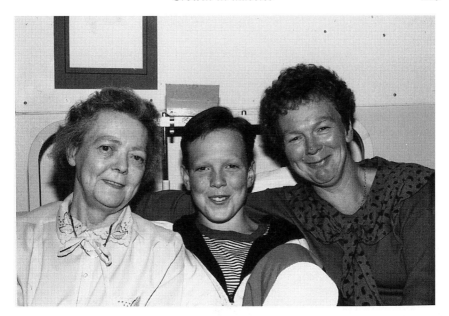

Figure 15.1. A teenager with newly diagnosed diabetes with hyperthyroid grandmother. (Reproduced with permission)

When a large British Children's Diabetes Clinic (*n*=191) in Oxfordshire, which at that time had no children diagnosed as hypothyroid, began an auto-antibody screening programme together with assessment of thyroid function, TMA screening was positive in 12%, AA were present in 2% and thyroid function studies showed five children to have biochemical evidence of thyroid failure, 25% of the TMA-positive individuals and 2.6% of the clinic population. No child was found to be hyperthyroid.

Monitoring of growth should provide an important clinical clue to thyroid disease but may be masked and confused by the effects IDDM has on growth in its own right, as discussed above. The clinical features of hypothyroid disease are subtle and difficult to detect. There is often little in the way of symptoms until thyroid failure is profound, and even the clinical signs are insidious and often masked to the clinical observer seeing the patient at regular and frequent intervals. None of these children had shown any evidence of growth failure despite three-monthly accurate measurement, and all were well controlled and asymptomatic. Although some of the facial and clinical features were present with the benefit of hindsight, regular review by the same team had not noted any change. In the case of one particular young lady, review of her notes showed that, at diagnosis, there were major concerns over her mother's ability to cope and a Health Visitor's note read 'called round at midday — mother still in bed'. The mother's thyroid function was also checked, she is now on replacement therapy and gets up at 7.30 a.m.!

A recently completed survey of the Yorkshire Region, to see the current situation regarding the prevalence of thyroid disease in children with diabetes and clinical practice regarding monitoring thyroid function and auto-antibody status, showed a child population of 724 900 in 17 health districts with 21 clinicians running Children's Diabetes Clinics. There were a total of 974 children aged 0–15 years with diabetes and, of these, 24 (2.5%) were currently known to have clinical thyroid disease. It is perhaps interesting to note that, with one exception, the highest rates of thyroid disease occurred in those clinics monitoring thyroid function and/or TMA status. Of the 24 children with known thyroid disease two were thyrotoxic at diagnosis and remained so and 22 were hypothyroid and on treatment. In terms of monitoring thyroid function, only 11/21 clinicians monitored thyroid function and only 10/21 on a regular basis. All 11 clinicians monitored TSH, but only eight in conjunction with fT4 and two with fT3. Only 3/21 clinicians monitored TMA at diagnosis and only one measured other auto-antibodies.

There is of course an interaction between thyroid function and insulin dependent diabetes — theoretically in both directions. Thyroid dysfunction has a number of effects on glucose homeostasis but, in practice, this is rarely clinically evident and usually explained as, primarily, an effect of the diabetes. Broadly speaking, hyperthyroidism increases and hypothyroidism decreases glucose intolerance. Intestinal absorption is increased in hyperthyroid disease, probably secondary to increased gastric emptying and increased intestinal hexokinase and phosphatase activity. The reverse is true in hypothyroid states. Glucagon secretion is increased in hyperthyroidism, both at basal levels and with failure to suppress in response to glucose and with a blunted response to stimulation, again the converse is true in hypothyroidism. Gluconeogenesis is increased in hyperthyroidism, as is glycogenolysis which leads to glycogen depletion in liver and other tissues. The glycogenolytic effect may be biphasic with an initial increase in glycogen stores at low levels of hyperactivity with subsequent depletion. Catecholamine gluco-regulatory response is potentiated in hyperthyroidism and probably suppressed in hypothyroidism. Growth hormone is increased in hyperthyroidism and decreased in hypothyroidism. Insulin resistance seems to be increased in hyperthyroid disease but it is not clear if this is a peripheral effect or due to enhanced degradation. Insulin secretion studies are inconclusive in both hyper- and hypothyroid states.

Similarly the normal physiology of TSH, fT4 and fT3 interaction is disturbed by changes in glucose homeostasis and ketoacidosis. This makes interpretation of thyroid function tests difficult, depending on exactly what is being measured and the disease state at the time. In addition there are measurable differences in thyroid function between non-diabetic controls and children with diabetes during puberty[9].

COELIAC DISEASE

Although not strictly an auto-immune disease, coeliac disease is often grouped along with these disorders and must be considered in the patient with IDDM.

Until recently the diagnosis and, in particular, monitoring for coeliac disease depended upon an invasive jejunal biopsy, but with the advent of screening using a combination of gliadin, reticulin and endomysial IgA antibodies surveillance of the diabetic population has become feasible.

Numerous studies have shown that children with diabetes have a prevalence of 3–5% of coeliac disease identified on antibody screening and confirmed on jejunal biopsy[10]. These patients were largely symptom-free and may otherwise be identifiable only by a marginal slow growth rate or low Body Mass Index.

Treatment of this group poses a particular problem as the super-imposition of a gluten-free diet means that it is difficult to continue to provide the recommended high-fibre high-carbohydrate diet, as the only source of fibre is in pulses or in added rice fibre. This often proves unacceptable and compliance is reported to be poor. Nevertheless, identification of this condition is important in terms of explaining variations in growth and blood glucose control and to at least offer advice regarding diet. There can be unexpected improvement in behaviour which can help with issues of compliance. Perhaps more importantly, there may be implications for the future development of malignancy but the data on this in the diabetes population compared to non-diabetics are not yet available.

SUMMARY

Regular (three- to four-monthly), accurate measurement of height and weight must form part of the diabetes management strategy and can often be used to explain and discuss a problem in management with the child/parent. Associated auto-immune conditions are not uncommon and 3–5% of the childhood diabetes population are likely to have or develop thyroid disease. Hyperthyroid disease is most likely at or before diagnosis of diabetes and is associated with a higher risk of adrenal auto-immune disease, whereas hypothyroid disease can occur at any time. Growth and symptoms of thyroid disease are poor and late clinical indicators; there are strong arguments, therefore, for identifying the high-risk sub-group by the measurement of autoantibodies, especially TMA, at diagnosis and probably at one to two years post-diagnosis and to check the family history for auto-immune disease. Consideration should be given to other family members who may also have undiagnosed thyroid disease. TMA is likely to be positive in about 25% of the diabetic population and up to a quarter of these will develop thyroid disease, the risk being particularly high in the female population. Thyroid function should be monitored annually in this high-risk group at or soon after diagnosis, with caution over interpretation in relation to blood glucose control and ketoacidosis, and yearly thereafter with measurement of TSH, fT4 and possibly fT3. In TMA-positive patients it is worth screening for other auto-antibodies to identify individuals at risk of other auto-immune disease. In addition, consideration should be given to the co-existence of coeliac disease, and many clinics now include a screen for gliadin, endomysial and reticulin antibodies at diagnosis and possibly at intervals thereafter, although the exact frequency of monitoring has not been established.

REFERENCES

1 Brown, M., Ahmed, M. L., Clayton, K. L., Dunger, D. B. Growth during childhood and final height in Type 1 diabetes. *Diabetic Medicine* 1994; **11**: 182–7.
2 Von Myenburg, H. Ueber 'insulitis' bei diabetes. *Schweizerische Medizinische Wochenschrift* 1940; **21**: 554–7.
3 Gepts, W. Pathologic anatomy of the pancreas in juvenile diabetes mellitus. *Diabetes* 1965; **14**: 619–33.
4 Bottazzo, G. F., Florin-Christensen, F., Doniach, D. Islet cell antibodies in diabetes mellitus with auto-immune polyendocrine deficiencies. *Lancet* 1974; **ii**: 1279–83.
5 MacCuish, A. C., Barnes, E. W., Irvine, W. J., Duncan, L. J. P. Antibodies to pancreatic islet cells in insulin dependent diabetics with co-existent auto-immune disease. *Lancet* 1974; **ii**: 1529–31.
6 Riley, W. J., MacLaren, N. K., Lezotte, D. C. Thyroid autoimmunity in insulin dependent diabetes. The case for routine screening. *Journal of Pediatrics* 1981; **98**: 350–4.
7 Riley, W. J., Winer, A., Goldstein, D. Coincident presence of thyrogastric autoimmunity at onset of type 1 (insulin dependent) diabetes. *Diabetologia* 1983; **24**: 418–21.
8 Hopwood, N. J., Rabin, B. S., Foley, T. P., Peake, R. L. Thyroid antibodies in children and adolescents with thyroid disorders. *Journal of Pediatrics* 1978; **93**: 57.
9 Dunger, D. B., Perkins, J. A., Jowett, J. P., Edwards, P. R., Cox, L. A., Preece, M. A., Ekins, R. P. A longitudinal study of total and free thyroid hormones and thyroid binding globulin during normal puberty. *Acta Endocrinologica* 1990; **123**: 305–10.
10 Sigurs, N., Johansson, C., Elfstrand, P. O., Viander, M., Lanner, A. Prevalence of coeliac disease in diabetic children and adolescents in Sweden. *Acta Paediatrica* 1993; **82(9)**: 748–51.

16

Diabetes in School

G. R. LAWSON AND S. COURT

INTRODUCTION

The prevalence of diabetes in the childhood population of the United Kingdom is increasing, with about 1 in 750 children under the age of 16 having this condition. The age at which children present with IDDM appears to be falling. Even so, the condition remains uncommon, and in a primary school (ages five to 11 years) of 300 children one might expect a new diabetic every four years, and therefore one or two diabetics in the school. Because of cumulative frequency and an increased incidence in older children, a secondary school may have three or four diabetic children.

The interface between chronic illness and education is one that has been neglected, and teachers can feel exposed, particularly as they are given little medical information as part of their teacher training. As a consequence they may be unclear as to the potential effects on school life of medical conditions including diabetes and are very dependent on information being provided by parents, children and, more recently, the Paediatric Diabetic Specialist Nurse (PDSN). Between the ages of five and 16 a child spends in the region of 15 000 hours at school. To allow children with diabetes to participate fully in school life and achieve their educational potential it seems reasonable to expect their teachers to have a basic working knowledge of those factors that may affect life at school, so that it becomes a safer and more tolerable environment for the diabetic child.

THE TEACHER'S ROLE

A model teacher's roles and responsibilities could be summarised as follows.

Childhood and Adolescent Diabetes. Edited by S. Court and B. Lamb.
© 1997 John Wiley & Sons, Ltd.

- Knowing that a child in the school/classroom has diabetes
- Knowing the potential educational effects of diabetes
- Understanding the psychological implications of diabetes to a child and family
- Understanding the basics of dietary management and how it can impinge on school life
- Recognising the signs and symptoms of altered blood glucose levels, particularly hypoglycaemia
- Knowing how to take care of the child with hypoglycaemia.

In order to fulfil this role schools and teachers need accessible and up-to-date information. In a study of 286 primary school teachers[1] the most common sources of information were friends, relatives and parents (see Figure 16.1) rather than the health professionals or leaflets provided by

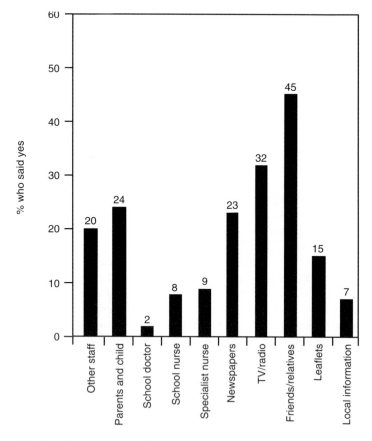

Figure 16.1. Teachers' sources of information on diabetes

Table 16.1. Teacher's knowledge of the special health needs of children with diabetes: a comparison of two studies

	Correct answer/ True or False	Bradbury[8] (Liverpool) (*n*=97) (%)	Gateshead[1] (*n*=286) (%)
Diabetic children need a special school lunch	F	31	22
Should diabetics have extra glucose before exercise?	T	46	39
If a diabetic develops thirst, tummy ache and vomits, is blood sugar HIGH or LOW?	HIGH	41	43
Can this be coped with at school?	NO	43	24
If a diabetic develops dizziness, sweating and confusion is the blood sugar HIGH or LOW	LOW	55	64
Can this be coped with at school?	YES	55	66
Insulin causes the blood sugar level to rise	F	40	36
Sugar/sweets should be available to eat in class at any time	T	54	72
Insulin is only given by injection	T	68	72

Values in columns 3 and 4 are percentages of teachers who gave the correct answer

voluntary agencies such as the British Diabetic Association (BDA). However, as more PDSNs are appointed and as the dissemination of the excellent information for schools produced by the BDA improves, this situation is likely to change[2].

That there is a need for better information in schools is evident from the results of direct enquiries. Table 16.1 gives a comparison of teachers' responses to questions about diabetes in two studies carried out in 1983 and 1994. Despite a gap of 11 years and all the input provided by the BDA and PDSNs, the level of knowledge is disappointing.

PSYCHO-EDUCATIONAL ASPECTS

Long before the discovery of insulin in 1921, Thomas Willis attributed the cause of diabetes to 'prolonged sorrow'. Anxiety and depression are commonly linked with diabetes and its management, which for children is a daily reminder that they are different. They are expected to do urine or blood testing at socially inconvenient times such as prior to the midday meal at school, as some new insulin regimes prescribe injections prior to the midday meal. As most children aim to avoid activities which differentiate them from their peers, the demands of diabetes will therefore tend to encourage non-compliance.

The psycho-educational aspects, however, are more subtle. It has long been recognised that adults with diabetes may have selective neuropsychological impairments that compromise sensory and memory abilities, as well as decreased mental and motor efficiency[3]. These impairments have been attributed to the cumulative effects of poor diabetic control where this may start in childhood. The intelligence of diabetic children falls within the normal spectrum. However, it may be compromised in selective subgroups, particularly those children developing diabetes under the age of five. The deficits most commonly observed include problems of visuo-spatial processing, verbal ability, visuo-motor abilities, memory and attention[4]. Translated into the classroom, the most commonly identified learning disability is that of reading and spelling[5,6]. Although learning difficulties may take a number of years to manifest and there are other factors that contribute, poor diabetic control is associated with educational difficulties. To improve this situation a tight collaborative approach is required between a number of professionals. This network of support for the child should include the PDSN, school nurse, dietitian, school doctor, psychologist, parents, paediatrician *and teacher*.

Hypoglycaemia is the most likely event of medical significance that may occur at school. It is important for the child that the serious manifestations are prevented if possible, or at least managed with confidence. If managed poorly such an episode can be disturbing for the class and further stigmatises the child. Thus the attitude of the school and the teachers within it are clearly immensely influential in determining the effect that diabetes has on a child at school and how this can be minimised.

TRAINING FOR TEACHERS

It would seem appropriate to include a short training in certain common medical conditions such as epilepsy, asthma and diabetes in the programmes for teachers in training. Unfortunately, to date the Teacher Training Agency has found itself unable to issue an unequivocal directive on this to Teacher Training colleges who are faced with many competing priorities for subjects to include in their courses. As a consequence the training received by teachers varies from rudimentary first aid to a complete course that gives details of medical conditions and the effects they can have on the educational process (University of Northumbria)[7]. Tables 16.2 and 16.3 describe the views of a group of primary school teachers on the effects of chronic childhood illness on the education process. Two different methods of assessment were used, a simple ranking of individual

Table 16.2. Ranking of condition against effect on education, the impact of individual diseases

Condition	Percentage	Rank
Dyslexia	88.0	1
Cystic fibrosis	75.5	2
Leukaemia	71.8	3
Congenital heart disease	48.7	4
Child protection register	47.8	5
Epilepsy	27.9	6
Grommets	24.1	7
Asthma	20.0	8
Diabetes	13.9	9

Each disease was ranked by effect from minimal to severe. The top two rankings were summated to give the above scores

disease or a ranking comparing diseases against each other. There is a consistency between the rankings, with diabetes being placed lowest in terms of effect on education. In this same study of 286 teachers only 8% had been given specific training relating to diabetes as part of initial training[1].

In schools there is pressure on time that limits the choice of subjects for training days and often precludes specific training for chronic medical conditions. Although the Department for Education and Employment (DEE) urges authorities and schools to work together in close partnership with parents to ensure proper support in schools for people with special medical needs, the same department emphasises that there is no legal or contractual duty on teachers to offer supervision of a child with such needs. This is a purely voluntary role. Nevertheless teachers and other school staff in charge of pupils have a common law duty to act 'as any reasonably

Table 16.3. Ranking of condition against effect on education, of each disease compared with the others

Condition	Percentage
Cystic fibrosis	48.3
Dyslexia	45.8
Leukaemia	44.0
Child protection register	17.4
Grommets	15.0
Congenital heart disease	12.8
Epilepsy	9.3
Asthma	5.4
Diabetes	3.8

prudent parent would' to make sure that pupils are healthy and safe whilst on school premises. This may, in certain circumstances, extend to administering medicine or taking action in an emergency.

The local council, as the employer, can indemnify staff against claims for alleged negligence 'whilst acting within the scope of their employment'. However, there are no national guidelines nor is there automatic indemnity covering the responsibility for the administration of medicine or dealing with a child with a known medical problem. Because of this some of the teachers' unions advise their members against administering medicines in schools, as do some local education authorities.

Thus in the final analysis a personal approach by parents to a teacher in order to gain their support is likely to be best. Many teachers are willing to learn about the management of hypoglycaemia, and a minority have expressed a willingness to undertake more invasive treatments, e.g. giving glucagon. This is clearly discretionary but may be important if diabetic children are to go with their peers on physically active school trips such as skiing.

GETTING BACK TO SCHOOL

It is important that, following the diagnosis of diabetes, children get back to school and normal routines quickly so that others can see they are not ill and can join in as before. However, parents may be apprehensive about the practical aspects and the handing over of care, and teachers may have a concern about accepting responsibility in this new situation. Indeed, sometimes roles can be reversed when parents find themselves teaching the teacher. The PDSN acts as a professional resource and should try to accompany parents when they are making the first post-diagnosis contacts with school. These are well described in the BDA school cards 1 and 2 (see Appendix 16.1).

Clearly the teachers in a school need to know the pupils that have diabetes and a system for informing them needs to be in place. Perhaps more particularly a mechanism for reminding them as the child moves through the school is important. Card 2 of the BDA pack outlines how this can be done, using a recent photograph and clear information as to how the school can contact parents and the local clinical team.

PRACTICAL ISSUES FOR SCHOOLS

This section tries to identify the aspects of care a teacher needs to understand and to put them into the context of the school environment.

THE BEGINNING AND THE END OF THE DAY

During the first days back at school many parents will want to go with their child to and from school until confidence is regained. The walk to school, good in terms of exercise, follows breakfast and is unlikely to generate a low blood glucose level. The return journey at the end of the day, however, once the 'honeymoon' period is over, can be a concern. This is often a time when many children head for the sweet shop on the way home. Diabetic children may need food at this time and hopefully can be persuaded to buy snacks rather than sweets, at least some of the time. This can be a difficult time, particularly in rural areas when the day ends in a long bus ride.

TELLING THE OTHERS

There are a number of issues that inevitably identify the new diabetic as different, such as wearing identification, the absolute need for snacks, easy access to toilets if diabetic control is less good, and the ever present concern about hypoglycaemia. Schools need to have strategies for all of these, but particularly for how the class is informed.

Depending on age, the responsibility will often lie with the young person to decide for themselves who should know, but friends do need to be told, and the PDSN can facilitate this. Keeping quiet is not an option as a 'buddy' system works well and protects older children on campus-style schools. For the younger age group it may be appropriate for the PDSN to talk to the class and explain why it may at times be necessary for a child to eat during lessons and go to the toilet more frequently. For the teacher this is information that should be passed on to parents as it may reflect periods of poor metabolic control. The sharing of this kind of information also helps to foster the concept of shared care.

SNACKS

Snacks can usually be eaten between lessons or at break times. Occasionally snacks become a tool for the child to wield over their peers; teachers need to realise that timing is rarely so crucial that they need to disrupt the lesson. One of us has had a patient who used to break up the snack in his pocket and surreptitiously eat the small pieces through the lesson, ostensibly to avoid his peers realising. In the event it repeatedly drew the attention of teachers and peers to him, and as such was perhaps successful as an attention-seeking device and served as a reflection of his high levels of anxiety at the time.

IDENTIFICATION

Identification bracelets and pendants are important items, but can fall foul of the school regulations concerning the wearing of jewellery. This issue needs to be clarified as part of the initial discussions. It is clearly sensible for these items to be removed during sporting activity. However, with the older child it is often difficult to persuade them to wear identification in the first place.

SCHOOL MEALS

School meals, exercise and hypoglycaemia may be interrelated or occur as separate problems in school. School meal times are important for a number of reasons. Teachers need to understand that children are eating to cover insulin that has already been given, although increasingly young people at secondary school may be using a basal bolus system which requires insulin to be given before lunch. This in itself also generates problems. Some of the issues are identified below.

1. In the timing of meals, consistency is important, so special arrangements may be necessary for the diabetic child if class meal times are staggered.
2. Both PDSN and dietitian should try to meet catering staff at the school to discuss appropriate food choices for a newly diagnosed child. It may be practical for staff to oversee a child's selection, but as children get older this can be resented. One approach is for school menus to be sent home for discussion; this allows the child to take increasing responsibility.
3. Meal times are social occasions and children may want to sit with, and eat similar food to, their friends. Now that schools commonly run a self-service menu, many children will go for the 'chips and burger' option. Unless the child has aspirations to sainthood, jacket potatoes will not be perceived as the 'cool' option.
4. The alternative of a packed lunch has some advantages as parents still have some input, although the option to barter the lunch box's contents still exists.
5. A growing practice is for adolescents to leave school at lunch time and go to a nearby sandwich bar where a sausage roll, packet of crisps, and a can of carbonated drink are more likely selections than a salad sandwich and an apple. 'Street credibility' rules; for one meal a day this probably does not matter unless it affects the selections made at other times.
6. For the school the fact that some diabetic students use a basal bolus regime and may have to carry insulin with them at school raises issues of safety.
7. For the student an appropriate environment to give insulin is important. The rule of 20 minutes before food is difficult, especially if they want to

sit with friends or gain an early place in the lunch queue. In these circumstances it is common for insulin to be given after food.

EXERCISE

Teachers need to understand the importance of exercise to children with diabetes and also its effect on blood glucose. There is a separate chapter on exercise, so what follows is a simple list of some of the issues for the school.

1. Diabetic young people should be encouraged to take part in all sports. There is considerable evidence that it can benefit this group, particularly in terms of their physical well-being, social skills, self-esteem and educational progress.
2. It should be recognised that exercise at break time does not usually require extra carbohydrate, and common sense needs to prevail in assessing the need for pre-exercise additional glucose. However, this should usually be taken prior to swimming.
3. Special arrangements will be necessary if training matches are held after school hours. This usually simply means an extra snack to cover the time until the next meal and the availability of fast-acting glucose (Dextrosol, Hypostop or a sugary drink). Purists might argue for blood monitoring, but testing at school is rarely appropriate unless there have been problems in these circumstances previously.
4. Before strenuous exercise extra food may be required during the school day. This needs to be accessible, and not locked away. Although many teachers would assume the young person would be responsible for managing this aspect of care, the handing over of fast-acting glucose to the teacher in charge for safe keeping also serves as a reminder of a diabetic child's presence.
5. Teachers need to recognise the relationship between a low blood glucose and behaviour which may become erratic, and performance which can deteriorate rapidly with impending hypoglycaemia. The response should be fast-acting glucose and not a 'punishment lap' round the field.

HYPOGLYCAEMIA

The following symptoms are indicators of hypoglycaemia in children. However, it must be emphasised that individual diabetic children can have particular symptoms.

- Hunger
- Sweating (usually cold and clammy)
- Drowsiness
- Pallor
- Glazed eyes

- Shaking or trembling
- Lack of concentration
- Irritability or naughtiness.

The BDA school card 2 allows for a description of these to be given to the school and also an account of appropriate fast-acting carbohydrate treatment response.

Teachers need:

— to understand that mild hypoglycaemia is not uncommon if control is tight, and that the child together with a teacher can manage this at school with little disruption.

— to have available a ready supply of biscuits and fast-acting glucose (Dextrosol, Hypostop, fruit juice or Lucozade). A child should not be sent off unaccompanied if emergency glucose supplies are held centrally within a school.

— to share information with parents if hypoglycaemia is occurring regularly at school so that food and insulin can be adjusted.

— to recognise that the likely time for a low glucose is just before lunch and at the end of the day before going home. If these times coincide with unusual behaviour, quietness, poor concentration or falling asleep it may relate to impending hypoglycaemia.

— to appreciate that severe hypoglycaemia can occur but is rare. They need to know that a child may become unconscious and can have a convulsion, that giving Hypostop or Dextrosol into the side of the mouth may be useful, that the child should be placed in the recovery position while medical help is being obtained, and that the child is not going to die.

— a plan of action, so that mild or severe hypoglycaemia can be dealt with confidently. This is important for the child but also for the class as it can be disturbing to see a child convulsing.

— to understand that a child may be embarrassed after a hypoglycaemic attack, because of things said and done. They and the class may need help with this.

— to recognise any bullying or isolation of a diabetic child that can occur if their condition has in some way interfered with class dynamics or opportunities. Self-esteem can be invaded by this condition and unpleasant 'name calling' is not uncommon.

MOVING UP THE SCHOOL

The time in junior school is usually not too problematic, particularly as the culture of such schools has a significant 'care' element. It is also a time when children can begin to assume increasing responsibility for their condition within a protected environment. Even so, with a new teacher each year it is important that information is passed on. In a recent study 40% of primary school teachers were not absolutely confident that they would know the name of a diabetic child in the school, and in the same study only 60% were actually identified by the schools concerned.

The move to the senior school is a time of concern. Transfer of information is more difficult due the numbers of teachers involved with a young person's education. Students have to take responsibility for their own care and they need to have the confidence to share details about diabetes with others at a time when, because of the physical and emotional influences of puberty, their natural inclination may be to minimise the condition and remain secretive about potential problems. It is a time when the network of parents, teachers, PDSN and paediatrician needs to be particularly sensitive to all the pressures being placed on the adolescent.

TRIPS AWAY FROM SCHOOL

Increasingly parents expect that children with medical conditions will rightly be included in school visits to other countries, outdoor pursuits centres, skiing, field trips, and school team away games. This can generate concern for teachers, who may feel unable to take on additional responsibility. For the child, however, it is potentially a time for being more independent, and also for bonding with the group as part of a 'joint adventure'. With sensible planning and liaison between school, clinic, parents, teachers, child and PDSN there should be no reason why a child should be excluded. Guidance is given in the BDA school card 5 and also in Chapter 18 as to how this can be undertaken safely.

EXAMINATIONS AND CAREER GUIDANCE

Although the purpose of this section has been to provide guidance to allow a diabetic child to experience all aspects of school life, the principal objective of school is to give young people the experience and qualifications that will allow them choices for their future.

Examinations are part of this process. For many these are extremely stressful and for the child with diabetes they can generate a period of poor control which in turn can affect academic performance. Schools and examination boards need to recognise this, and letters of support from paediatricians should be asked for if it becomes clear that a student is underperforming either because of disturbed nights or overt problems during an exam. It may also be necessary for young people to eat during the exams or use toilet facilities more frequently, and medical advice to this effect should be offered.

Increasingly young people are being encouraged to take up 'work placements' for short periods of time before leaving school as part of career guidance. There are a number of advantages to this as it allows them to develop strategies of approach with potential employers in relation to their diabetes. However, some careers in the UK are not open to diabetic young adults. These include the armed forces, the police and fire services and driving heavy goods or public service vehicles. It is important that schools career officers have up-to-date information about the suitability of work options, but as a general comment all other occupations can be readily undertaken by diabetic young people with the appropriate qualifications. Despite this they can be disadvantaged by the prejudice which sadly still exists.

PRACTICE POINTS

☞ A teacher's involvement is mainly voluntary.
☞ A personal approach is usually best in achieving co-operation between parents and teachers.
☞ Teachers need information on:
— diabetes and its management
— the effect diabetes can have on the educational process
— the relevance of diet and exercise to the diabetic child
— the recognition and treatment of hypoglycaemia.
☞ A clear plan of action for emergencies needs to be in place.
☞ Children of different ages and different school settings have very different needs.
☞ Parents need to appreciate that new teachers are as fearful as they were at the time of first diagnosis.
☞ Children and young people with diabetes need to know that their carers are confident in the management of diabetes.

REFERENCES

1 Court, S. The Health Education boundary. MSc Dissertation, Public Health Medicine, Newcastle Upon Tyne University, 1994.
2 BDA. *Guidance for teachers and school staff.* London: BDA, 1996.
3 Bale, R. N. Brain damage in diabetes mellitus. *British Journal of Psychiatry* 1973; **122:** 337–41.
4 Rovet, J. F., Ehrlich, R. M., Czuchtad, D. Intellectual characteristics of diabetic children at diagnosis and one year later on. *Journal of Paediatric Psychology* 1990; **15:** 775–88.

5 Gath, A., Smith, M., Baum, J. D. Emotional disorders in diabetic children. *Archives of Disease in Childhood* 1980; **55:** 371–5.
6 Rovet, J. F., Ehrlich, R. M., Czuchtad, D., Ackler, M. Psychoeducational characteristics of children and adolescents with insulin dependent diabetes mellitus. *Journal of Learning Disabilities* 1993; **26:** 7–22.
7 Health awareness in schools. Primary BEd Programme, 1994, Department of Education Studies, University of Northumbria at Newcastle.
8 Bradbury, A. J., Smith, C. S. An assessment of the diabetes knowledge of schoolteachers. *Archives of Disease in Childhood* 1983; **53:** 692–6.

FURTHER READING

Using medicines in school. *Drug and Therapeutics Bulletin* 1994; **32:** 81–3.
Taking drugs to school. *Which Way to Health.* Hertford: Consumers Association, December 1994.
Supporting Pupils With Medical Needs In School. Circular 14/96. London: Department for Education and Employment/Department of Health, 1996.

Appendix 16.1

School 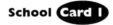 Card 1

PLANNING FOR THE CHILD WITH DIABETES

This card explains the important preparation and planning that is needed to ensure that staff are fully briefed about diabetes.

Meeting the child's parents

Personal contact between the school and parents is essential. It is important that a meeting is arranged between the parents, the head teacher and the class teacher or tutor before the child joins or returns to school. At this meeting the parents can give you information about their child's diabetes and they can complete the details on the attached School Cards. The parents may be able to attend with a diabetes specialist nurse. Close liaison with the child's medical team, especially the diabetes specialist nurse, is important. The parents will have the telephone number.

This meeting will be an opportunity for the parents to describe the child's diabetes care. In particular you should cover:

Hypoglycaemia: *symptoms and individual treatment.*

Meal and snack times: *what should be eaten and when.*

Exercise and activity: *what preparation is necessary before and during physical activity.*

Emergency contacts: *who should be contacted in the event of emergencies.*

Explaining diabetes: *how to explain to the class that the child has diabetes and why snacks need to be eaten.*

Informing school staff

After meeting the parents, an early meeting of relevant school staff should be arranged to inform them about the child with diabetes. At this meeting, questions can be answered and decisions made regarding the care for the child at school. It may be helpful to invite the child's diabetes specialist nurse to this meeting.

In this meeting, the following should be covered:

❶ Ensure that all staff know about the child with diabetes in the school. Place the Diabetes Record Card (School Card 2) in the staff room where it can be seen, and make photocopies for staff who need them.

❷ Establish where supplies of fast acting sugar are to be kept (to treat hypoglycaemia) and ensure that these supplies are clearly marked and accessible at all times. Establish whether the child will carry sugar themselves to treat early symptoms of hypoglycaemia. Ensure that staff are aware of the symptoms and treatment of hypoglycaemia.

School 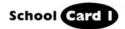 Card 1

❸ Ensure that staff know the importance of NOT sending the child out of the classroom or anywhere alone to treat hypoglycaemia.

❹ Ensure that staff are aware that the child can be fully involved in all school activities, including school trips. Consult the child's family if there are any particular questions.

❺ Inform your colleagues that the child may well have a good understanding of the management of their diabetes, and will usually be aware of their own needs. If you have any questions or concerns, contact the family.

❻ Discuss how diabetes can be explained to the rest of the children and why the child may need to eat snacks in class.

How to use the rest of this pack
There are four other School Cards which cover detailed aspects of the child's care and provide important information for staff:

SCHOOL CARD 2 - Diabetes Record Card
This card should be completed when meeting the child's parents and updated as necessary. Each member of school staff who supervises the child should be given a photocopy of this card.

SCHOOL CARD 3 - Food
This card explains the child's food requirements. It should be given to the staff who prepare and supervise school lunch breaks.

SCHOOL CARD 4 - Physical Activity
This card explains how exercise and activity can affect diabetes and the preparation required before, during and after games or activities. It should be given to staff responsible for physical education.

SCHOOL CARD 5 - Trips Away From Home
This card is to be used for outings, trips and holidays. It should be given to staff who are responsible for the organisation of trips. The sheet needs to be completed by the parents of the child.

PLANNING FOR THE CHILD WITH DIABETES

School **Card 2**

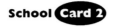

THIS CHILD HAS DIABETES

PHOTO

Name: _____

Date of Birth: _____

Current year/Class

If s/he has a low blood sugar (hypoglycaemia), you will need to take the action described on the back of this card.

In case of medical emergency, use the contact numbers below.

If the parent(s) are not available, or you need to speak to a medical professional, the telephone numbers of the child's GP and hospital clinic are also given below.

CONTACT INFORMATION

Family Contact 1

Name: _____

Phone: _____

Relationship: _____

Family Contact 2

Name: _____

Phone: _____

Relationship: _____

Clinic Contact

Name: _____

Phone: _____

GP

Name: _____

Phone: _____

Please turn over to find information on hypoglycaemia and treatment.

DIABETES RECORD CARD

School 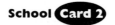 **Card 2**

Hypoglycaemia

Children with diabetes may experience low blood glucose (hypoglycaemia).

Look out for the following symptoms:
Hunger
Sweating
Drowsiness
Pallor
Glazed Eyes
Shaking
Mood Changes or Lack of Concentration

Typical symptoms for this child are: *(to be completed in consultation with the parents)*

Fast acting sugar should be given immediately. Examples of these are:

Lucozade; sugary drink eg Coke, Tango, Fanta (not diet drinks); mini chocolate bars eg Mars, Milky Way; fresh fruit juice; glucose tablets; honey or jam.

For this child, give (details from parents):

Fast acting sugar	Quantity

Recovery should be in 10 - 15 minutes. The child may feel nauseous, tired or have a headache.

When the child has recovered, follow up the fast acting sugar with some slower acting starchy food such as two biscuits and a glass of milk or a sandwich.

If the child is unconscious, do not give anything to swallow. Rub some jam, honey or Hypo Stop (a special glucose gel which the parents can supply) inside the cheek where it can be absorbed. Place the child in the recovery position and call an ambulance.

DIABETES RECORD CARD

School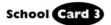

FOOD

*This card is for lunch-time supervisors, catering staff and other
people who supervise a child with diabetes
during meal times.*

If you are supervising or preparing food for a child with diabetes, you may be
worried that s/he is eating the wrong kinds of food. There is no need to worry:
the food recommended for children with diabetes is no different from that
recommended for children in the general population. There is no special
diabetic diet. However, a regular intake of starchy foods at meals and snack
times is important.

There are two important aspects to consider:

● the quantity of starchy or carbohydrate foods eaten
● the importance of regular meals and snacks

Types and quantity of foods eaten
The diet for children with diabetes is based on the healthy diet recommended
for the general population, a diet which is low in sugar and fat and high in fibre.

The child will have seen a dietitian at the hospital, who will have given her/him
a basic food plan on which daily choices can be based. Most importantly the
child will have been advised to eat a certain amount of starchy or carbohydrate
food at each meal. S/he will probably know how much should be eaten. Please
check this with the parents.

Carbohydrate foods are important because the child will need to eat enough
of these to maintain near normal blood glucose levels. These foods can be
roughly divided into slow acting and fast acting carbohydrates. Slow acting
carbohydrates are starchy foods, pulses (eg beans) and fruit. Fast acting
carbohydrates are sugary foods.

Slow acting carbohydrates help to maintain near normal blood glucose levels.
They can be found in the following foods, at least one of which should be eaten
at every meal:

   potatoes, rice, bread, chapatis, pasta, breakfast cereal.

The faster acting sugary foods are useful for raising the blood sugar quickly (as
in treating hypoglycaemia), but should be limited in the day to day food intake.
These foods include:

   **fizzy drinks eg, Coke, Fanta, lemonade etc. (not diet varieties),
   puddings, sweets, chocolates, fudge, iced cakes, syrups, sugars,
   treacles, squash, jams**

Ordinary sweets and chocolates may be incorporated into the diet, either
before exercise when extra energy is required or after a meal as a treat.
Likewise, the occasional sweet pudding or dessert will not do any harm as part
of an overall healthy diet.

School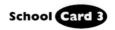

FOOD

Timing of meals and snacks

Meals and snacks should be eaten at regular intervals, following a plan drawn up by the family and the dietitian. It is important for the child with diabetes to eat at regular times in order to maintain blood glucose levels. A missed or delayed meal or snack could lead to low blood glucose (hypoglycaemia).

It is important for you to know the times when the child needs to eat and ensure that these times are kept to by the child. S/he may need to be near the front of the queue (and at the same sitting each day) for the midday meal. The times that this child needs to eat are:

Name of child

	Morning snack	Lunch	Afternoon snack
TIME			

Why snacks?

The child with diabetes will need to have mid morning and mid afternoon snacks, such as fruit or crisps or a cereal bar, which the parents should give to the child to bring to school. These snacks are needed to maintain the blood glucose at a sufficient level between meals. Snacks may need to be eaten in class, but are best taken at break time.

The child's choice of foods

Learning to trust the child with diabetes with their choice of foods is important for staff. If you have concerns about the child's eating habits or choice of foods, speak to their parents.

If you would like further information about food and diabetes, contact Diet Information Services on the *Careline* at the British Diabetic Association. 0171 636 6112. (Monday - Friday 9.00am - 5.00pm).

School 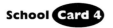 Card 4

This card is for staff supervising exercise and activity sessions. This includes games lessons, swimming, gymnastics, dancing, walks and other activities that use up energy.

Diabetes is no bar to enjoying activity or indeed sporting excellence. In addition to thousands of people who enjoy sports, there are successful footballers, ballet dancers, golfers and marathon runners with diabetes; people with diabetes have competed in and succeeded in top level sports at national and international levels. Therefore, there is no reason why children with diabetes should not join in all school sports, or be selected to represent school and other teams providing they have made some simple preparations.

These preparations are needed because all forms of extra strenuous activity, such as swimming, football, dancing, gymnastics and long walks, use up glucose. If the child with diabetes uses too much glucose or does not eat enough before starting activity, the blood glucose will fall too low, and the child will experience hypoglycaemia.

Preparing for activity
It is important for the child with diabetes to eat some extra glucose before vigorous activity. Some things s/he may eat are;
- mini chocolate bar
- cereal snack bar
- 2 biscuits.

This will provide the extra glucose needed for the activity. The more strenuous and prolonged the activity, the more food will be needed before (and possibly during) the activity.

Tottenham and England footballer Gary Mabbutt, who has diabetes, drinks a bottle of Lucozade before a match, and more if needed at half time. This covers his own requirements during a match.

During activity
During activity sessions, it is important to have glucose tablets or a sugary drink nearby (ie on the side of the pool or in the goalmouth on the pitch or in an accessible rucksack on a nature hike) in case the child's blood glucose levels drops too low (hypoglycaemia).

During activities or sports, teachers keep watch over all the children. The child with diabetes need not be singled out for special attention. This will make the child feel different and may lead to embarrassment.

After activity
After particularly strenuous activity, the child may need to eat some more food. This depends on the timing of the activity and the level of exercise undertaken.

Hypoglycaemia
Hypoglycaemia (Hypo) means low blood glucose. It is important to know how to identify and treat a hypo.

Symptoms of a hypo
The symptoms of a hypo can include hunger, sweating, drowsiness, pallor, glazed eyes,

School 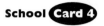 Card 4

shaking, lack of concentration. The symptoms are different for every child.

Symptoms for (name of child) _____ are:

Hypo symptoms:

Treating a Hypo

If a hypo occurs during sport or activity, fast acting sugar needs to be given immediately. This should be followed by some slower acting carbohydrate such as a sandwich or two biscuits and a glass of milk. The fast acting sugar will raise the blood glucose levels quickly.

Fast acting sugars include Lucozade, sugary drink such as Coke, Fanta, Tango (not diet drinks); mini Mars Bar or Milky Way, glucose tablets, or fresh fruit juice. The child will often be aware that s/he is going hypo and will take appropriate action.

Give this child: (details from parents)　　　　　　　Amount:

When the child has recovered, give a longer-acting carbohydrate such as a sandwich or two biscuits and a glass of milk. This will keep the blood glucose levels up until the next meal or snack. Depending on the response of the child, let them continue with the activity.

Unconscious

In the unlikely event of the child losing consciousness, do not give anything to swallow. Instead, try rubbing jam, honey or Hypo Stop (a special glucose gel which the parents will be able to supply) inside the cheek where it can be absorbed. Place the child in the recovery position (on their side with the chin tilted back). Call an ambulance. If the child does lose consciousness, s/he will come round eventually and should not come to any immediate harm.

And finally...

A final word to raise the issue of children using excuses to avoid games or activities. Most children love joining in activities, but some less favoured activities, such as cross country running, may elicit a range of excuses from some children. We hope the child with diabetes will not use their diabetes as an excuse for not participating. If this does occur regularly, speak to the child's family to find out more about the individual situation. Diabetes should not be an excuse for opting out out of school activities.

For further information about diabetes, contact the *Careline* at the British Diabetic Association on 0171 636 6112

School 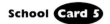 Card 5

This card is for staff organising a trip away. It covers the preparation that is needed before a trip is made.

Planning for the child with diabetes needs to be considered. Before the first trip, a meeting with the staff involved and the parents is necessary.

Day outings
These should pose few problems, as the routine will be much like that at school. Remember to take along a copy of the Diabetes Record Card (card 2 in this series) and some extra food, such as fruit or sandwiches in case of unexpected delays. In addition, children should take their insulin and injection kit, just in case the delay continues over their usual injection time.

Overnight stays and longer trips in Britain
In the case of overnight stays, these will include injection routines and blood glucose monitoring. You will need to be confident that the child is able to do their own injections or that there is a member of staff who is willing to take responsibility for helping with injections and blood glucose testing.

If their child is not doing their own injections, most parents, quite sensibly, would not consider letting them go away at this stage.

Before the trip, use the checklist below to ensure that the child has packed their insulin, injection device and blood testing equipment and supplies to treat hypogly-caemia. These can all too easily be left behind in the excitement of the departure. A spare pack should be carried by the teacher in case of loss. If s/he has forgotten medical equipment, contact the paediatric department at the nearest large hospital, who will be able to help.

Trips abroad and exchange visits
In addition to the above, if you are travelling outside Britain you will find the BDA travel packs useful. These packs contain information, such as availability of emergency supplies, food facts and translations of phrases in the local language(s). These are available from the BDA.

Checklist for trips/holidays

Child should take:

- **Glucose in case of hypos**
  eg *fizzy drink (not diet drinks), sugar, glucose tablets*

- **Food for journeys**
  eg *sandwiches in case of delayed travel*

- **Personal identification**
  eg *BDA identification card, 'I have diabetes' card or SOS bracelet*

- **Insulin(s)**

- **Syringes or insulin pen and needles**

- **Blood testing equipment and spare strip**

Staff should take:

- **Diabetes Record Card**
  (card 2 in this series)

- **School trip information**

- **Glucose in case of hypos**

School 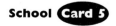 Card 5

School trip information

Name of child: _____

Date of birth: _____

Insulin injections

Type(s) of insulin	Breakfast dose	Lunch dose	Dinner dose	Bed-time dose

Further Useful Information:

Information about the treatment of hypoglycaemia and emergency contact numbers can be found on the Diabetes Record Card, a copy of which should be attached to this card.

If you would like further information about diabetes, contact the *Careline* at the British Diabetic Association on 0171 636 6112.

TRIPS AWAY FROM HOME

17

Exercise and Diabetes

MOHAMMED KIBIRIGE AND SIMON COURT

INTRODUCTION

The *Concise Oxford Dictionary* defines 'exercise' as the 'exertion of muscles, and limbs especially for health's sake, (bodily, mental or spiritual training)'; 'sport' is defined as a 'pastime, game or outdoor pastime'. 'Physical training', on the other hand, is defined as becoming 'physically fit where training means coming to physical efficiency by exercise and diet' (Figure 17.1).

These definitions are important to all children, but particularly those with insulin dependent diabetes mellitus (IDDM). Understanding the purpose of exercise by children, adolescents and particularly parents can influence whether exercise done sporadically develops into a family routine that can be carried forward into adult life by young people with diabetes. The views and attitudes of parents cannot be underestimated, as they are probably the most important determining factor. Children need to be encouraged and often transported to the ground, pool or sports hall where they are competing, or practising their sport. There are, however, some general comments that can be made about exercise in children.

UNDER-FIVES

Exercise under the age of five years tends to be spontaneous, expending a lot of energy simply running around. The seasons of the year influence patterns and types of exercise undertaken, and school programmes change. Playing out during the lighter evenings is replaced by playing computer

Childhood and Adolescent Diabetes. Edited by S. Court and B. Lamb.
© 1997 John Wiley & Sons, Ltd.

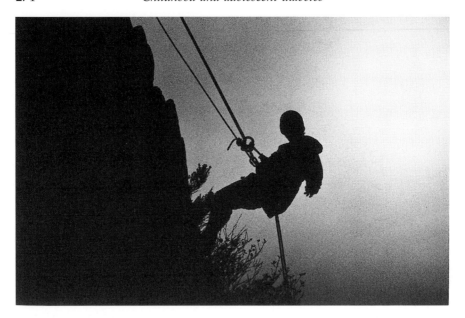

Figure 17.1. Abseiling

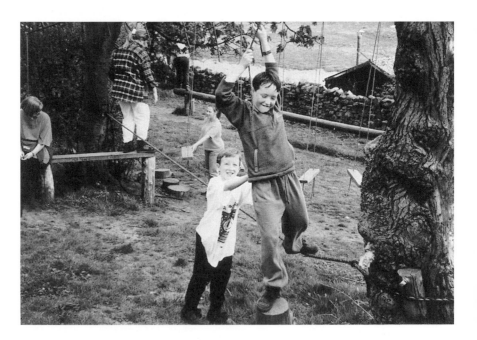

Figure 17.2. Tackling an assault course

Table 17.1. Calories burnt in different types of exercise

Activity	kcal/min	kcal/hour
Walking (3 mph)		
Golf, pulling cart	4–5	240–300
Cycling (6 mph)		
Bowling		
Cycling (8 mph)		
Volley ball	5–6	300–360
Tennis, doubles		
Golf, carrying clubs		
Walking (4 mph)		
Ice or roller skating	6–7	360–420
Cycling (10 mph)		
Walking (5 mph)		
Cycling (11 mph)	7–8	420–480
Water skiing		
Tennis, singles		
Jogging (5 mph)		
Cycling (12 mph)	8–10	480–600
Downhill skiing		
Running (5½ mph)		
Aerobics	10–11	600–660
Cycling (13 mph)		
Running (6 mph)	11 or more	660 or more
Swimming		
Football	These are team games and the calorie per minute	
Hockey	or calorie per hour requirements depend on how	
Netball	active the individuals involved in the team game	
Rugby	are and what positions they play in.	

mph—miles per hour (1 mph=1.6 km/hour)

games inside in the winter. Some of the 'control' effects are mediated through changing diet, from summer salads to winter puddings (Figure 17.2).

FIVE- TO TEN-YEAR-OLDS

Children between the ages of five and 10 years will have prescribed physical education (PE) lessons at school in addition to normal play. A small percentage will also have physical training as members of school teams, particularly as they become older. PE lessons may be affected by the weather, so it is not always practical to make adjustments to insulin or diet on the day of the lesson, as the actual exercise done by each individual child in the lesson may vary. The energy utilised is difficult to gauge and therefore the calories required to cover particular exercise can only be estimated (see Table 17.1). Physical training for various sports is more predictable and allows an experimental approach, i.e. blood glucose testing before and after to measure effects; planning may then be possible. Dietary planning, however, is very dependent on compliance.

OVER 10s

Children over the age of 10 years will have the choice of similar activities to those aged between five and 10 years. They, however, are entering puberty with the associated metabolic demands of growth. Although some may be involved in serious competitive sport, many are distracted by the other pressures of adolescence and the views of their peers. Even so, for boys of this age sport is acceptable and they tend to be more active than girls, which

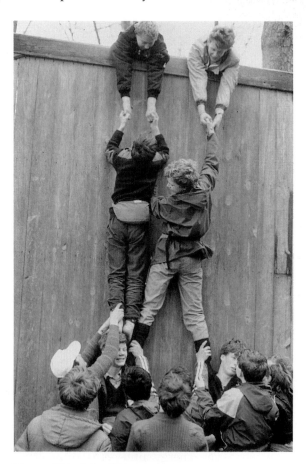

Figure 17.3. A 'wall' game for teams

Table 17.2. Determinants of the type of exercise available to a child

---

- Parental attitudes
- Age
- State of health
- Physical ability
- Psychological well-being
- Facilities (local authority or private)
- School attitudes
- Weather
- Political (local and national, e.g. selling of school fields for building)
- Economics (family and national, e.g. sports scholarship, car ownership, club membership)
- Ability to obtain appropriate insurance

---

may contribute to their better glycaemic control as a group (Figure 17.3). In general, however, children and adolescents spend little time on exercise[1]. There is some evidence that diabetics as a group are less involved in team games, perhaps as a consequence of a degree of social isolation or because the effects of exercise can be unpredictable and therefore generate anxiety (see Table 17.2). The ripples of concern following a significant hypoglycaemic episode can last a long time.

BENEFITS OF EXERCISE

Arguably the benefits and importance of exercise for all are self-evident. The British government's Departments of Health and Education have, in the past, highlighted the need for exercise. Recommendations to improve well-being of all children were devised[2-5]. It was recommended that all pupils should have a minimum of two hours of curriculum time each week devoted to physical education (including sport). In 1987 it was found that 40% of state school pupils of 14 years of age had less than two hours. Unfortunately in most state schools the downward trend continues, and in some the playing fields have been seen as a financial asset to be sold off. There are provisions for extracurricular activities and sport but they are expensive and often depend on the willingness of teachers to give up spare time and of parents to underwrite costs — clearly this can be discriminatory but does potentially allow voluntary agencies to subsidise individual children.

In this country PE lessons usually last between 30 and 40 minutes, during which children can undertake a broad spectrum of sporting activity: for example, netball, gymnastics, hockey, football or athletics. Individual schools may place very different levels of emphasis on sport and have

Table 17.3. Factors to be taken into account in assessment of energy requirements

- Type (swimming, running, cycling etc.) (see Table 17.1)
- Duration of exercise
- Severity
- Team or individual ('striker or goalkeeper')
- Temperature
- Physique
- Level of training

changing programmes as children progress through the school. This places a significant demand on parents, teachers and the paediatric diabetes specialist nurse (PDSN) to keep in good communication if a diabetic child is going to compete on equal terms.

The national sports of countries also vary, although football is becoming universal. For children in the UK cricket and rugby have become almost the exclusive preserve of the independent schools. In other countries with colder climates winter sports are of greater relevance, although dry ski slopes are becoming more common in the UK. The novice skier uses up a great deal of energy (Table 17.1).

Although the social and health benefits of exercise are discussed in the clinics and at school, some parents still discourage their diabetic children from active exercise for fear of hypoglycaemia. The remainder of this chapter is given over to a description of the physiological and metabolic events that take place with exercise, where diabetes 'makes waves', and some practical guidelines on how individuals and families might cope.

BLOOD GLUCOSE RESPONSE TO EXERCISE

Blood glucose levels during exercise are influenced by many factors (Tables 17.1, 17.2 and 17.3). It is important to have a clear understanding of the biochemical processes in the non-diabetic and how these can vary considerably in children with IDDM, depending on insulin status.

EXERCISE IN A NON-DIABETIC SUBJECT

During moderate exercise, insulin plays a major role in regulating fuel homeostasis. In moderate exercise ($<60\%$ of maximum oxygen consumption) glucose regulation is tightly controlled, with hepatic glucose production (glycogenolysis) rising by 2.5-fold to match precisely the increased utilisation in muscle. The glucagon/insulin molar ratio is the main regulator of hepatic glucose production. Euglycaemia is maintained because of feedback signals from glucose sensors that pick up any blood glucose fall consequent on the increase in peripheral glucose utilisation. Matching of hepatic glucose production with exercise-induced glucose utilisation is mediated through neuroendocrine pathways[6].

In very intense, short-duration exercise (e.g. 100 metre sprint or >85% oxygen consumption) to exhaustion, glucose regulation differs in several important respects. During 100% oxygen consumption there is a seven- to eight-fold increment in hepatic glucose production, considerably greater than the four-fold increment in glucose disappearance from the circulation — glucose levels therefore rise. Plasma insulin concentrations remain unchanged or decline very slowly and those of peripheral glucagon increase by at most 50%[6,7]. Plasma levels of adrenaline rise with exercise, resulting in increased gluconeogenesis. Cortisol and growth hormone also rise, and with falling insulin levels this produces an increase in lipolysis generating free fatty acids (FFA) from triglyceride (TG) as an energy source.

Insulin sensitivity is increased by endurance exercise and training. This is believed to be through increased number and activity of adipocytes and myocytes, leading to an increase in insulin-stimulated glucose transport into those cells following exercise. The effect of reducing insulin resistance may persist for as long as 24 hours after prolonged exercise. If exercise is discontinued insulin sensitivity starts to decrease after three days[8].

EXERCISE IN PEOPLE WITH IDDM

The hormonal balance that maintains normal blood glucose levels following food or exercise as described for the non-diabetic is lost in IDDM. The major problem in the child with diabetes is the lack of regulation of insulin once injected. Insulin levels are only loosely related to food intake. If insulin delivery is mismatched, the consequences will depend on the bio-availability of insulin and whether a child is over- or under-insulinised (see Tables 17.4 and 17.5).

The effects of exercise in these two situations differ. In the low insulin situation, with raised blood glucose levels at the start of exercise, hypoglycaemia does not occur and ketoacidosis can be accelerated. With insulin lack glycogenolysis and lipolysis are not switched off. In the presence of insulin hypoglycaemia needs to be anticipated even though the counter-regulatory hormones are acting to maintain glucose levels. In this situation it is the insulin effect that cannot be switched off.

In a well controlled diabetic child appropriate adjustments can be effected to deal with the problems that may arise. In practical terms, however, it is difficult to make appropriate predictions[9]. However, insulin can more easily be adjusted when monitoring is done regularly and accurately. It is difficult to produce general guidelines that are applicable to

Table 17.4. The effects of exercise on hormone levels and energy sources in non-diabetic and diabetic children

	Non-diabetic	Diabetic	
		Well insulinised	Insulin-deficient
Insulin	Down	Increased	No change
Glucose	No change	Down	Up
Ketones	Down	Down	Up
Glucagon	Up	Up	Up
Catecholamines	Up	Up	Up
Growth hormone	Up	Up	Up
Cortisol	Up	Up	Up

every individual in all situations. Insulin dose has to be tailored to the individual child, on the basis of experience, hopefully more by 'trial' than 'error'.

HYPOGLYCAEMIA AND HOW TO AVOID IT

As suggested before, parental concern about exercise very largely relates to the perceived risk of hypoglycaemia occurring at a time or in a situation that precludes easy administration of glucose. For the child it is the

Table 17.5. Metabolic and hormonal responses to exercise in muscle

Time	At rest	2–3 min	Next few min	1–2 hours	Longer
Energy source	**FFA** (fat oxidation)	**ATP** (muscle)	**Muscle glycogen** (rapidly depleted)	**Glucose** (from body stores, e.g. liver glyco-gen)	**Fat** *Muscle* TG *Blood* LCF TG Glycerol βOHButy-rate
Hormonal control	Insulin (down) Glucagon (up)			Glucagon Adrenaline	Cortisol, growth hormone

FFA: free fatty acids, TG: triglycerides, LCF: long-chain fatty acids nuisance of carrying glucose in some shape or form, making them different, and the unpleasant feeling of 'going hypo' together with the 'embarrassment' of such an episode in front of their friends. Clearly a simple answer is to eat easily available glucose before exercise, but if we are trying to encourage parents and children to have a better understanding of the influences that dictate glucose levels at and around the time of exercise then the following factors need to be considered.

1. The state of diabetic control at the time:

- Insulin bio-availability (the response will differ, see above)
- Insulin reduction not usually necessary unless exercise severe, e.g. skiing, or dangerous by virtue of site, e.g. long-distance swimming
- Pre-exercise glucose levels give a baseline.

2. The temporal relationship to a meal:

- Try to avoid severe exercise just before meals

3. The calories, fibre and fast-acting glucose content of the meal:

- High-fibre starchy foods prior to exercise help to provide stable glucose levels
- There may be a need to supplement with easily available glucose (Dextrosol, sweets, cola)
- Glucose may be needed quickly (keep in a pocket, bum bag or with adult carer)
- Do not keep glucose locked up in the changing rooms.

4. The timing and process of insulin administration:

- Try to avoid exercise soon after injection
- Try to avoid intramuscular injection
- Try to avoid sites involved in exercise (probably does not make a big difference).

5. The type, severity, duration of exercise being undertaken:

- How 'fit' is the child?
- How accomplished are they at the sport?

6. The presence of complications:

- Can the child recognise hypoglycaemic symptoms?

7. Is the weather going to influence outcome?

- The temperature may fall
- The duration of exercise may be extended
- The game may be cancelled.

8. Is the child old enough to take responsibility?

- Should there be a 'buddy' as back up (friend or adult *in loco parentis*)[10]?

Although the above list looks some what daunting, much of it is common sense. Pre- and post-exercise glucose monitoring is very important if hypoglycaemia is to be avoided and diabetic control is to remain good.

ADVANTAGES OF EXERCISE TO CHILDREN WITH DIABETES

There are a number of well defined benefits of exercise for the diabetic child and there are some that are perhaps more theoretical than practical. There is evidence for improved glycaemic control following an eight-week programme of exercise[11]; the evidence, however, that sustained programmes of training inevitably lead to improved metabolic control is lacking. There is good evidence that physical training can lead to increased insulin sensitivity through an increase in insulin receptors, and the daily dose of insulin may need reducing. Exercise increases the ability of muscles to take up and oxidise free fatty acids during exercise and also increases the activity of lipoprotein lipase in muscle. Training causes a fall in cholesterol levels and a rise in the protective high-density lipoproteins. This in turn may decrease the risk of coronary heart disease[12]. There is some evidence to suggest that physical activity may also be associated with a lower risk of diabetic retinopathy[13]. The effect of exercise on the general well-being and level of obesity in the general population also applies to diabetic children. Physical fitness may improve cognitive performance and alertness, though evidence for this is mainly anecdotal. Early morning activity has been shown to have an association with improved glycaemic control and lower fructosamine levels. Sackay and Jefferson[14] described a group of diabetic children who were encouraged to undertake an early morning paper delivery round, in whom improved metabolic control was found. A possible confounding factor, however, is that this activity may be a marker of generally increased responsibility.

The guidelines and information from the British Diabetic Association (BDA)[15] summarise this well.

> Exercise helps keep your heart in good shape by improving your circulation, reducing blood pressure, and reducing levels of fat such as cholesterol and triglycerides. It improves your stamina and flexibility, and gives you a general feeling of well being.

PERCEPTION AND VIEWS—CHILDREN, PARENTS AND THE CLINIC

There seems little doubt that the attitude of parents plays a key role in the involvement of children in sport and exercise in general. On the whole this is a positive influence, although there is a negative aspect when parents are living their sporting aspirations through their children. This is particularly poignant if the child in question is not being very successful; sport then simply adds to the stress, or even worse, diabetes is recruited as the reason.

The clinic can help in a number of ways to help the profile of exercise being presented to parents and children.

1. The health professionals involved can lead by example!
2. The clinic can develop outdoor activities/camps etc. (see Chapter 18).
3. Advertise the BDA camps.
4. Have a picture board with photographs of successful children, or pin up certificates.
5. Send accounts of particular achievements plus a photograph to the BDA magazine.
6. Use local media to highlight sporting success.
7. Have an anti-smoking strategy.
8. Use exercise as a focus for 'education discussion'.

AN EXERCISE ON EXERCISE

In 1996, as part of our regular education programme within the children's diabetic clinic, we carried out a discussion exercise with groups of parents (n=68). This was entitled 'An exercise on exercise'. The format of the questions is given below, together with some of the answers generated by parents.

1. What is exercise, can you define it?
- 71% of parents were able to give a reasonable definition.

2. List the exercise that children of the same age as your child regularly do.
- Swimming 85%
- Football 62%
- Running 52%
- PE /school 51%
- Cycling 38%

3. How often should children exercise? How often do they?
- A majority felt that school was the place for sport, and this occurred once or twice a week. In addition, 71% of children were exercising regularly out of school.

4. Are there forms of exercise that are better than others for children?

- Swimming was seen as the best, with football and walking 'runners up'.

5. When do you consider exercise portions, i.e. extra food, and what factors influence your decisions?

- 100% used extra carbohydrate, mainly prior to focused exercise.

6. In your family what do you use as an exercise portion?

- The majority used sweets/chocolate biscuits, i.e. took the opportunity to relax the 'rules'.

7. When should the exercise portion be eaten?

- The majority failed to recognise the potential for late post-exercise hypoglycemia and therefore few considered the need for extra carbohydrate prior to bed.

8. Are there practical difficulties with exercise portions?

- No problems if sweets being used!

9. Do you think exercise portions are very important, important, or not very important?

- The majority felt they were very important.

10. What advice about exercise do you give other adults looking after your child?

- 30% asked for blood glucose to be done
- 67% gave advice about hypoglycaemia
- 57% gave advice on food types
- 33% gave advice on insulin reduction.

(It should be recognised that these responses are from parents of differing experience.)

11. Do girls do less exercise than boys?

- 'It depends on age.'

12. Should we try to prescribe exercise?

- NO.

13. Should there be a specific exercise box in the hand held record to be filled in?

- NO.

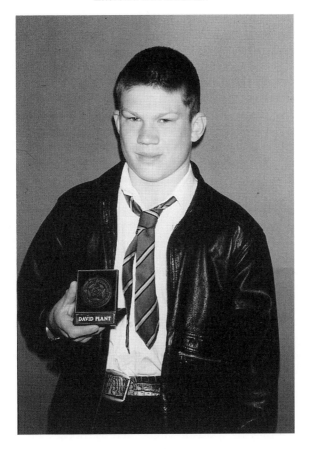

Figure 17.4. A karate champion. (Reproduced with permission)

It is always difficult to know if discussions of this kind make a difference, but it seems reasonable to include this kind of process in the clinic. If repeated, it would provide a measure of educational audit.

SUMMARY

An age-appropriate programme of exercise should be discussed with families as a basic health promotion strategy for all diabetic children and their parents. Responsibility and independence should be encouraged in the appropriate age groups. Self-monitoring of blood glucose before, during and after exercise should be highlighted as the most reliable way of dealing with and avoiding hypoglycaemia. Ingestion of carbohydrate before, during and after exercise should be dependent on results of blood glucose monitoring and types of exercise. Insulin dose reduction should be used where appropriate, depending on adequate monitoring. In choosing injection sites, one should avoid those areas that involve maximum muscular activity. The benefits of exercise include general well-being, improved metabolic control, lowering of lipids, lowering of hypertension, reduced risk of coronary heart disease and reduced risk of diabetic retinopathy. All diabetic children should be reminded of the performances of diabetic individuals who have excelled in their respective sports: Garry Mabbut — footballer (soccer); William Taabert, Hamilton Richardson and Lennart Berelin — tennis in the 1950s; Dominique Garde — cycling (1987 Tour de France). In our clinics we have young girls and boys who have excelled in their respective sports (judo, golf, hockey, football and netball); their success should be profiled in the clinic (Figure 17.4). The traditional basis of diabetic management depends on insulin, food and exercise; the last of these seems to be neglected by many people, perhaps due to lack of understanding and fear of hypoglycaemia.

PRACTICE POINTS

☞ Good metabolic control is the main basis and should also be the starting point. Avoid hyperglycaemia and ketonuria.
☞ Always monitor blood glucose before exercise.
☞ Always carry some sugar:

— for people playing football, rugby, tennis, hockey or cricket, glucose drinks can be kept on the touchline
— for golf, cycling, cross-country running, skiing, glucose can be carried in a waist pocket container (bum bag)
— goalkeepers can keep glucose at the back of the net
— swimmers must always be observed/accompanied and glucose kept at the side of the pool.

☞ The intensity and duration of exercise should be progressive, giving a chance to practise monitoring.
☞ If exercise is spontaneous, as in the majority of children under five years of age, glucose ingestion should be regulated to avoid hypoglycaemia without inducing hyperglycaemia and ketosis. As it is difficult to determine the intensity and duration in this group, monitoring is important. Common sense should prevail to ensure not only safety but also that children do not interpret this as punishment, thus avoiding exercise in the future.

☞ Where exercise is spontaneous but duration and intensity are known, ingestion of carbohydrate before, during and after exercise should be based on previous experience and post-exercise monitoring.
☞ Where activity is planned:

— consider decreasing the dose of insulin prior to severe exercise, e.g. the novice skier. The decrease needed varies from one person to another, and also depends on the intensity of the exercise; it is prudent to reduce insulin by 10–15%. The reduction can be adjusted after monitoring the effect
— avoid muscles of maximum activity as sites of injections
— physical activity should be avoided at the peak of insulin action
— usually one to one and a half hours post prandial is a good time to exercise
— where endurance is required, e.g. cross-country running or skiing, ingestion of glucose just before the start is advised; this can be repeated every 30–40 minutes
— physical activity with natural breaks (e.g. football half-time) can be used to monitor and give extra glucose as required.

☞ The monitoring kit should always contain Glucagon.
☞ All modifications on insulin or food should be evaluated.

— this in itself is an educational exercise.

☞ An accompanying person needs to know about the modifications.
☞ Some activities are dangerous to diabetic and non-diabetic people alike, and some have medicolegal constraints so should be avoided. These include skydiving, boxing, scuba diving, hang-gliding and motorcycle racing.

REFERENCES

1   Riddoch, C., Savage, J. M., Murphy, N., Cran, G. W., Boreham C. Long term health implications of fitness and physical activity patterns. *Arch Dis Child* 1991; **66(12):** 1426–33.
2   Fentem, P. H. Benefits of exercise in health and disease. *BMJ* 1994; **308:** 1291–5.
3   Boreham, C., Savage, J. M., Primrose, D., Cran, G., Strain, J. Coronary risk factors in school children. *Arch Dis Child* 1993; **68(2):** 182–6.
4   *The Teaching and Learning of Physical Education: Aspects of Primary Education.* London: HMSO, 1991: 9–22.
5   Education, Science and Arts Committee. *Sport in Schools.* London: HMSO, 1990: HC 155–11, volume II.

6 Sigal, R. J., Purdon, C., Fisher, S. J., Halter, J. B., Vranic, M., Marliss, E. B. Hyperinsulinaemia prevents prolonged hyperglycaemia after intense exercise in insulin dependent diabetic subjects. *J Clin Endocr Metabol* 1994; **79(4):** 1049–57.
7 Purdon, C., Brousson, M., Nyvgeen, S. L., Miles, P. D., Hatten, J. B., Vranic, M., Marliss, E. B. The role of insulin and catecholamines in the regulatory response during intense exercise and early recovery in insulin dependent and diabetic control subjects. *J Clin Endocr Metabol* 1993; **76(3):** 566–73.
8 Bell, D. S. H. Exercise for patients with diabetes. *Postgrad Med* 1992; **92(1):** 183–98.
9 Hauser, T., Campbell, L. V., Kraegen, E. L. O., Chisholm, D. J. Application of physician's predictions of meal and exercise effects on blood glucose control to a computer simulation. *Diabet Med* 1993; **10(8):** 744–50.
10 Wasserman, D. H., Zinman, B. Exercise in individuals with IDDM. *Diabet Care* 1994; **17(8):** 925–37.
11 Stratton, R., Wilson, D. P., Endres, R. K., Goldstein, D. E. Improved glycaemic control after supervised 8 week exercise program in insulin dependent diabetic adolescents. *Diabet Care* 1987; **10(5):** 589–93.
12 Austin, A., Warty, V., Janosky, J., Arslanian, S. The relationship of physical fitness to lipid and lipoprotein (a) levels in adolescents with IDDM. *Diabet Care* 1993; **16(2):** 421–5.
13 Cruickshanks, K. J., Moss, S. E., Klein, R., Klein, B. E. K. Physical activity and proliferative retinopathy in people diagnosed with diabetes before age 30 yr. *Diabet Care* 1992; **15(10):** 1267–72.
14 Sackay, A. H., Jefferson, I. G. Physical activity and glycaemic control in diabetes (Abstract). *Br Soc Paediatr Endocrinol* 1995; **September.**
15 Anonymous. In: L. Hallett (ed.) *Balance for Beginners.* London: BDA, 1995–1996: 75–6.

FURTHER READING

Darcy, H., Portmans, J. Sport and the diabetic child. *Sports Med* 1989; **7:** 248–62.
Kelnar, C. J. H. (ed.). *Child and Adolescent Diabetes.* London: Chapman and Hall Medical, 1995.
Maynard, T. Exercise part II. Translating the exercise prescription. Review. *Diabet Educ* 1991; **17(5):** 384–93.
Ritcher, E. A., Turcotte, L., Hespel, P., Kliens, B. Metabolic responses to exercise. *Diabet Care* 1992; **15:** 1767–75.
Ryder, O., Johnsson, P., Nevander, L., Sjobland, S., Westbom, L. Co-operation between parents in caring for diabetic children: relations to metabolic control and parents' field dependence–independence. *Diabet Res Clin Pract* 1993; **20(3):** 223–9.

18

Activities beyond the Clinic

SIMON COURT

INTRODUCTION

When first seeking the references for this chapter, I used the key words 'children', 'camps' and 'diabetes'. The Medline response was surprising, throwing up references relating to the care of children in Bosnian refugee camps, cAMP and numerous articles where children at camps had been used in a variety of research studies. Although there were references from all parts of the world—China, Japan, Australia, USA and Europe— suggesting that the principle of holding camps for diabetic children was widespread and presumably felt to be worthwhile, there was surprisingly little about the purpose of camps or indeed other out-of-clinic activities.

Since the 1930s the British Diabetic Association (BDA) has been organising camps of different kinds (Figure 18.1). Initially these were to provide a healthy, safe break for diabetic children from less privileged families. Since those early beginnings the holidays have continued to evolve and now provide a wide range of different opportunities for any diabetic child from five to 18 years of age, being held all over the British Isles and in France. Such holidays not only provide opportunities for young people but also health professionals who have been able to cut their organisational teeth by going as 'staff' with the BDA and seeing how it can be done[1].

In this chapter examples are described and a case made for the local development of 'camps', which can function as a 'protected' stepping off point for children and young people with diabetes, before they embark on a BDA holiday for which children are recruited nationally, or simply a holiday with friends. It can represent an opportunity to practise being away

Childhood and Adolescent Diabetes. Edited by S. Court and B. Lamb.
© 1997 John Wiley & Sons, Ltd.

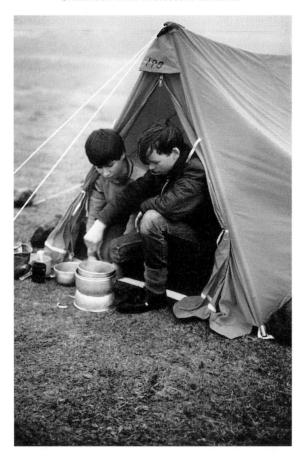

Figure 18.1. Camping out

from home in a safe environment. There are also advantages for others, including parents, siblings and clinic staff. The main objective of this chapter, however, is to describe some of the practical issues involved in setting up and running opportunities of this kind.

The aims and objectives of such holidays are several (see Table 18.1). Much of the evidence that these objectives are met is anecdotal, and it is not really surprising that evidence of sustained behavioural change after a two-week 'educational' holiday is difficult to find. Limited scientific evaluation suggests that benefits for the child relate to improved self-confidence and independence in diabetic self-care, where testing and improved recognition of hypoglycaemia were the two principal outcome measures[2]. Equally, where parents and children share the experiences of a 'diabetic' educational

Table 18.1. The aims and objectives of holidays for children with diabetes

For young people

- To have a good holiday
- To meet with other diabetic peers
- To learn more about their condition in a safe caring environment
- To share experiences
- To begin taking responsibility for self care
- To learn how to cope safely with activities
- To leave home perhaps for the first time

For parents and siblings

- To have a break from the 24-hour routine of care
- Providing space for themselves and other family members
- To initiate the transfer of self care to their child
- To appreciate that their child can cope

For staff

- To experience the role of *in loco parentis* with all its concerns, giving practical insight into the worries of parents
- Practical experience in the management of hypoglycaemia in non-clinical circumstances (e.g. in the top bunk or in a canoe)
- A chance to develop a more open relationship with patients

weekend away, there is evidence of improved parental confidence in management of the condition, which was sustained over time[3].

Benefits for staff need to be experienced, but when different professionals involved in varying patterns of 'camp' describe the same positive feeling (stories of problems dealt with, hypoglycaemic conundrums surmounted, patient partnerships made or reinforced), anecdote takes on the quality of evidence. Many different examples of local initiatives from across the country have now been described, and the next section draws on these accounts. It also describes personal involvement in the Eskdale outward bound British Diabetic camp, our own local outdoor pursuits camp based in Yorkshire, and other shorter but equally 'interesting' adventures.

HOW TO START

We started 16 years ago when two doctors said to their respective Diabetes Specialist Nurses (DSNs), 'Why don't we take some diabetic kids away?' It seemed like a good idea—we knew of the BDA holidays, and the suggestion coincided with increasing opportunities within mainstream

Table 18.2. Key elements for success and safety

Choice of holiday centre
Planning/staff meetings
Written communication
Ratio of staff to children
Right skill mix of staff
Appropriate mix of children
General and personal medical KIT list
The activity programme of the day
The diabetic programme
Medical equipment
Plan for the unexpected

schools for children to have adventure holidays. There was at that time a certain reluctance to include children with diabetes in these holidays, which in some measure still exists today. In retrospect we were pretty cavalier, and took what would now be regarded as unacceptable risks. By good fortune, common sense and rudimentary knowledge, we made some key decisions that proved correct and have stood the test of time, and to date we have not had any major preventable incidents.

CHOOSING A CENTRE

Since we started there has been an explosion in outdoor pursuit centres (ODPCs), giving a wide choice. Look before you leap and ask about the centre's reputation. Centres now have to be accredited and have in place clear policy guidelines, fire drill, etc. You should ascertain that centre staff members have their own specific qualifications to lead groups down caves, sailing, canoeing, etc. and that the centre carries its own insurance.

The centre that we originally chose was becoming popular with many schools. It was not set up to take diabetic children, but it had the advantage that food was prepared on site, allowing the dietitian to influence meals and produce 'in house flapjack', that well known 'hypo' preventer. We have in the main stayed with the same centre. This has a number of advantages — the centre staff develop a good understanding of diabetes and all its nuances, and we gain a continuing appreciation of the effects of various elements of the activity programme on diabetic management, i.e. where and when the 'hypos' are likely to occur. Perhaps more particularly, we gain an understanding of how young urban children cope with the different elements of the programme, what they enjoy, how well they perform and when and where to look out for the 'clumsy' child. Although the

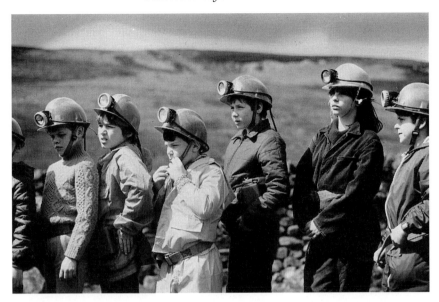

Figure 18.2. Caving: before going in

programme changes, knowing the local geography helps us stay one foot ahead of the children.

Obviously centre staff do change, but hopefully not too frequently, as friendships made the year before help enormously and allow diabetic update rather than re-education for the centre staff. The importance of this aspect depends on the staffing levels and the environment. In a cave, for example, children may not be near 'medical staff', so the activity leader needs to be able to recognise hypoglycaemia in a cold, wet and tired child, and must have the right equipment and know-how to administer glucose tablets and Hypostop (Figures 18.2 and 18.3). The medical staff (doctors and nurses) clearly have a responsibility to ensure that the centre staff have appropriate levels of knowledge. It makes sense to put this specific training into the context of a broader awareness of the consequences of diabetes to a child. In some circumstances knowing how to perform a blood test may be relevant — allowing the staff to test themselves encourages a better understanding. We should encourage as many lay people as possible to understand the consequences to children of diabetes.

It is very important that there is a clear demarcation of responsibility between centre staff, who have absolute control during the activity programme, and the health staff who have responsibility for medical matters and during the 'time off' periods. One trick is to have a mixed programme without too much 'hanging loose' time.

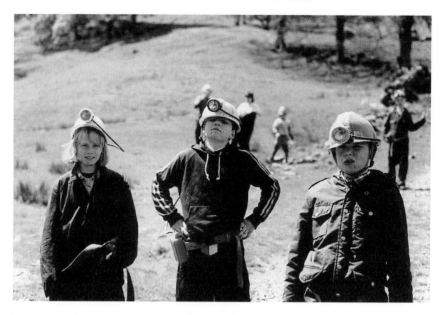

Figure 18.3. Caving: wet, dirty and triumphant

On the whole ODPCs are distanced from the 'illicit' pleasures obtainable in shops (sweets, cigarettes and alcohol), but, depending on the age of the group, some or all of these will be secreted in the baggage. You may find that the centre has rules that make life easier, particularly concerning smoking and alcohol, but there is often a stall selling T-shirts and other mementoes — and sweets. A discreet word to remove serious temptation is usually enough. 'In house' shops, however, are important to the finances of such centres, and some children seem to have inordinate amounts of money burning holes in their pockets. Depending on age they need to be encouraged to spend wisely, leaving enough for a present for mum and dad!

PLANNING

We have learned from experience that time spent planning is time well spent. It initially involves the development of a number of documents.

1. A description of the holiday aims and objectives, details of the centre with photographs of the activities.
2. A document to provide medical information about the child with particular reference to recent concerns (Appendix 18.1).

3. A clear application form for parents.
4. A check-list of personal diabetic requirements (Appendix 18.2).
5. A check-list of appropriate clothes and other items (Appendix 18.2).

As our groups are made up of children from different health districts within the Northern region of the UK, we had to negotiate a base district. Their pharmacy makes up the medical packs (see below), and their finance office deals with paying the ODPC. A single payment is made which is then reimbursed by the separate districts, where the money is collected by a named individual member of staff in each district, usually the DSN or doctor.

Plans, systems and information documents need to be regularly reviewed. It should also be recognised that, if an ODPC is popular, bookings may need to be made several years ahead, and a deposit is often needed.

Since children come from different health districts within the region, we have argued that they can only be included if a staff member comes with them (DSN or doctor). As a consequence all children are known well by at least one member of staff who has specific responsibilities to oversee their care, particularly at injection times (depending on age). This gives real insight into problems and concerns and allows an easy opportunity for informal education. Although we originally included formal education elements in the overall programme, we have increasingly moved to an opportunistic approach. However, we retain quizzes and competitive games, with prizes for the younger age groups.

Over recent years an additional concern has emerged relating to child protection guidelines for staff. Guidance on this issue is provided in Ref. 1 and Appendix 18.3. As it may be necessary for medical and nursing staff to do things of a personal nature, particularly for children with additional medical problems, explicit consent should be obtained from parents, over and above the general parental consent asked for on the application form.

GENERAL MEDICAL SUPPLIES

We held lengthy discussions about the provision of additional medical supplies. There are several examples in the literature of lists of equipment and drugs that should be taken on activity holidays, e.g. BDA staff guidelines[1]. Our list is detailed in Appendix 18.4.

There is always some child who forgets to bring their diabetic box, so a reasonable selection of insulin, delivery systems and testing equipment is appropriate; however, many hospital pharmacies will not accept insulin back once dispensed. In practice a consensus reflecting local practice emerges as to which analgesics, antihistamines, antibiotics, anti-emetics and anti-diarrhoeals are included — it is in the miscellaneous section that scope is given for individual choice or eccentricity.

I have had more anxious times with asthma than diabetic problems, and I have in the past carried a foot pump nebuliser across the mountains in order to be able to treat exercise-induced asthma. It is clearly important to know your patients: an inhaler plus 'spacing device' is a sensible precaution. A mobile phone is valuable if an expedition takes you away from the centre overnight, since it is better to be able to call in help than to take a 'field hospital' with you.

What to take out for the day's programme requires careful consideration. Staff members and children should each have a portable 'hypo kit', most conveniently placed in a 'bum bag'. This should include simple blood-testing equipment and glucose tablets (Dextrosol); the medical staff should also carry glucagon, Hypostop (oral glucose gel), 25% glucose for injection, the preferred giving system plus securing tape (NB: take care with rate of injection and amount given — rarely required), a selection of Elastoplast tape and analgesics. It is sensible for at least one of the leaders to carry a watertight medical box containing the same items.

CHILDREN AND STAFF

Holidays of this kind should naturally be open to all children with diabetes, irrespective of background and financial circumstances. It has usually proved possible partially to subsidise children across the board, but where serious deprivation exists the whole cost may need to be met, and kit may have to be provided so that particular children have comparable anoraks, trainers, etc.

It is clearly appropriate to age band the holidays, allowing suitable programmes to be developed. At present we are trying to run a short break each year for age groups 8–11 years and 12–15 years, and a long weekend for young people of 16 years and over. We usually have about 30 children from six districts, although this is expanding. The BDA guidance on ratio of staff to young children is 1:2, but some are assistants rather than health professionals. In our camps there is a minimum of two doctors (usually three, where one is a junior doctor in training), three DSNs, a dietitian and often a spouse or medical student. In addition to the ODPCs staff, two health professionals are usually allocated to each of the activities, allowing three to be run at the same time. We have also used older diabetic teenagers, known to the staff as extra helpers. This gives a ratio similar to the BDA guidance of 1:2 or 3, whatever the age range. Others have included interested parents and some have developed a 'buddy' system where clear responsibilities are given to adolescents to look after each other, particularly relevant if camping is in two-person tents and food has to be self-prepared (BDA outward bound camp).

As we use a local camp we can usually include the most difficult/ complex young people because we are within an hour's drive of home if there are major problems of a social or medical kind. There is no doubt that it is very important to have a balance between well adjusted and more problematic children. To date we have only needed to hospitalise two children, one because of vomiting and the other following a scald. We have never had to return a child because of anti-social or behavioural problems (for example, homesickness). Unfortunately, we have so far been unable to persuade our psychology colleagues to come on the camps, although we feel that this would be a good idea.

In some respects it is advantageous to have some staff who independently have outdoor pursuit experience and can offer support to children who are trying everything, and others who are happy to support the children that find some of the activities too hard. Children may decide at the mouth of the cave, the bottom of the hill or the side of the lake, that this activity is not for them, so there must be staff available to stay with them or accompany them back to the centre.

THE FIRST DAY

With everyone arriving at once, it is easy for the shy child to feel left out; assigning staff to small groups of children makes this less likely to happen. It is important that all staff know of complex children, and time should be set aside to go through the details provided on every child, so that those with asthma, non-swimmers, those who do not do their own injections, and so on can be identified.When children are not known to the staff before the camp, it is important for each child to be seen by 'their' member of staff— recent diabetic concerns can be identified, their 'hypo' symptoms recorded and, if the camp is particularly demanding, appropriate adjustments made to insulin and eating regimens. In most situations of this kind a reduction of 10–15% of the total dose of insulin and doubling of snack portions is reasonable. With twice-daily monitoring plus troubleshooting 'bloods', serious hypoglycaemia can be avoided. In less arduous camps a more pragmatic approach can be taken. Significant and recurrent hypoglycaemia is a common phenomenon at camps[4] and is discussed later. At mealtimes staff can identify those children who, for whatever reason, are not eating and are therefore putting themselves at risk of hypoglycaemia. They may be ill or simply missing home cooking; in either case they need some acceptable form of carbohydrate.

It will usually be appropriate at the start of the holiday to have all participants meet together so that introductions can be made, but more particularly the ground rules of the camp explained. Rotas of duties for staff and young people need to be set out and groups arranged for the next day's activities.

Although it is important to give young people space/free time to explore, 'ice-breaking' activities at the start help to generate camaraderie. An activity where all, including the staff, are involved helps to break down barriers and get people talking. A 'night line' is one useful ice-breaking activity: all the participants are blindfolded and asked to follow a previously laid out rope that may go through wooded, uneven ground in a tortuous way such that people bump into each other, or have to crawl through pipes, climb over obstacles or go through water. By the end everyone has a better repertoire of swear words and has discovered bits of anatomy they had forgotten about!

I suspect that most parents of diabetic children check that their children are fine at the time they themselves go to bed, and when functioning *in loco parentis* a 'hypo' round seems a proper thing to do, assuming that you have persuaded the children to go to sleep in the first place. Excitement does not always send blood sugars up, especially if associated with extra activity.

ACTIVITIES

These clearly relate to the age range of the group; an example of one of our programmes is given in Appendix 18.5. For the older groups more serious climbing, caving, gorge walking and mountain biking are available. There are ball games for all, a rope assault course and zip wire. With each new set of centre staff, variants of tried and tested activities are used. One recent application of orienteering and map-reading skills involved finding a ladder some miles away from the centre, carrying it across country to a tree where the 'drugs' were hidden and returning to base. Meanwhile, the other group, the 'Cops', set off in a different direction to find the same location and ambush the 'Robbers'.

Using other local ODP groups allows different activities to be experienced: for us this has included sailing, pony trekking, night orienteering in a forest location ending with an abseil from a railway bridge, and skiing. All of these have required a planning phase to foresee problems, and appropriate staffing numbers. Groups from other districts have undertaken similar adventures both in this country and abroad, and have written up their experiences, describing slightly different approaches but with common themes[5–8].

One set of mothers argued that we did things for the older children but nothing for the younger children, ages five to eight. Duly chastened, we set up some simpler activities, lasting only a day. The first was a picnic in the hospital grounds using the children's play area, not on the face of it very adventurous, but in fact most successful as it included insulin injections before tea, which was for many of the adults the first time they had seen other parents battling with injections. This was the first occasion on which we asked parents to be involved in the planning and execution of an event. From this we progressed to beach picnics with games, a sports day along the lines of *It's a Knockout*, where each district sent in teams of competitors of different ages (obstacle races, ducking for apples, running in custard-filled boots, etc.) and barbecues on the beach. Other districts have organised days out to Theme Parks and Water Parks.

Although we have not involved parents to a great extent with the longer holidays, some groups have included parents very successfully in developing activities, fund-raising and taking part[6,7]. For others parental involvement has been limited to the planning and evaluation elements only[9].

PLANNING FOR THE UNEXPECTED

In all the literature accounts referred to, details of unexpected problems are described. Although we have not had major problems, we have had genuine accidents, including a fall from a horse resulting in a broken wrist, and a fall from a balcony while staff were distracted, producing a winded but otherwise unhurt adolescent. The scald mentioned previously generated a change in procedures for carrying teapots in the centre, and a review of the insurance cover for both the centre and ourselves. There have been other cuts, bumps and bruises, but the main concern remains the unexpected severe hypoglycaemic episode. It is clearly important to have in place robust systems that aim to prevent hypoglycaemia.

1. Know the children in your care.
   - Do they recognise low glucose levels?
   - What are their symptoms?
   - Is there a pattern of delayed hypoglycaemia with exercise?
   - Is there evidence of serious manipulative behaviour in the past?
   - Do they appear to be on a high dose of insulin (> 0.7 u/kg pre-pubertal; > 1.5 u/kg post-pubertal)?
2. Try to gauge the severity of the exercise being set (Figure 18.4).
   - What are the intensity and duration?
   - Will it be COLD and WET?

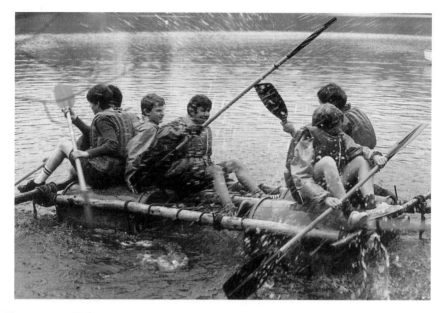

Figure 18.4. Rafting

- Is there a potential for it to run over time (if the weather changes or a child proves slower than expected)?
- Is the exercise intrinsically more 'dangerous' because of geography (i.e. down a cave, in a canoe or on a multiple pitched climb)?
3. Consider alterations in INSULIN and DIET before the start.
4. Convince or cajole participants into an increased pattern of monitoring and to record results in order to readjust insulin.
5. Make sure that staff and children have appropriate supplies of readily available glucose.
6. Try to make sure that the 'group' has a joint responsibility for all its members and knows what to do if a member is 'hypo'.
- Report to staff if hypoglycaemia is suspected
- Start treatment if practical (appropriate age group)
- Consider an explicit 'buddy' system if children are likely to participate as a pair.

It is common to underestimate the amounts of food required. In one study 38 children generated 85 clinical episodes of hypoglycaemia during the first weeks of two consecutive camps[4].

We have had the experience of members of a group all approaching hypoglycaemia simultaneously as a consequence of misjudging the distance

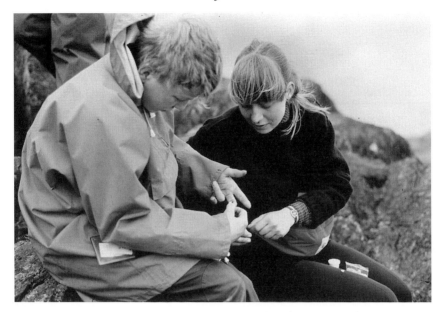

Figure 18.5. Dealing with a hypo: 1. (Reproduced with permission)

of the walk, the time taken and being caught out by the weather. Supplies of glucose were beginning to run short and sleet and mist obscured the van where food and hot drinks were available. Others have described the consequences of a puncture during mountain biking: some of the group became separated and one of them developed hypoglycaemia.

In the main, hypoglycaemic episodes are mild and easily treated, but severe episodes presenting with a convulsion are not especially uncommon. Dealing with the obtunded hypoglycaemic child in a tent, on a mountain or on a top bunk with 10 onlookers is best prevented; the experience does, however, give the professional carers real insight into the fears of parents who usually have the 24-hour responsibility for support and care (Figures 18.5 and 18.6).

ALCOHOL

It is difficult, especially when skiing abroad, to stop teenagers drinking. Hot sweet spiced wine has many attractions when you have fallen off your skis for the tenth time. Local wine is an essential part of the celebratory final meal out, and why not? However, alcohol can generate and mask significant hypoglycaemia, so care and attention are needed — doing

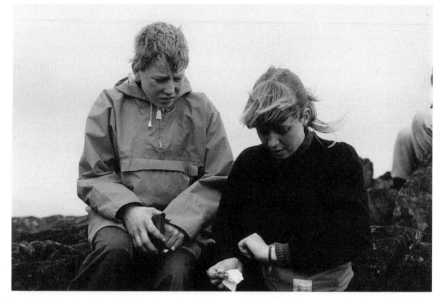

Figure 18.6. Dealing with a hypo: 2. (Reproduced with permission)

blood monitoring at 3 a.m. on some unfortunate with his head down the toilet is an experience to avoid, even if there is a certain logic in young diabetics experimenting with alcohol when doctors and DSNs are dancing in attendance. Sadly, everyone only seems to learn by their own experience in these matters.

If staff members are tempted to bring out the wine when they have finally got the young people to bed, it is a good idea to have a duty rota, so that those on duty for the night do not drink.

BDA CAMPS

In many cases, doctors and nurses start a local camp or activity after initiation at a BDA camp. My own first such experiences were the Eskdale outward bound camp and skiing in France. Encouraging a very deprived teenager from the north-east of England, who happens to have diabetes, to go skiing in the French Alps on a trip sponsored by the BDA, seems a very proper use of funds. The commitment to educational activity and children's and young people's holidays has been a tenet of the BDA since the 1930s. This has evolved over the years, and in 1996 the Youth Education Project was established, by which the BDA can help the development of local initiatives by providing the following.

- Advice — the BDA staff guidelines[1] can be recommended
- Guidance — specifically related to arranging shorter educational activities
- Shared funding — up to 50% of the total gross cost
- Support — in the provision of experienced staff to help initially.

More information can be obtained from the Youth and Family services department of the BDA.

CONCLUSIONS

I have a memory from the Eskdale camp of the arrival of a disparate bunch of young people with diabetes from all over the country. They stayed together in order to compete against other non-diabetic groups, as was the style of the Outward Bound experience. Each group activity, from cleaning bedrooms to climbing mountains, was evaluated and grades plus marks for the overtly competitive elements were added together. Needless to say this group came out on top, and they were on the summit of Scafell Pike as the dawn came up. These are achievements that cannot be measured in terms of blood glucose or HbA1c. Within this kind of experience young people with diabetes get a chance to show that they can cope well in difficult physical and complex social circumstances.

I remain convinced that there are very significant gains to be had for young people with diabetes and those with the responsibility to help them, from involvement in local activities and camps of this kind. Relationships in the clinic are immeasurably improved, with a more natural and honest dialogue emerging during the camp that inevitably influences the clinic exchanges. The aims and objectives set out at the start of this chapter are in my view consistently met.

PRACTICE POINTS

☞ Take the first step.
☞ Start small.
☞ Go on a BDA camp first.
☞ Look at the BDA guidelines (for example, on staff numbers).
☞ Plan.
☞ Have good documentation.

☞ Arrange insurance (e.g. British Activity Holiday Insurance Services: see useful addresses in Appendix 2).
☞ Choose a good ODPC (check it out).
☞ Have a robust hypoglycaemia policy.
☞ Have a child/staff protection policy.
☞ Make sure the food is good.
☞ Have a good time.

REFERENCES

1 *Young Peoples Holidays 1996 Staff Guidelines, British Diabetic Association Publication (Youth and Family Services).* British Diabetic Association, 10 Queen Anne Street, London, W1M 0BD.
2 Vyas, S., Mullee, M. A., Kinmonth, A. L. British Diabetic Association Holidays, What are they worth? *Diabetic Medicine* 1988; **5:** 89–92.
3 Marteau, T. M., Gilespie, C., Swift, P. G. F. Evaluation of a weekend group for parents of children with diabetes. *Diabetic Medicine* 1987; **4:** 488–90.
4 Frost, G. J., Hodges, S., Swift, P. G. F. Dietary carbohydrate deficits and hypoglycaemia in the young diabetic on holiday. *Diabetic Medicine* 1986; **3:** 250–2.
5 Newton-Young, C. A. The Calshot experience. *Diabetic Medicine (Innovative Care)* 1991; **8:** 594–5.
6 Chadwick, J., Brown, K. G. E. A party of forty three young people with diabetes go skiing. *Diabetic Medicine (Innovative Care)* 1992; **9:** 671–3.
7 Swift, P. G. F., Waldron, S. 'Have diabetes — will travel'. *Practical Diabetes* 1990; **7(3):** 101–4.
8 Hilson, R. *Diabetes — A Beyond Basic Guide.* London: MacDonald, 1987.
9 Hatcher, T. Residential weekend for children with diabetes. *Diabetic Medicine (Innovative Care)* 1990; **7:** 175–7.

Appendix 18.1

MARRICK PRIORITY HOLIDAY

NAME: DATE OF BIRTH:

ADDRESS:

TELEPHONE CONTACT NUMBER:

ADDRESS OF PARENT/GUARDIAN (IF DIFFERENT FROM ABOVE)

NAME AND ADDRESS OF FAMILY DOCTOR:

DIABETES CLINIC

CONSULTANT:

HOSPITAL:

PRESENT INSULIN REGIME:

FOOD PLAN: BREAKFAST   SNACK: LUNCH:

SNACK: EVENING MEAL: SUPPER:

ANY SPECIAL COMMENTS ABOUT DIABETIC CONTROL

ARE SYMPTOMS OF HYPOS (LOW BLOOD SUGAR) RECOGNISED?

HAVE YOU EVER HAD A HYPO WITHOUT WARNING?

DO YOU HAVE NIGHT TIME HYPOS?

HOW MANY HYPOS HAVE YOU HAD IN THE PAST MONTH AND AT WHAT TIME
OF DAY?

HAVE YOU HAD ANY HOSPITAL ADMISSIONS IN THE PAST YEAR – IF SO WHEN AND WHY?

DO YOU HAVE ANY OTHER CONDITIONS APART FROM DIABETES – IF SO WHAT?

IF "YES" TO THE ABOVE, WHAT TREATMENT (IF ANY) IS USED?

HAVE YOU EVER HAD A FIT (INCLUDING HYPOGLYCAEMIC FITS)?

DO YOU HAVE ANY ALLERGIES – IF SO WHAT?

DO YOU TAKE PART IN REGULAR SPORT AND EXERCISE – IF SO WHAT?

ANY OTHER COMMENTS

**COULD PARENT/GUARDIAN PLEASE SIGN THE FOLLOWING STATEMENT:

I..PARENT/GUARDIAN OF

....GIVE MY CONSENT FOR HIM/HER

TO TAKE PART IN THE ACTIVITIES DURING THE HOLIDAY AT MARRICK

PRIORY FOR CHILDREN WITH DIABETES, FROM

SIGNATURE... DATE.................................

Appendix 18.2
Activity Holiday — Kit List

DIABETES KIT:

Insulins, insulin pens or syringes
Identification card or disc
Dextrosol × 3 pkts
Cotton wool
Blood-testing pen and lancets
Blood-testing strips and monitor
Monitoring diary

GENERAL KIT:

Washing kit and towel
Night wear
All bed linen is provided

INDOOR CLOTHING:

Trainers or sandshoes
Tracksuits, leggings; T-shirts are ideal

OUTDOOR CLOTHING:

Walking boots/strong lace-up shoes, woollen socks to wear with walking boots/shoes
Windproof anorak or cagoule
Warm trousers (not jeans which are difficult to dry when wet)
One or two warm jumpers, T-shirts, polo shirts
Gloves, hat, scarf (essential on the fells in cold weather, or for use in dry slope skiing)
Swimming costume
Old trainers/sandshoes (useful for canoeing or rafting)
Very old top and trousers which may get spoilt during pot-holing/caving

ESSENTIAL: **1 × Plastic water bottle (approx 500 ml)**
                              A small rucksack and bumbag (to carry your
                              daily packed lunch/drink and essentials)
                              A small torch

USEFUL
BUT NOT ESSENTIAL: Waterproof overtrousers

MONEY: Please do not bring too much!
                              There is a small gift shop which sells T-shirts,
                              sweatshirts, stationery, e.g. pens,
                              pencils, key rings, etc.
                              The following activities may be available and
                              cost approx £5.00 each — Dry-ski slope, Horse
                              riding

**PLEASE BRING A SNACK WITH YOU IN CASE OUR ARRIVAL AT
MARRICK IS DELAYED BY THE TRAFFIC**

ALL OTHER MEALS ARE PROVIDED

Appendix 18.3

Pointers to Remember when Working with Children and Young People

1. Welcome and be friendly towards each child, particularly those who may feel left out. Treat children and young people as individuals. Get to know each child and familiarise yourself with their Health Form and capabilities.
2. Try not to exclude any child from group activities or organise programme activities that undermine someone's ability or confidence.
3. Be careful about physical contact, and do not allow rough, hurtful or sexually provocative games or activities. Be alert to bullying, scapegoating, ridiculing, rejecting and mockery. Do not allow it. Never use abusive language or behaviour yourself.
4. Do not assume that it is right to touch a child.
   Do not assume that it is wrong to touch a child.
5. Be aware that for some children physical contact can be inappropriately sexualised.
6. Avoid being alone with any child or young person. If, in exceptional circumstances, you are alone with one—or with a group—make sure that you are only seconds and an open door away from another authorised leader or helper.
7. With this in mind, however, make sure that each child or young person can privately voice any worries that they may have with someone they trust.

8. Stop and think before you criticise a child's behaviour. If something is wrong with a child's behaviour something may be wrong with the child, or with their circumstances.

9. Be aware. Be alert. Consider what you see, hear and feel. Encourage discussion of what is appropriate behaviour for the group and leaders. Trust your own instincts and seek advice if you are worried about the behaviour of any child or adult in your group. Know the name and telephone number of people you can contact if you are concerned for the safety of any child or young person you know. If you are unsure about how to behave yourself, talk to someone with more experience.

10. Only breach these guidelines if you are sure that to do so is for the greater good of the child or young person you are with. If possible discuss it with another leader first.

11. Remember that you are responsible for your actions, and that the welfare of the child is paramount.

Appendix 18.4

Suggested Contents List for Camp Medical Boxes

Diabetic Equipment and Drugs	Blood-testing equipment, including supplies of BM glycaemic strips Glucolet pricking device or equivalent (enough for each staff member) Keto Diabur strips Hypostop Glucagon 25% Dextrose (ampoules for IV injection) 25 ml 21 g Butterfly needles 23 g Butterfly needles Securing tape
Insulin	Short-acting and intermediate-acting insulin where the type and system of delivery relates to the group BD and Novopen plus Cartridges — short-acting and intermediate-acting insulin
Equipment for Intravenous Fluid Replacement	IV Giving Set with paediatric burette Range of IV cannulae with securing tape and bandages (splints) IV fluids to include dextrose 10%, dextrose 5%, sodium chloride 0.9% Mediswabs and Savlon solution Dressing pack × 2 Gauze swabs

Cotton wool balls
Assorted syringes 2–10 ml
Normal saline ampoules for injection

Dressings   Crepe bandages (5 and 10 cm)
Micropore tape
Melolin dressings
Assorted Band Aid plasters
Triangular bandage

Drugs
Diarrhoea and vomiting: Metoclopramide (for oral and IV use)
Loperamide anti-diarrhoea mixture (simple kaolin)

Analgesia: DF118
Paracetamol tablets and syrup
NSAI (Brufen or equivalent)

Antihistamines: Piriton, oral and for IV use
Antibiotics: Penicillin V
Erythromycin
Amoxicillin
Flucloxacillin

Drugs—*others*:   Prednisolone (treatment of asthma)
Stesolid tubes (10 mg and 5 mg)
Becotide and Ventolin Inhalers with spacer
Pulmicort, Ventolin Nebuliser solutions with foot nebuliser
Hydrocortisone (for IV use)
Epinephrine, 1 in 10 000

Other Miscellaneous   Lignocaine 2% local anaesthetic with stitch set
Oral airways
Throat lozenges
Calamine lotion
Topical antiseptic
Mediswabs
Dextrasol

Appendix 18.5

Sample Programme

PROGRAMME FOR

MON: April 4

FRI: April 8

GROUP: Northern Diabetic Group

AVERAGE AGE: 8–12 years

NUMBERS: 31

PURPOSE OF VISIT: education/holiday

	MORNING	AFTERNOON	EVENING
MON		Arrive (Not before 1 p.m.) Volley ball Local walk	Evening meal: Night line
TUES	Breakfast 8.30 a.m. Archery Zip wire Assault course	Canoeing or Orienteering	Evening meal: Table tennis Indoor climbing wall
WED	Breakfast 8.30 a.m. Canoeing Bridge building	Caving or Climbing/abseiling	Evening meal: Night ride (mountain bikes) Indoor climbing wall
THURS	Breakfast 8.30 a.m. Archery Indoor skiing	Canoeing or Swimming	Evening meal: Indoor games/Quiz 'Disco'
FRI	Breakfast 8.30 a.m. Clean up Depart 10–10.30 a.m.		

Programme Proforma

PROGRAMME FOR

MON:
FRI:

GROUP:

AVERAGE AGE:

NUMBERS:

PURPOSE OF VISIT:

	MORNING	AFTERNOON	EVENING
MON			
TUES			
WED			
THURS			
FRI			

19

Psychological Factors, Stigma and Family Consequences

ALAN ENGLISH AND MICHAEL SILLS

INTRODUCTION

In Chapter 5, we endeavoured to describe the importance of a 'holistic approach' to the management of diabetes in middle childhood and the start of puberty. The essence of this approach relies on consideration of a variety of factors in understanding and managing diabetes. Of particular importance in this approach are emotional and psychological factors, and in this present chapter we will attempt to consider these issues more fully.

We will also try to consider a number of issues relating to the stigma that children with diabetes and their families experience or perceive and identify ways of reducing this.

Finally, we will look at some of the consequences for the family of having a child with diabetes and also try to consider issues relating to multiple pathology in some children with diabetes.

EMOTIONAL AND PSYCHOLOGICAL FACTORS

All physicians with an interest in diabetes know that good control is important in both the short and the long term, but how to ensure this is less well understood. Initial emphasis on medical management is essential, as are monitoring, education and encouragement, but perhaps there are other

Childhood and Adolescent Diabetes. Edited by S. Court and B. Lamb.
© 1997 John Wiley & Sons, Ltd.

actions that can be taken to ensure optimal control and a fully rounded and well adjusted individual. While physicians working in the field will often know instinctively who in their caseload will do well and who badly, it is more difficult to identify what factors need to be addressed to bring about change.

How, then, is it possible to identify the best climate within which children with diabetes can grow? What are the factors that can help them enjoy a reasonably normal childhood, experience a relatively non-traumatic adolescence and emerge as independent contributing adults, well used to achieving excellent control of their diabetes in order to put themselves into a low-risk group for long-term complications?

It is generally accepted that emotional and psychological factors can influence diabetes but how to predict and manage these forces remains, to many, something of a mystery. The sheer number of non-physical factors that can alter blood sugar regulation can often seem quite daunting.

The importance of psychological factors in diabetes has long been recognised. Thomas Willis in 1684 stated that he believed that the disease was the result of 'prolonged sorrow'. When psychologists became interested in diabetes in the 1940s and 1950s, their initial quest was to identify the 'diabetic personality' and reflected general approaches at that time. Needless to say, they did not succeed, and although the work in this area has declined, many investigators such as Swift *et al.*[1] suggest that the incidence of behavioural and psychological problems in people with diabetes is higher than in the population generally. Later work focused on the role of education and knowledge in relation to biochemical control. Here, researchers found generally, to their surprise, that there appeared to be little relationship between the two.

With the development of health psychology and the interest in how attitudes, beliefs and attributions play a part in a patient's compliance, there were a variety of studies of these areas in relation to diabetes. Much of this early work is annotated by Bennett-Johnson[2]. She suggests that:

> On the whole, however, further work in which children with diabetes are compared to 'normal' controls on one or more personality measures does not seem warranted. There is little doubt that *some* children with diabetes have psychological problems. Some of these problems may have existed prior to the onset of diabetes, others after. The currently available data do not shed any light on this distinction. Perhaps a more fruitful approach would be to study the multivariate conditions (e.g. family characteristics, cultural factors, and the course of the disease) under which psychological disturbance or psychological health is associated with a chronic disease such as diabetes.

Exploration of the more recent literature on the psychological dimensions of diabetes produces some interesting findings. Studies aimed at looking at the time around initial diagnosis have suggested certain advantages in reducing or avoiding hospitalisation. Simell *et al.*[3,4], focusing on the effect of reduced initial hospital admission, have shown shorter hospital stays to be associated with significantly better subsequent family functioning, and also that such stays are cheaper in the long run and no less effective. In the UK Swift and colleagues[5] have documented the effectiveness of keeping selected individuals at home after diagnosis in reducing subsequent admissions. It is now the practice of many UK teams to keep children at home after diagnosis where possible.

There has been much written about the influence of family factors on diabetes control. Ryden *et al.*[6] compared the families of children with optimal metabolic control with those with poor psychological adaptation. They showed that families with poor psychological adaptation had parents who were less appreciative of each other, did not agree on diabetic care and did not encourage independence and integrity in their children. In these families, mothers were more likely to be discontented and the children took less responsibility and were less confident. They also showed that family therapy was more effective than conventional therapy in improving diabetes control in a group with poor metabolic control. In families with an adolescent daughter with diabetes Dashiff[7] showed that diabetes tended to draw families closer together but negatively affected the spousal relationship. Overstreet *et al.*[8] looked at the effect of different family environments and showed that, compared with control families, families with a child with diabetes showed less expressiveness. In non-traditional (single-parent or blended) families, where there was a child with diabetes, there was less cohesion, more behavioural difficulties and poorer metabolic control. Levers *et al.*[9] looked at child-rearing behaviour and found that mothers of children with a chronic illness such as diabetes were less likely to set limits for their children but otherwise did not behave differently from controls.

Of particular interest has been the relationship between biochemical control and psychological factors. Dumont *et al.*[10] investigated the psychological factors associated with acute complications and showed that family conflict, and low levels of family organisation and of expressiveness were associated with reduced social competence in the children, more behaviour problems and recurrent admissions for diabetic ketoacidosis. Kovacs *et al.*[11] looked at the psychological factors associated with multiple diabetes-related admissions and found four significant factors — higher levels of glycosylated haemoglobin, increased behaviour problems and externalisation of symptoms, younger age at diagnosis and lower socio-economic status. Challen *et al.*[12] also looked at reasons for admission and found that those readmitted were more likely to have emotional difficulties and a negative attitude to their diabetes. Auslander *et al.*[13] showed poor metabolic control to be related to increased levels of family stress and reduced family resources — they wondered if there was a case for social work intervention in families with a child with recent onset diabetes. Miller-Johnson *et al.*[14] showed poor metabolic control to be associated with increased parent–child conflict. Weist *et al.*[15] discovered that a higher level of parental involvement in children and adolescents with diabetes was associated with better metabolic control. Jacobson *et al.*[16] showed that the ability of families to express feelings freely was linked positively to better metabolic control.

Other researchers have looked at issues of adjustment in children with diabetes. Nassau and Drotar[17] looked at social competence in children with diabetes and found no measurable difference in levels of social competence as compared with controls. Looking particularly at adolescent issues, Kovacs *et al.*[18] suggested that non-compliance with diabetes tended to emerge in middle adolescence and predisposed to later psychiatric disorder. La Greca *et al.*[19] looked at support from family and friends and showed that whilst families provided support for injections, blood tests and meals, friends provided more emotional support for adolescents — better family support was associated with younger age, shorter duration of diabetes and better adherence to treatment. The question as to whether the adopted roles of family and friends could be blended with advantage has been raised.

There has also been increasing concern about eating disorders in children with diabetes; there has been a suggestion that these are more common and relate to factors associated with poor control. Striegal-Moore *et al.*[20] found that adolescent girls with diabetes were more likely than controls to have eating disorder symptoms and that this was associated with dissatisfaction about the diabetes and its impact on their lives. However, they did not show a significant increase in eating disorders as such.

Peveler *et al.*[21] also found that clinical eating disorders were no more prevalent in adolescents with diabetes than in controls, but adolescent girls were frequently identified to be dieting to control their weight and to be misusing their insulin to achieve weight loss. Pollock *et al.*[22] showed that by the mean age of 21 years, 11.4% of adolescents of both sexes had 'eating problems' with severe dietary indiscretion and repeated insulin omission, boys with eating problems were nine times more likely to have psychiatric problems than their controls, and had a significantly higher rate of non-compliance with their medical treatment.

In contrast to eating disorders, smoking in young people with diabetes has been little studied. Shaw *et al.*[23] showed that although the prevalence of smoking in teenagers with diabetes was low at 9%, the prevalence in a young adult clinic was much higher at 48%, indicating the importance of early education and identifying the increase as, perhaps, the result of peer pressure.

While much of the psychological research has concentrated on emotional, behavioural and family issues in relation to adjustment and control, several groups have also looked at cognitive function. Jyothi *et al.*[24], using psychometric methods, observed poor cognitive task performance in children with diabetes. The children with diabetes had much lower scores than controls, which did not seem to be related to age of onset. Holmes *et al.*[25] showed that children with diabetes performed less well with visual discrimination tasks and they postulated that this might be a sign of early mild visual neuropathy.

Holmes *et al.*[26] showed in their study that 24% of children with diabetes experienced learning difficulties as compared to 13% of controls. Closer scrutiny of the group with diabetes showed that whereas 40% of boys displayed difficulties, this was true for only 16% of girls. Furthermore, the boys were significantly more distractible.

Rovet *et al.*[27], in a review of research evidence, suggested that selective neurophysiological impairment associated with insulin dependent diabetes in childhood was more likely when the onset of the diabetes was before the age of five, and that those who had experienced severe hypo- and hyperglycaemia or who had frequent episodes of mild to moderate hypoglycaemia were at increased risk. Westeman[28] found significant changes in verbal functioning associated with the duration of the illness and indicated that girls were particularly vulnerable. Gschwend *et al.*[29] looked at cognitive function under conditions of hyperglycaemia, normoglycaemia and controlled mild hypoglycaemia (3.3 mmol/l). There was no change in cognitive function during hyperglycaemia but there was a significant decline in performance on all cognitive tests during mild hypoglycaemia, confirming that even mild hypoglycaemia causes transient decrements in cognitive function. This might explain why it has been reported occasionally that children with optimal glycaemic control some-times perform less well at school.

In conclusion, from the evidence cited above, it can be seen that poor metabolic control is associated with families who are disorganised, function poorly, do not easily express feelings and do not give themselves or their children with diabetes continuing support. There is an association with low socio-economic status, and children and adolescents with poor control are more likely to have emotional and behaviour difficulties, eating difficulties and problems complying with treatment as well as an increased likelihood of admission to hospital and diabetic ketoacidosis.

Much of this information has contributed to our approach. However, sometimes it is difficult to know if the problems in families are the cause or the result of the problems with the diabetes. It may be that although the way people are programmed to operate by their personality and back-ground will affect how well they cope with diabetes in the family, this does not mean that appropriate intervention to support families and their children is any less worthwhile.

For the individual children who have their lives with diabetes ahead of them, it is perhaps as important, if not more important, to address the complex psychological issues as just to get the insulin dose right. If the emotional and psychological issues are well attended to then everything else will fall into place more easily, including insulin dose and metabolic control.

The issue of cognitive function is also extremely important, and it certainly appears that problems with cognitive function are the result of hypoglycaemia, which can cause short- and long-term effects. The potential danger for children of even mild hypoglycaemia also needs to be considered. It is of concern that striving for better and better metabolic control to improve the long-term outcome may give rise to other problems in the short and medium term, due to hypoglycaemia, which may have lasting consequences. In our own clinic, we have seen children with strange patterns of learning disability which may well have been due to recurrent moderately severe hypoglycaemia.

Finally, it can be seen from this limited review of psychological research that issues of diabetes management and metabolic control should never be considered without thinking about the non-physical factors involved. Clinicians need to be aware of the importance of family functioning and relationships, the emotional climate for the child, the child's own adjustment and beliefs as well as those of the family, and the possible consequences of aggressive management on long-term cognitive functioning.

Most physicians with an interest in childhood diabetes have only limited training in psychology and may therefore often find it easier to ignore such issues. Ideally, it would be advantageous for all teams to have access to the services of a member of staff specifically trained in this field, and this view is stressed in many of the recent guidelines produced in the wake of the St Vincent Declaration[30]. Unfortunately, due to staffing shortages and funding constraints, this is not always possible.

STIGMA

When anyone develops an illness, especially one which is chronic, there are usually problems of adjustment. This is particularly so for both the family and the child with diabetes. In Chapter 5 we identified some of the issues around the time of diagnosis—a time to grieve, the importance of consistency of advice, and most importantly, the need for being a child to come first. However, it is also necessary for the child and the family to understand, and overcome, the stigma attached to the illness.

Stigma associated with illness is usually a result of either ignorance or fear. It can lead to alienation, which can be damaging to self-esteem and social competence. While adults are often ignorant of the cause and course of an illness, this is much more of a problem for children. There has been much research on the child's perception about bodies and illness. Whilst Boyle[31] found that the majority of his adult sample could not correctly locate a variety of internal organs, Eiser and Patterson[32] found the drawings by seven-year-olds of the insides of bodies liberally decorated with slices of apple pie, and chicken and chips!

Eiser[33], in a review of work on the development of sick children's ideas about illness, reports that early work on the child's perception of the cause of illness concluded that children tend to apportion blame to themselves for the illness and see it and its treatment as a form of punishment. They were also more likely to see its cause as a result of contagion, and it was only as they reached puberty that they began to recognise other possible causes.

Despite the prevalence of diabetes, especially Type II, there is a lack of understanding in the general population, and often in the caring professions, of the illness. Many myths still surround the cause of diabetes, such as that it is the result of eating too much sugar or the result of a shock, and despite the educational attempts of organisations such as the British Diabetic Association (BDA) to dispel these, they continue. Indeed, a fairly recent fund-raising campaign by the BDA in which they depicted a child 'under the shadow of diabetes' did little to overcome the stigma associated with the illness.

Many parents, once they have begun to understand their child's diabetes and dealt with their own unnecessary guilt, find the responses from members of their extended family to their child's illness rather bewildering and upsetting. Grandparents can find it particularly difficult to accept the illness, especially as they often have the strongest misconceptions about its cause. It is at this time that parents greatly need support, but in some cases even their friends may react in an adverse manner. It is not unknown for other parents to prevent their children from playing with the newly diagnosed child, for fear of contagion. It is, therefore, not surprising that many newly diagnosed children experience responses from their peers that are disturbing. It is not uncommon for younger children to avoid contact because of the fear they might 'catch' diabetes. Many older children find that the relationship between injections and drug misuse leads to comments and ridicule from their peers. These responses can result in both families and the child with diabetes 'hiding' the illness for fear of the consequences. There is a danger that, if others find out, this will then lead to alienation, social isolation and low self-esteem.

Thus, the clinic team has a responsibility to try to address these issues, first by ensuring that their educational programme is geared to identify misconceptions in parents and put them right, and also to recognise the developmental stage of the child and modify their input accordingly.

Their task in the wider environment is rather more difficult. Encouraging parents to share their knowledge with their families and friends is important, and providing them with appropriate literature to give to others is useful, but this will still not solve the problem for the hardened disbeliever. It is also important that, as the child spends a large part of their time in school, efforts are made to address issues there, perhaps by discussions in personal and social education classes or in other class group settings. The role of the diabetes liaison nurse in this area is crucial. Most clinics encourage children to share information about their illness with their peers, but need to be aware that there are times when this can go wrong and be prepared to help the child through this. There is no doubt that the role of organisations such as the BDA in the general education of the public is crucial.

In conclusion, while there is a risk that the stigma associated with having a chronic illness can be damaging for the family and child, good education and social support can lessen its effects. By encouraging parents and carers that life can go on as normal and giving them the tools to achieve this, the effects of stigma can be removed.

FAMILY CONSEQUENCES

As with all chronic illnesses, the diagnosis of diabetes in a child will cause disruption to the nature of family life. Although diabetes can be considered to be one of the 'safer' chronic conditions, it still has the potential to be life-threatening and this will necessitate a number of changes in the family's functioning. The family has to learn to accommodate changes in diet and eating patterns, life must be organised around the routines of testing and injections, and strategies must be developed for coping when things go wrong. Balancing the requirements of the child with diabetes and those of the rest of the family is not an easy task.

The initial impact of diagnosis is obviously a traumatic experience for the family with issues of denial, self-blame and anxiety predominating, and there is often a period of 'mourning' the loss of good health. This is usually fairly short and families quickly begin to develop coping strategies, yet there is evidence that a number of mothers remain depressed one year after diagnosis.

Research has identified some of the critical factors in families that may hinder the successful management of the child's diabetes. In general, there is evidence that those families which showed dysfunctional characteristics prior to diagnosis, particularly in areas of marital adjustment, continue to have difficulties which were often made worse by the diagnosis of the diabetic child[34,35]. In the first section of this chapter, the importance of good psychological adaptation in families was identified.

What then can be done to lessen the adverse consequences on the family? First, it would seem important to try to understand how individual families function and have an interest in them and what they do, not just in their diabetes. This will take time and effort, but is advantageous, if it enables them to be a normal family with normal family problems and a child with diabetes — rather than a 'diabetic family', who can only get help and support to function through the diabetes. This 'normalisation' is important and will help families to feel more successful. While this role may be taken on by non-medical members of the diabetes team, it is important that the lead physician is also interested in the family as a whole and not totally diabetes-centred in approach.

Families can be encouraged and empowered to take control of the diabetes at a level they can manage, and not become controlled by it. Families can be helped to be proactive and forward-thinking and to come to terms with feelings of guilt, self-blame and resentment. Helping families feel more normal and successful has positive advantages for their self-image and functioning. Obviously, families will differ in their amenability to intervention, and it is important that the timing is right for them. The sheer number of professionals involved may in fact be threatening and become a barrier if attempts to befriend are made too broadly or too early. As in life, most friendships and long-term relationships take a little while to consolidate and mutual trust and understanding are required.

It is essential to encourage the child or young person not to feel different. It would appear that young people with diabetes resent this the most and often far more than the intensive injections and blood tests. Eating regularly and healthily should be encouraged in families and a lead can be given by pressurising hospitals and schools to adopt a healthy eating policy. Exercise should be encouraged and all children with diabetes should be allowed to take full part in activities, both at school and at home. The positive value of role models from the world of sport, who have succeeded despite their diabetes, should not be underestimated.

There is still a tendency not to allow children with diabetes sufficient carbohydrate for their daily needs, and a general lack of appreciation of just how much carbohydrate may be needed to cover vigorous exercise. Sweets and quick-acting carbohydrates should be allowed, especially to cover such exercise periods, as this will help the child to feel more like their peers.

Minimising the time spent in hospital or, where facilities and safety allow, not admitting children at all, will lessen the feeling of being different.

Ensuring a quick return to school will also reduce the chance of a child feeling different or being seen as strange. It will also avoid an excessive interest in their diabetes being developed which overtakes their other achievements. Children with diabetes should be encouraged to take part in all out-of-school activities if they wish.

The family as a whole can be encouraged to experiment with the diabetes and by doing so learn how they can best cope with certain situations so that they remain in control. Their success can be praised and celebrated or used as example and encouragement to others.

Whilst encouragement and empowerment are helpful for the child with diabetes, other family members must not be forgotten. Parents need time together — diabetes can test marriages and other relationships, some it will strengthen, some it will damage, especially if the mother is allowed to plough too much of her energy into 'sorting out' the diabetes. A healthy relationship between parents and carers can be a very important force in ensuring that diabetes within the family is contained and sensibly and effectively approached. Non-diabetic siblings will need attention too, and behaviour difficulties can arise if this is not addressed. Extended family may wish to help — but as with new babies, these family members should not be allowed or encouraged to take over. Similarly a child's peers can be a source of support, especially if exposed appropriately to the organisational aspects of diabetes (injections, blood tests, meals), but equally, they should not become parents' allies or spies at school!

If normalisation can be encouraged and children and families enabled to succeed and take control, then self-esteem will be improved and this will lead to increased self-confidence and greater success. Once this has been achieved, families can begin to realise that not only does good control make children with diabetes feel better but also can help improve the long-term outlook. This will help to reduce anxieties about the long term which many parents experience.

It may be necessary to review expectations of glycaemic control with individual families in the light of what they are capable of achieving. If too high expectations are set, this can be a barrier to success, and taking smaller steps towards an agreed goal is more likely to work. Similarly with families who are coping well it would seem logical to encourage them to continue to improve and edge towards normoglycaemia. Not only does nothing succeed like success, but also lack of it can lead to feelings of inadequacy which may stop people even trying. It is essential that all members of the clinic team find and praise success at all levels and use their relationship with families to find areas which can be improved and developed.

Further, when talking with families it is important not to underestimate the power of optimism and enthusiasm. It is important to recognise the progress in diabetes care since the introduction of insulin, and to be optimistic for future developments in the hope that children will continue to thrive, that control will improve and that the long-term outlook may not be too bleak. It may be that before too long some better form of treatment will come along. It is imperative to continue to review clinical practice and not be afraid to innovate and develop, in ways which will better help those who cause concern.

While the above suggestions may go far in addressing some of the family consequences from the development of diabetes, it is important to remember that the condition does not exist in isolation. Emphasis in this chapter has been on the psychological and social sequelae of the illness, but it must be recognised that there is often other pathology in the client group.

Consideration of multiple pathology in our own clinic reveals the following pattern (Table 19.1) at the start of 1996. (The clinic population is 81 of a population of 43 000 children in the district served.)

In some individual children there is multiple pathology, but overall 17 out of 81 now have, or have had, some significant medical condition, in addition to their diabetes. Although this has not been tested out with age- and sex-matched controls, it appears that there is more pathology than expected in this group of children with diabetes. However, at the very least, this does illustrate the need to look at conditions other than the diabetes

Table 19.1. Additional significant conditions identified in children with diabetes in one paediatric clinic

Condition or problem	Number
Hypothyroidism	5
Down's syndrome	1
Coeliac disease	3
Asthma	2
Remission from neoplasm	1
Idiopathic thrombocytopenic purpura	2
Myalgic encephalomyelitis	1
Mild prolonged fatigue	3
Cerebral palsy	1
Severe hearing impairment	1 (sibling also)
Moderate learning disability	1
Severe learning disability	1
Dyslexia	1
Sibling with diabetes	2
Parent with diabetes	6 (3 fathers, 3 mothers)
Recurrent admission with DKA	6 (2 boys, 4 girls)
Portacaths for venous access	2 (both girls with DKA)
In care	2
Birth parents not together	14
Parent deceased	1

from time to time, and that these may be medical issues as well as psychological ones. It further emphasises the difficulties some families can face in bringing up their children.

In conclusion, Chapter 5 outlined the view that childhood is a journey from total dependence towards controlled independence which parents and carers have to manage. Difficulties can occur if parents and carers either hang on too long to the reins of control, or absolve themselves of responsibility too early. In this chapter, the emphasis has been on the psycho-social aspects of diabetes. The need to recognise and intervene where there are emotional difficulties cannot be underestimated and the importance of understanding the functioning of the family should always be considered.

REFERENCES

1   Swift, C. R., Seindman, F., Stein, H. Adjustment problems in juvenile diabetes. *Psychosomatic Medicine* 1967; **29(6):** 555–71.
2   Bennett-Johnson, S. Psychosocial factors in juvenile diabetes; a review. *Journal of Behavioural Medicine* 1980; **3(1):** 95–116.
3   Simell, T., Moren, R., Keltikangas-Jarvinen, L., Hakalax, J., Simell, O. Short term and long term initial stay in hospital of children with insulin dependent diabetes; adjustment of families after two years. *Acta Paediatrica* 1995; **84(1):** 41–50.
4   Simell, T., Simell, O., Sintonen, H. The first two years of type 1 diabetes in children; length of the initial hospital stay affects costs but not effectiveness of care. *Diabetic Medicine* 1993; **10(9):** 855–62.
5   Swift, P. G., Hearnshaw, J. R., Botha, J. L., Wright, G., Raymond, N. T., Jamieson, K. F. A decade of diabetes: keeping children out of hospital. *BMJ* 1993; **307:** 96–8.
6   Ryden, O., Nevander, L., Johnsson, P., Hansson, K., Kronvall, P., Sjoblad, S., Westborn, L. Family therapy in poorly controlled juvenile IDDM: effects on diabetic control, self evaluation and behavioural symptoms. *Acta Paediatrica* 1994; **83(3):** 285–91.
7   Dashiff, C. J. Parents' perceptions of diabetes in adolescent daughters and its impact on the family. *Journal of Paediatric Nursing* 1993; **8(6):** 361–9.
8   Overstreet, S., Goins, J., Chen, R. S., Holmes, C. S., Greer, T., Dunlap, W. P., Frentz, J. Family environment and the interrelation of family structure, child behaviour, and metabolic control for children with diabetes. *Journal of Paediatric Psychology* 1995; **20(4):** 435–47.
9   Levers, C. E., Drotar, D., Dahms, W. T., Doershuk, C. F., Stern, R. C. Maternal child-rearing behaviour in three groups: cystic fibrosis, insulin dependent diabetes mellitus, and healthy children. *Journal of Paediatric Psychology* 1994; **19(6):** 681–7.
10 Dumont, R. H., Jacobson, A. M., Cole, C., Hauser, S. T., Wolfsdorf, J. I., Willett, J. B., Milley, J. E., Wertlieb, D. Psychosocial predictors of acute complications of diabetes in youth. *Diabetic Medicine* 1995; **12(7):** 612–18.
11 Kovacs, M., Charron-Prochownik, D., Obrosky, D. S. A longitudinal study of biomedical and psychosocial predictors of multiple hospitalisations among

young people with insulin dependent diabetes mellitus. *Diabetic Medicine* 1995; **12(2):** 142–8.

12 Challen, A. H., Davies, A. G., Williams, R. J., Baum, J. D. Hospital admissions of adolescent patients with diabetes. *Diabetic Medicine* 1992; **9(9):** 850–4.

13 Auslander, W. F., Bubb, J., Rogge, M., Santiago, J. V. Family stress and resources; potential areas of intervention in children recently diagnosed with diabetes. *Health and Social Work* 1993; **18(2):** 101–13. (Published erratum appears in *Health and Social Work* 1993; **18(3):** 194.)

14 Miller-Johnson, S., Emery, R. E., Marvin, R. S., Clarke, W., Lovinger, R., Martin, M. Parent child relationships and the management of insulin dependent diabetes mellitus. *Journal of Consulting and Clinical Psychology* 1994; **62(3):** 603–10.

15 Weist, M. D., Finney, J. W., Barnard, M. U., Davis, C. D., Ollendick, T. H. Empirical selection of psychosocial treatment targets for children and adolescents with diabetes. *Journal of Paediatric Psychology* 1993; **18(1):** 11–28.

16 Jacobson, A. M., Hauser, S. T., Lavori, P., Willett, J. B., Cole, C. F., Wolfsdorf, J. I., Dumont, R. H., Wertlieb, D. Family environment and glycaemic control; a four year prospective study of children and adolescents with insulin dependent diabetes mellitus. *Psychosomatic Medicine* 1994; **56(5):** 4401–9.

17 Nassau, J. H., Drotar, D. Social competence in children with IDDM and asthma; child, teacher, and parents' reports of children's social adjustment, social performance, and social skills. *Journal of Paediatric Psychology* 1995; **20(2):** 187–204.

18 Kovacs, M., Goldston, D., Obrosky, D. S., Iyengar, S. Prevalence and predictors of pervasive noncompliance with medical treatment among youths with insulin dependent diabetes mellitus. *Journal of the American Academy of Child and Adolescent Psychiatry* 1992; **31(6):** 1112–19.

19 La Greca, A. M., Auslander, W. F., Greco, P., Spetter, D., Fisher, E. B. Jr, Santiago, J. V. I get by with a little help from my family and friends: adolescents' support for diabetes care. *Journal of Paediatric Psychology* 1995; **20(4):** 449–76.

20 Striegal-Moore, R. H., Nicholson, T. J., Tamborlane, W. V. Prevalence of eating disorder symptoms in preadolescent and adolescent girls with IDDM. *Diabetes Care* 1992; **15(10):** 1361–8.

21 Peveler, R. C., Fairburn, C. G., Boller, I., Dunger, D. Eating disorders in adolescents with IDDM. A controlled study. *Diabetes Care* 1992; **15(10):** 1356–60.

22 Pollock, M., Kovacs, M., Charron-Prochownik, D. Eating disorders and maladaptive dietary/insulin management among youths with childhood onset insulin dependent diabetes mellitus. *Journal of the American Academy of Child and Adolescent Psychiatry* 1995; **34(3):** 291–6.

23 Shaw, N. J., McClure, R. J., Kerr, S., Lawton, K., Smith, G. S. Smoking in diabetic teenagers. *Diabetic Medicine* 1993; **10(3):** 275–7.

24 Jyothi, K., Susheela, S., Kodali, V. R., Balakrishnan, S., Seshaiah, V. Poor cognitive task performance of insulin dependent diabetic children (6–12 years) in India. *Diabetes Research and Clinical Practice* 1993; **20(3):** 209–13.

25 Holmes, C. S., Dunlap, W. P., Chen, R. S., Cornwell, J., Weissman, L., Obach, M., Frentz, J. Postpubertal disease status in diabetes and factor structure anomaly on the WISC-R. *Journal of Clinical and Experimental Neuropsychology* 1993; **15(5):** 843–8.

26   Holmes, C. S., Dunlap, W. P., Chen, R. S., Cornwell, J. M. Gender differences in the learning status of diabetic children. *Journal of Consulting & Clinical Psychology* 1992; **15(5):** 698–704.

27   Rovet, J. F., Ehrlich, R. M., Czuchta, D., Akler, M. Psychoeducational characteristics of children and adolescents with insulin dependent diabetes mellitus (see comments) (Review). *Journal of Learning Disabilities* 1993; **26(1):** 7–22. (Comment in *Journal of Learning Disabilities* 1993; **26(7):** 426–7; Comment in: *Journal of Learning Disabilities* 1993; **26(9):** 571.)

28   Westeman, K. A preliminary investigation of cognitive functioning in children with insulin dependent diabetes mellitus. Unpublished MSc thesis, University of Leeds, UK, 1990.

29   Gschwend, S., Ryan, C., Atchison, J., Arslanian, S., Becker, D. Effects of acute hyperglycaemia on mental efficiency and counter regulatory hormones in adolescents with insulin dependent diabetes mellitus. *Journal of Paediatrics* 1995; **126(2):** 178–84.

30   St Vincent Joint Task Force for Diabetes. *The Principles of Good Practice for the Care of Young People with Diabetes, Report of the Sub-group.* London: British Diabetic Association, 1994.

31   Boyle, C. M. Differences between doctors' and patients' interpretations of some common medical terms. *British Medical Journal* 1970; **ii:** 286–9.

32   Eiser, C., Patterson, D. "Slugs and snails and puppies dogs tails". Childrens ideas about the insides of their bodies. *Child Care, Health and Development* 1983; **9:** 233–40.

33   Eiser, C. *The Psychology of Childhood Illness.* New York: Springer Verlag, 1985.

34   Kovacs, M. The psychosocial sequelae of the diagnosis of juvenile diabetes on the parents of youngsters. Paper presented at 5th International Beilinson Symposium, Israel, 1981.

35   Crain, A. R., Sussman, M. B., Weil, W. B. Effect of a diabetic child on marital integration and related measures of family functioning. *Journal of Health and Human Behaviour* 1966; **7:** 122–7.

20

Parents and Children — Stories, Pictures and Explanations

INTRODUCTION

In a book that is about the management of diabetes in children, it seemed right that a section was given over to them and to their parents. The accounts vary in length and content but have been left unchanged. In the main they describe the feelings at diagnosis and the time in hospital. Some go on into the early weeks and some reflect a longer time-frame. Although we try to listen to children and parents, sometimes other pressures squeeze out these opportunities. One alternative is to ask children to write down their feelings and thoughts. We have found this helpful, amusing, sometimes sad, but informative and always giving fresh insight into our own strategies and failings. For both parents and children it may be too difficult at first, as to write such detail demands an acceptance of the change that has taken place when diabetes is diagnosed.

Drawing provides opportunities to discuss blood testing and injections with younger children (Figures 20.1, 20.2 and 20.3). We use drawing in the education process both on a one-to-one basis and during the group education clinics. Figure 20.4 shows the internal anatomy, lungs, heart, the stomach with food; the pancreas has been crossed out, beyond this I am less certain!

In Figures 20.5 and 20.6 hypoglycaemia has been drawn and the feelings described. In Figure 20.7, written comments were asked for after the child

Childhood and Adolescent Diabetes. Edited by S. Court and B. Lamb.
© 1997 John Wiley & Sons, Ltd.

had seen one of the commercially available videos in which Frank is the diabetic. Whatever the vehicle, the object is to allow children space to express their feelings:

> People could help him by not calling him names here dose not show eny sign of hurtnes but it hurts him in side.

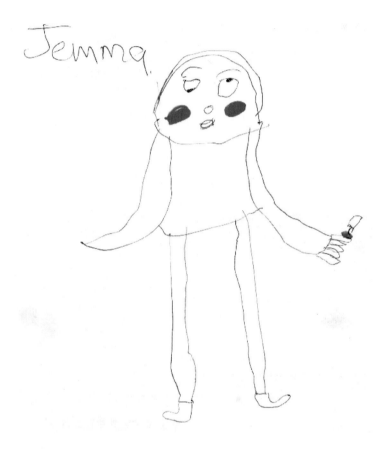

Figure 20.1. Jemma, aged about seven years

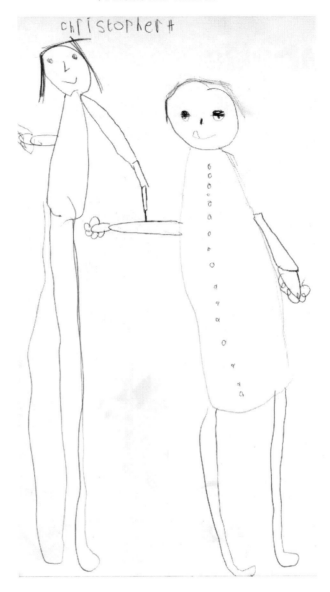

Figure 20.2. Christopher, aged eight years

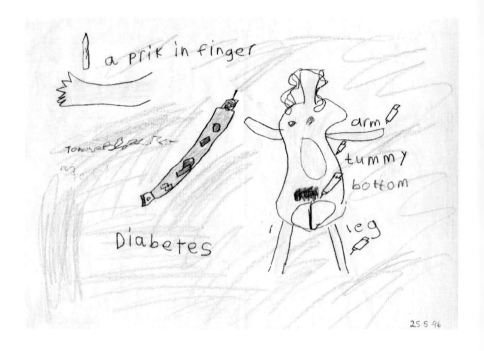

Figure 20.3. John, aged seven years

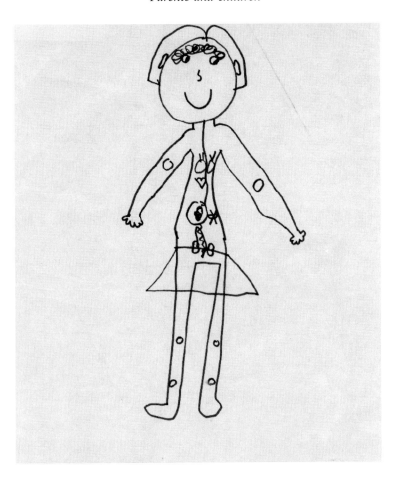

Figure 20.4. Laura, aged about eight years

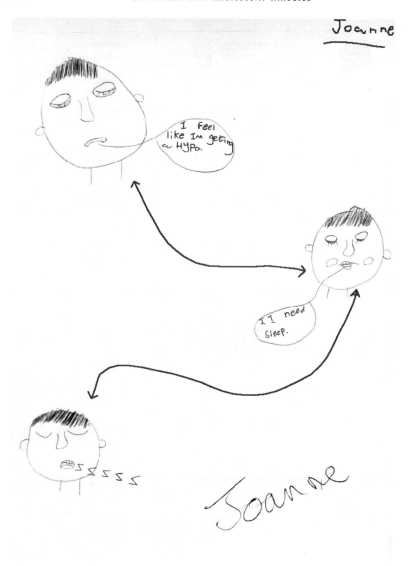

Figure 20.5. Joanne, aged about nine years

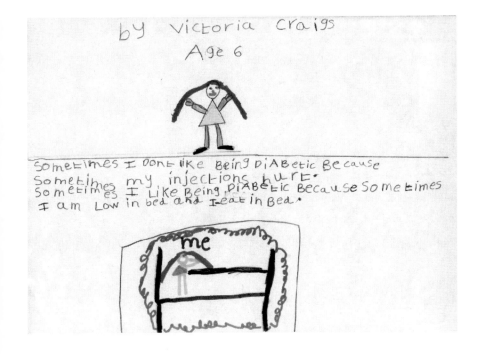

by Victoria Craigs
Age 6

Sometimes I Dont like Being Diabetic Because
Sometimes my injections hurt.
Sometimes I Like Being Diabetic Because Sometimes
I am Low in bed and I eat in Bed.

me

Figure 20.6. Victoria, aged about six years

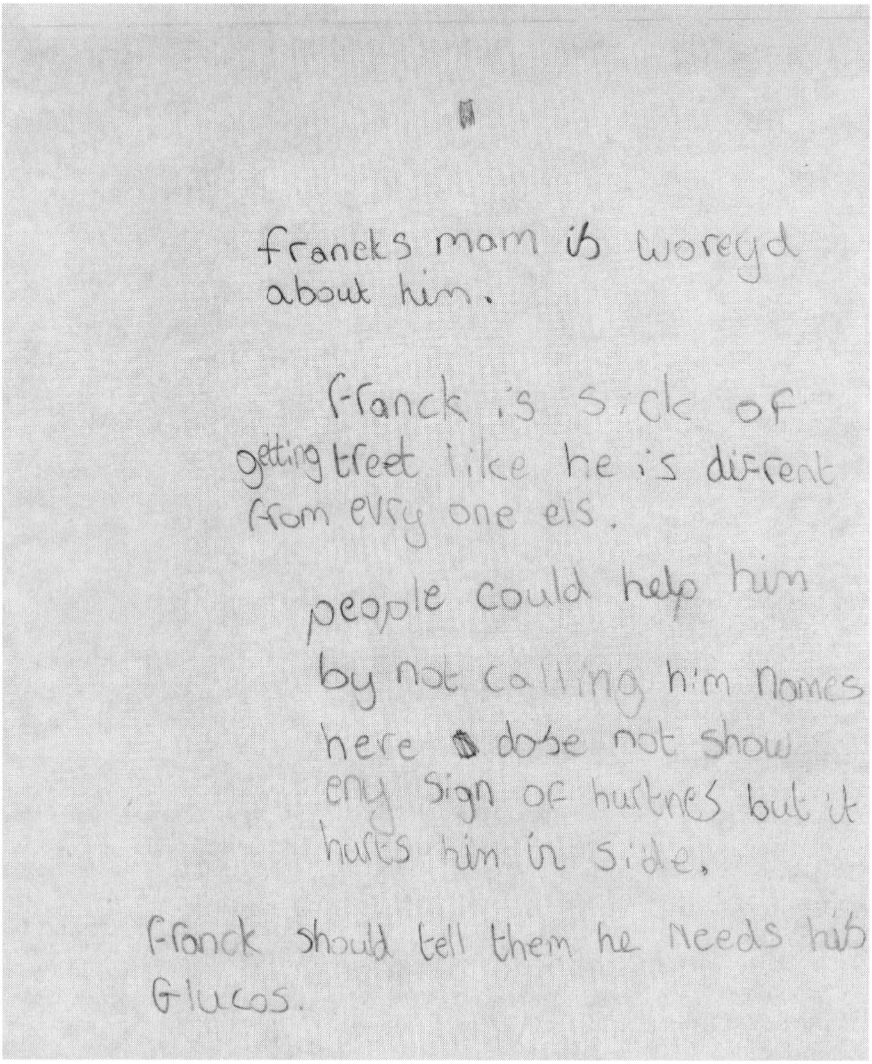

francks mom is woreyd about him.

franck is sick of getting treet like he is difrent from evry one els.

people could help him by not calling him names here dose not show eny sign of hurtnes but it hurts him in side.

franck should tell them he needs his Glucos.

Figure 20.7. Michael, aged 10 years

DIABETES

Introduction

Having Diabetes is not very nice, but eventually you get used to it. My name is David M********* and I am a newly diagnosed Diabetic. I was diagnosed as having Diabetes in January 1996. I have begun to come to terms with my Diabetes and am now (a month or so later) starting to get back to my old way of living which includes playing football, running, playing badminton, swimming, playing tennis, and many other sports!!!

Having Diabetes can be very hard. I sometimes get angry, and think 'why me', but I know it won't change anything, and I will just have to get on with it.

I hope this book will help the families and friends of the Diabetic patient, cope with Diabetes.

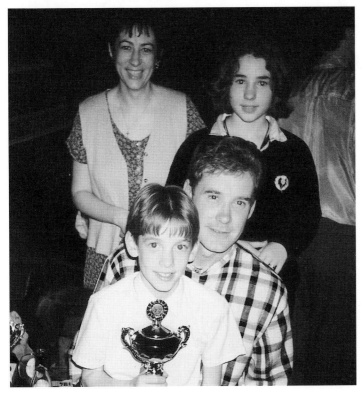

This is me with my dad. The photograph was taken after I had won runner up Manager's Player of the Year for my football team — Cramlington Juniors. (Photograph reproduced with permission)

DIABETES

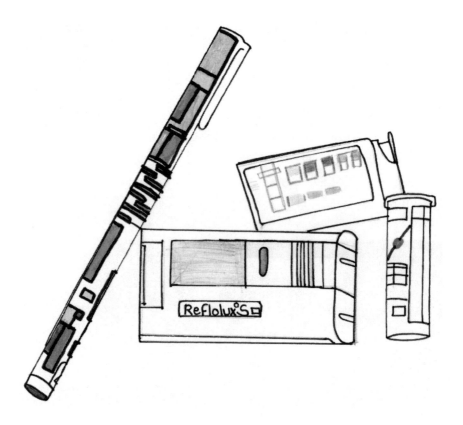

DAVID M*********   AGE 11

HAVING DIABETES
MY DIARY

At about 9.30 in the morning I went to the doctor's with my mam because during the last week I had been drinking a *lot*. I had been taking bottles of water to school with me and getting up through the night to drink and I was also going to the toilet a lot more than usual. I was very tired too, but we thought that this was because I had been getting up such a lot through the night — I was so tired in fact that yesterday I could hardly put my shirt on for school!

My mam and dad knew that this could be diabetes but hoped it wasn't and didn't tell me anyway in case it was a false alarm. The doctor asked for a sample of urine, so I went to the toilet and brought one back in a small bottle. At this time I was a bit worried, though we did not know what lay ahead! Dr Dove dipped a strip of paper called a keto-stick into my urine and said he had found what he thought he was going to find — I had DIABETES.

He telephoned the RVI in Newcastle, described my condition and asked if there was a bed available for me. He wrote a letter for me to take. I was afraid and upset at this time — it was just like my worst nightmare, and I could not believe what was happening to me. I asked Dr Dove if I was going to die, and even though he said I was not, I still felt very frightened. My mam and I went home and packed some clothes for my stay in hospital and my dad and sister Kirstin said they wanted to come with us.

We got to the RVI about 1200. I walked up to Ward 6 and met a funny male nurse called David. We went into a consulting room and talked about diabetes. I had my blood pressure taken (which squeezed my arm a lot), my temperature taken, my height and weight measured, and my blood sugars checked. This was done by a pin prick and did not hurt — much.

A bit later I talked to a doctor called Mary and she explained about what diabetes is and answered all my questions. My question to her was — was I going to die? — and my second question was — will I still be able to play football?

Mary was very nice and after I had talked to her I began to feel a bit better about having diabetes. She said that if I look after myself well by taking my insulin injections, and eat the right amount and type of food, I will still be able to do all the things I could do before. I didn't feel so frightened now.

At about 6 o'clock at night it was time for my first insulin injection and I felt quite worried about it. The nurse who was looking after me, Sharon, gave me it. She squeezed the skin at the top of my leg so there was some soft tissue to inject into. The injection did not hurt at all and it was all over in a few seconds. In fact it did not hurt as much as the pin prick to test my blood sugar level!

I felt really strange after all that had happened to me in one day and although I was very tired, it took me a long time to get to sleep as I had lots of things buzzing around in my mind. The ward had videos and televisions and I had some football magazines to read, but I could not concentrate on any of these for long. One of the things I was thinking about was the football match I was supposed to be playing in on Sunday afternoon as my team does not have a sub-goalkeeper and it was a cup game against Wallsend! In fact I was wondering if I would be able to play football ever again. I was also thinking about how my friends at school would react to my diabetes, and if I would ever get the hang of testing my blood level and giving my own injections.

My dad stayed with me overnight — he had to sleep in the chair — and I was glad he was there with me.

Life was never going to be the same for me again!!!

Food and Diabetes

I like most foods, and I also like chocolate. I don't love it, but I like it.

When I first found out I had Diabetes I thought I would never be able to have chocolate ever again, but now I am allowed to have some now and again, as long as I am careful to balance it with the rest of my food.

I fortunately am a boy who loves playing sports, and that means I can have chocolate before my games, which is brilliant. If you are not sure, ask your dietician (mine's called Shirley) and she will give you good advice.

Carbohydrates

Counting carbohydrates is difficult to begin with, and I know my mum and dad took a lot longer to do the shopping and getting my meals ready at first, but now my family and I have got used to it, you will too, but first I have some tips for you. . . .

Tips!!!

My tips on counting carbohydrates are . . .

- To always read the labels on packets of food, and if possible, see how much sugar there is in them, it always helps.
- If you are going to have something sweet, try to save it until the end of a meal.
- Learn as quickly as you can to work out some of the carbohydrate values of things you eat a lot of like bowls of cereal, packets of crisps, slices of toast, chips, and yoghurts.

Injections

Not all Diabetics take injections, but in my case and many other people's cases, we have to. Before I found out that I had Diabetes I thought it would be horrible to have to inject myself everyday, but now, I don't think that. I still don't like having injections, but I know that they keep me alive, so I just get on with it.

Advice!!!

Needles
My advice is to do everything the doctor tells you, and for injections, use the small needles, if like me you haven't got much fat!! I find them a lot better, I hope you do.

New cartridges
For new cartridges when you get them from the fridge leave them out for a bit so they can warm up. Oh and don't forget to prime your needle when you renew your cartridge!!!

Having your injection
When you are having your injection, hold your needle at 90 degrees, then make sure all the Insulin has been injected in. Count to three before you pull the needle out, and take it out carefully. Don't worry if you see a spot of blood when you take the needle out, you have just popped a capillary [a tiny blood vessel] and it will heal over in a very short time!!! I worried about that when it first happened to me!

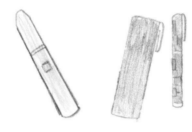

Diabetics need

Insulin injections

And must

Balance this with the amount of

Exercise they

Take, and the food they

Eat to

Stay healthy

P. M********* (David's Mum)

Dr Simon Court
Children's Diabetic Clinic
RVI

Dear Simon

You may recall that at the last educational morning, I briefly
mentioned that Elizabeth had been writing 'her story' about life with
diabetes. I'm enclosing a copy for you to read. This is Elizabeth's own
work and we haven't altered it apart from correcting the odd spelling
mistake (hope we haven't missed too many!)

Although she doesn't cover all aspects of having diabetes, we feel it is
a big step forward for Elizabeth as she has been reluctant to discuss
how she felt when she was diagnosed as diabetic.

Best wishes.

Yours sincerely

Maureen D******

Maureen D*****

MY STORY

I can remember it like it was yesterday except it wasn't. It was three years and five months ago. Here is my story of my three years and five months of being a diabetic.

Monday 21 December 1992; I was 10 years of age. I was staying at may grandma's and my grand-ad's with my brother and sister. I had been drinking a lot of water, pop, tea, etc. My gran had noticed so when my mum came to pick us up she mentioned it to my mum. 'Yes, I had noticed it before she came to stay,' said mum. We went out the next day with my Uncle Jim to a restau-rant, just my mum, uncle, Catherine, Michael and me. We sat down for some food and my mum started talking to my uncle saying how much had I drunk and how tired I looked. 'I've made an appointment with the doctor for tonight' my mum said. 'No, there's nothing wrong with me'. The more I protested the more convinced my mum became. I'd been going to the toilet a lot so that added to the reason for going to the doctors.

My mum and I drove to the doctor's on Tuesday night. 'Elizabeth D******' my name came over the speaker. We went in and sat down. My mum explained to the doctor about me drinking lots, feeling tired and needing the toilet all of the time. He did a blood test which scared me, my hands were sweating then. I also had to do a urine test. I came back into the doctor's room then he very calmly told my mum and me that I had diabetes. My mum started to cry with tears rolling down her cheeks. The doctor and my mum tried to explain to me what diabetes was. 'You will be giving your self injections for the rest of your life', the doctor told me.

'No' I said and started to cry. The doctor gave my mum some information on diabetes and told us that we would have to go to the hospital for some treatment. We said goodbye to the doctor and my mum thanked him for his help then we left. We got in the car and drove home. My mum told me it was all right to cry as it was good for you. We arrived home and my dad, Catherine and Michael were in. My mum told dad and she got all upset again and so did my dad. My brother was supposed to be sleeping next door so my dad went across to see the parents and explained what had happened and said that Michael would stay another time.

Wednesday 23 December came and my mum dad and I set off to the hospital. We met a number of doctors and nurses. They all did tests on me. We were in a room on a ward but that wasn't the ward that I would be staying in. Even my grandad phoned to ask if I was all right. One of the questions that I asked was 'Will I be going home for Christmas?' 'We'll see', replied a doctor called Doctor Gregory. For my lunch my mum took me to the hospital canteen. I had an omel-ette and chips but I didn't like the omelette, so I just had the chips. I then went back to see the doctors and nurses. A nurse called Carol showed me and mum my ward and bed. Carol showed me a menu and I had to choose some food off it for my dinner.

The nurses told me that they would be around during the night to give me a blood test. I was very apprehensive about that because I was scared of needles. So my mum asked them if it was really necessary to do one during the night. The nurse said no, so I tried to go to sleep. Then about 2.00 a.m. I felt someone touch my hand so I woke up in a sweat. 'Don't worry, it won't hurt' as the nurse took a blood test. Two girls were still talking with the big light on, and one girl was attached to a machine that went off nearly every half hour. I eventually went back to sleep. The noise woke me up and I went to the toilet and to see my mum because she was talking to the nurses about the girls making lots of noise so that herself and other mothers on the ward couldn't get to sleep. It took me a while to get back to sleep but eventually I managed to.

Then around about 7.00 a.m. the cleaners came with their big vacuum cleaners. Then came breakfast. I can't remember what I had but I didn't like it! Then they all started to pour in . . . the visitors. They all gathered around my hospital bed (even I could have thought of a better way to spend Christmas Eve). I wouldn't have minded but they all asked the same thing. 'Are you all right?' 'How are you doing?' I got a bit sick of it.

After they all went home my mum and I were moved to our own room so that we could get some sleep at night because of the girls making the noise. When I was settled in my new bed in came the Priest. He gave us Holy Communion (because we knew him and we didn't know if we were going to be able to go to church in the hospital in the morning). The nurses told me that I was able to go home on Christmas Day but I had to be back for half past six and to bring some sandwiches as I would have missed tea at the hospital.

So around about 11.00 p.m. I went off to sleep. About half an hour later mum woke me up saying that people were coming round to sing Christmas carols so I got up to listen to them. Then came Santa Claus. He popped in to see the little babies then went off to different wards. I went back to bed and then around half past two in the morning I woke up and there were two presents on my bed. I told my mum and asked if I could open them. She said 'Yes, they were from the hospital'. I got a watch and a game board of scrabble. I went back to sleep and woke up when the nurses came in to give me my injection of insulin. Later on my mum and I went to mass. I was supposed to be doing the offertory at St Charles (our church) but since I was in hospital I couldn't. Then about 11.30 a.m. in came my dad, brother and sister. They had all come to collect me and take me home. I went off to get a can of coke but when you are a diabetic you have to drink diet drinks or drinks without sugar to control my sugar level (I haven't had a normal drink without it being diet or sugar-free for nearly $3\frac{1}{2}$ years now). 'Dad wouldn't let us open any presents until you got home but we managed to persuade him to let us open one', Michael said as we were getting in the car to go home. When I arrived home my grandad and grandma were there helping around the house with Catherine and Michael and the housework.

I opened some presents then went next door to give them their presents. They asked me how I was and I showed them the little holes in my fingers from all the blood tests that I'd done in hospital. I stayed there a while then I went home and put all my presents on show for everyone to see. I remember my grandma giving me a tube of fruit pastilles but I couldn't take them as they were covered in sugar (the enemy). The very last present that we all got to open was the computer. Catherine took a rage because she didn't want a computer but my dad explained it would come in useful for her work and that she could do all sorts on it. I wanted my dad to try and set it up before I had to go back to the hospital but he was busy.

We had lunch — it was the first proper meal that I'd had since I had been in hospital. In the afternoon I just played with my toys then I packed a plastic bag with things for the hospital, I took some videos and some other things.

I said goodbye to every one and got in the car. My mum had made some sandwiches just in case I got hungry. We got to the hospital and I said goodbye to my dad and off he went. In my hospital room I had a television, video machine and a wardrobe with a little set of drawers on which the television sat. My bed was against the wall and my mum and dad took it in turns to stay overnight as it wasn't fair on one person. My mum and dad hadn't got used to doing the injection and I certainly hadn't!

The next day my sister Catherine came in with her friend Laura. Laura had brought a present with her from her family. It was a teddy bear sitting in a basket with some writing paper and two pencils. Then my uncle popped in to see me. Then Mary popped in, she was a friend of the family. They all came because they cared for me.

I settled down for the night with my mum on the Z-bed, I woke up and in came the nurses, 'Time for your injection, would you like to do it'? 'Er . . . no thanks'. Then they turned to my mum. 'Would you like to give your daughter her injection?', the nurse asked my mum. 'Er — yeh, I mean yes'. So the nurse showed my mum how it was done. The needle went in, it hurt a bit but not too much. Some times when the needle came out so did blood. The nurse explained that only a little blood vessel had been hit. The blood came pouring out so the nurse handed me a piece of cotton wool. My mum had done my injection for the first time. I thought great, now we can go home; I was wrong. The next day my dad came to stay with me and my mum went home. Once again I settled down to sleep at night after watching some TV. I said to my dad 'In the morning could I do my own blood test', and my dad replied 'Yes, of course you can'. So when the morning came I did my own blood test and I felt very proud of myself.

So I could do my own blood test but that was it, I couldn't bring myself to do my own insulin injections. My dad did them as well as my mum. I was nearly ready to go home and get back to school when mum and dad told me that I would need to take it slowly so that I could adjust myself to life at home with diabetes. I would also have to ease myself into school; so I had Monday and Tuesday off then Wednesday and Thursday I would go in for half a day and Friday would be my first full day. On Tuesday my mum and dad and I went into school to see my class and headteacher to tell them how things went and what to do if something did happen.

So the next week came and I did my blood test in the classroom and everyone sat and stared but I didn't mind too much. Then the class had their dinner at 12.30 p.m. but I had to have mine at 12.00 in the classroom in front of everyone. I guess they got used to it, like I did, but I used to get the odd 'oh she's having her lunch, can I have mine?' Also I had to have a snack in the class at mid-morning and afternoon so they got a bit jealous and they would easily forget and groan as to why I had to have this snack.

That year I was supposed to be going to High Close in the Lake District but I didn't want to go as I didn't let anyone else do my insulin injections except my mum and dad.

After having diabetes for a while my family found out more about it and so did I in turn. In October 1993 my mum, dad and I went to the Springfield Hotel for a weekend to learn more about diabetes, which had been organised by The British Diabetic Association. I met lots of new people and we went swimming and on a mystery tour which eventually turned out to be the illuminations at Sunderland. It was good fun. One of the BDA helpers was Fraser Richmond from Glasgow and he still sends me a copy of The Insulin Dependent, which is a newsletter for children with diabetes.

When I found out that I had diabetes it 'knocked me for six'. I would never talk about it, especially how I felt. So in 1994 my mum decided that I needed to talk about how I felt so she got in touch with the hospital who arranged for me to see Ann Trewick. I would go and see her with my mum but I would not talk about diabetes. I would burst into tears and cuddle my mum. Then Ann suggested that I talked to her on my own so I agreed. I did little exercises which sort of helped me to understand about diabetes. Then I would have to wait while my mum talked to Ann by herself. We went to see Ann for about a year and then we all agreed that I wasn't getting anywhere so we decided to stop the . . . well, the counselling, that's what I would call it. I sort of grasped the purpose of going to see Ann and looking back it helped me because when people ask me about being a diabetic, I don't get 'uptight' like I used to.

I go to the hospital for check ups every three months and once a year for an education lesson; they are all right.

I think the best year for me having diabetes was in 1995. It was the Thursday before Father's day and it was a school day. It was also six days before my birthday so I decided that it would be the best Father's Day present for my dad (and also my mum). So I did my own injection for the first time since I had been diagnosed as a diabetic. I went in to my mum and dad's bedroom and said 'I've done it'. 'Done what?' my mum asked. 'My own injection' I said with a big smile on my face. My mum and dad were really pleased for me. It had taken me from December 1992 until 13 June 1995 to do my own injections.

Some months later while I was in my bedroom with two of my friends I was putting some blood monitoring strips away. My friend said I was brave because I have to inject twice a day on Humulin M1. I have 21 units of it in the morning and 15 in the afternoon, about 20 to 30 minutes before my breakfast or evening meal. I didn't realise that people could be scared of needles but my friend wouldn't even hold a needle.

When I think about it, three years and five months ago I thought that I wouldn't be able to inject myself twice a day then do blood tests whenever necessary, but I can and only because of people who care for me and have helped me through my difficult times when I needed help.

I don't think that I could have got through it without my family and friends, so thank you.

Elizabeth D******
May 1996

Things were very difficult when Michelle was first diagnosed as a diabetic. The worst parts were meal times and injection times. Michelle was too young to understand why she would need to have daily injections for the rest of her life, so trying to inject her was difficult, not only for her but for us too.

From a parent's point of view things do get easier as your child gets older, and starts to take more control over injections, blood glucose monitoring, etc.

One thing that did bother us, though, was that not enough information about dealing with Hypoglycaemias is published to school teachers and the few times Michelle went hypo at school no one knew what to do. Most parents have probably found this to be the case, simply because diabetes is not publicised enough in schools.

Over the past sixteen years, the technology concerned with diabetes has improved 100% which has made all our lives easier.

Even though Michelle is almost completely independent now, we still worry about her diabetes and the long-term effects of high blood sugars. Things do definitely get easier for parents partly because it becomes second nature and partly because once your child reaches their teens they become more responsible for themselves and their diabetes.

H. F**** and J. F**** (parents)

I was diagnosed as a diabetic when I was almost 2 years old, but living with diabetes wasn't a problem until I was about 10 years old and started going out with friends after school.

While they were eating chocolate & crisps, I was stuck with an apple or a bar of diabetic chocolate (which is absolutely disgusting). I thought life was unfair and I began to rebel against diabetes.

Within a few weeks, my diabetic control had gone out of the window and it stayed that way until I was about 15.

I realise that diabetes was a big part of me, so in the long run, the only person I'm hurting is myself.

I'm almost 17 now, and already suffering from eye problems due to bad control. Your life doesn't suddenly stop because you have diabetes — I learnt the hard way.

Michelle F**** (17)

Claire D**** age 5 — Berwick

Claire was diagnosed as diabetic when she was three years old. At first I was devastated, as a single mum having to deal with this can be very frightening.

I couldn't believe that someone as young could have this condition, I always thought it was something you get when you are old. I also thought she'll not be able to eat sweets, crisps, all the things other children eat, but this isn't exactly true. Everything in moderation doesn't do any harm. I try to give Claire as much variation as possible, she has sweets but just now and again.

Claire is very good and copes very well. I can't say that it's not hard, but when I look around at what some other young children have to cope with I realise how lucky we are as Claire's condition is at least controllable and if looked after properly Claire can lead a very normal life. In fact if we were all diabetic we would all have a much healthier lifestyle.

(Mother)

CARING FOR A SIX YEAR OLD GIRL WITH DIABETES
A DAY IN THE LIFE OF A MOTHER

7.00 a.m.   Drag children from their beds — well, it is a school day! No trouble at weekends.
Daddy takes them downstairs to give eldest injection and start breakfast. Mummy takes chance of fifteen minutes 'peace' to wake up.

8.00 a.m.   Daddy makes up packed lunches — decisions, decisions, is it crisps and sweets with the sandwiches or custard, or fruit? Bingo! fifty carbohydrates. Don't forget the snack — decisions again — two rich tea or a digestive?

8.45 a.m.   Still trying to get eldest ready (don't forget to pick up the mobile phone and testing kit).

9.00 a.m.   Late again for school. With any luck they will think we had to stop for a blood test or to finish breakfast! Off to Toddlers with youngest. Eldest safely ensconced in the capable hands of the teacher.

12.20 p.m. Shopping in Adams when mobile phone rings, answer it nonchalantly, to look as normal as possible while flicking through underwear and talking to oneself. Forgot to pack a drink in the packed lunch, DRAT, head informs me child won't have juice out of emergency kit — sensible girl. Nowhere in town sells sugar-free juice — luckily there is a carton left in the car by mistake — luckily I have the car. Leave youngest at Toddler group with friend having lunch and mercy dash to school. Didn't think to say just give her water! but there again she doesn't like water.

12.55 p.m. Take youngest to Nursery. Spare time!!!!!!!

3.00 p.m.   Collect youngest

3.15 p.m.   Collect eldest, pay the forty pence it cost the school to phone. (It is the first time in a year they have had to use it.)

3.30 p.m.   Home and snack time.

4.00 p.m.   Children have mad hour — is she high? low? or just letting off steam? retire to the kitchen and await developments.

5.05 p.m.   Remember to do a blood test — running a bit high, had a few of those, try to remember to phone Hilary and Jen tomorrow.

5.10 p.m.   So busy with dinner nearly forgot to give injection. It has been known to forget it altogether!

5.35 p.m.   Dinner.

7.30 p.m.   Supper and bed.

3.00 a.m.   Awakened to the cry of 'I don't feel well'. Groan, stagger out of bed (the days of leaping out are long past, it's been two years now, we are old hands!) Testing kit downstairs, of course, and if really unlucky forgot to refill the lancets. Down to 3.1. Reach for the 'umbongo' and a tin of rice pudding — thank goodness for Ambrosia. Settle down again.

4.00 a.m.   Youngest at side of bed, throws back covers and with a 'move over' and cold feet settles himself down. Ah well, it only goes to prove there's no rest for the parents!

RICHARD'S STORY

Richard was diagnosed as having diabetes six months ago at the age of six and we've all had a lot of adjustments to make. Initially, he was hysterical at the very idea of blood tests and insulin injections. His emotions at the time of diagnosis ranged from rage and aggressive outbursts to being very weepy and withdrawn. He seemed preoccupied with his diabetes and at his lowest point, sobbed saying 'I'm not in charge of my body anymore'.

Richard's acceptance of his diabetes has been gradual. Initially, he immersed himself in trying to understand as much about the medical aspects of his condition as possible, and words like 'pancreas' and 'carbohydrate' appeared in his stories at school. We sent off for information from the BDA and have read the material together. It has been important for Richard to have some understanding of his condition to help him make sense of it all, and for him to accept blood tests and injections as a necessary part of life for him.

It has been helpful to Richard to be seen as an active member of the Diabetic team and not as 'the patient'. Hilary, the Diabetic Nurse and Shirley, the Dietician have listened to him and sought his views. He gets the opportunity to express for himself how he feels things are going, without us as parents being relied upon to interpret his views second-hand. Richard feels strongly about his place in the Diabetic team, and has co-opted his teacher and his Granny Ann, whom he feels should also have a place there.

When we first came home from hospital, we had a few problems with food. Richard couldn't understand why he was asked to eat a fun-sized Mars bar before he did P.E. or swimming, but was then denied one at other times. He was quite annoyed by this, so with the help of his brother and sister (Richard is a triplet) he helped himself to them whenever he liked and the others covered up for him! At first, we were panic-stricken at the high BMs, as we didn't know what was wrong. However, this only lasted a few weeks as Richard soon got tired of additional soluble insulin injections, feeling ill and wetting the bed. Shirley explained to both Richard and his brother at the next clinic visit how this wasn't a very wise thing to do, and it has not happened since.

About eight weeks ago, a breakthrough occurred for us all when Richard overcame his fears and learnt to do his own blood tests and to inject himself. We were all so proud of him that we had a family outing to celebrate. He has also won celebrity status amongst his faint hearted friends to whom he has demonstrated his skills. We had to call a halt to the blood test side shows in particular as some of his friends felt ill and he got too much blood on the carpet! Nevertheless, he has the admiration of all his friends who could never imagine being able to do such things to themselves.

Six months on from the point of diagnosis, life has returned to normal. As a family, I think we all cope very well with Richard's diabetes, although it must be said we will always have anxieties about him but we manage the best we can. Richard has only had three fairly minor hypos so far, so we have still to encounter a serious one. On a day-to-day basis, I worry about this less than I did at first.

My biggest concern lies in the future and about the possibility of Richard developing complications, but I don't dwell on my fears. What's the point? We try to do all we can to prevent them so we get on with life. I want Richard to enjoy his life now and constant worries about the future would spoil it. I also worry about our other children. Richard has an older brother, and as a triplet, has an identical brother, and a sister. Will they develop diabetes too? For peace of mind, we test their urine every so often.

Richard's diabetes hasn't stopped us doing any of the things we have always done as a family, but we do have to give our preparations a little more thought. We still go hill walking and swimming and we still have the odd meal out. Richard has been to lots of birthday parties and has survived the cakes and party bags unscathed. This summer, we are off to Disney Paris.

Having spent a week in hospital with Richard, I can see there are far worse conditions to live with, and provided his diabetes is properly controlled, there is no reason why he shouldn't have a normal happy life.

Dorothy D.******

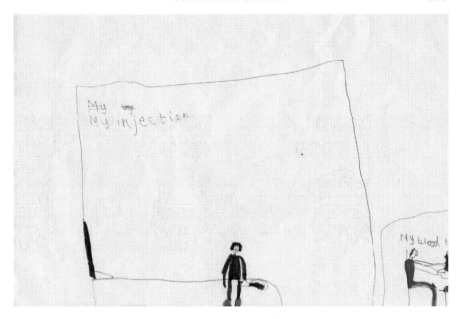

Figure 20.8. Richard, aged about six years

Appendix 1

The St Vincent Declaration

Representatives of government health departments and patients' organisations from all European countries met diabetes experts under the aegis of the WRO Regional Offices for Europe and the International Diabetes Federation in St Vincent, Italy, on 10–12 October 1989. They unanimously agreed on the following recommendations, and urged that they should be presented in all countries throughout Europe for implementation.

Diabetes mellitus is a major and growing European health problem, a problem at all ages and in all countries. It causes prolonged ill health and early death. It threatens at least ten million European citizens.

It is within the power of national governments and health departments to create conditions in which a major reduction in this heavy burden of disease and death can be achieved. Countries should give formal recognition to the diabetes problem and deploy resources for its solution. Plans for the prevention, identification and treatment of diabetes, and in particular its complications (blindness, renal failure, gangrene and amputation, aggravated coronary heart disease and stroke) should be formulated at local, national and European regional levels. Investment now will earn great dividends in the reduction of human misery and in massive savings of human and material resources.

The general goals and five-year targets listed below can be achieved by the organized activities of the medical services in active partnership with diabetic citizens, their families, friends, and workmates and their organizations; in the management of their own diabetes and education for it; in the planning, provision and quality audit of health care; in national, regional and international organizations for disseminating information about health maintenance; and in promoting and applying research.

GENERAL GOALS FOR PEOPLE — CHILDREN AND ADULTS — WITH DIABETES

- Sustained improvement in health experience and a life approaching normal expectation in quality and quantity.
- Prevention and cure of diabetes and its complications through an intensification of the research effort.

Appendix 1

FIVE-YEAR TARGETS

Elaborate, initiate and evaluate comprehensive programmes for detection and control of diabetes and its complications, with self-care and community support as major components.

Raise awareness in the population and among health care professionals of the current opportunities and the future needs for prevention of the complications of diabetes and of diabetes itself.

Organise training and teaching in diabetes management and care for people of all ages with diabetes, for their families, friends and working associates and for the health care team.

Ensure that care for children with diabetes is provided by individuals and teams specialised both in the management of diabetes and of children, and that families with a diabetic child get the necessary social, economic and emotional support.

Reinforce existing centres of excellence in diabetes care, education and research.

Create new centres where the need and potential exist.

Promote independence, equity and self-sufficiency for all people with diabetes — children, adolescents, people of working age and the elderly.

Remove hindrances to the fullest possible integration of the diabetic citizen into society.

Implement effective measures for the prevention of costly complications:

- Reduce new blindness due to diabetes by one-third or more.
- Reduce the numbers of people entering end-stage diabetic renal failure by at least one-third.
- Reduce the rate of limb amputations for diabetic gangrene by a half.
- Cut morbidity and mortality from coronary heart disease in the diabetic by vigorous programmes of risk factor reduction.
- Achieve pregnancy outcome in diabetic women that approximates to that of non-diabetic women.

Establish monitoring and control systems using state-of-the-art information technology for quality assurance of diabetes health care provision and for laboratory and technical procedures in diabetes diagnosis treatment and self-management.

Promote European and international collaboration in programmes of diabetes research and development through national, regional and WHO agencies and in active partnership with diabetes patients' organisations.

Take urgent action in the spirit of the WHO programme 'Health for All' to establish joint machinery between WHO and the European branch of the IDF to initiate, accelerate and facilitate the implementation of these recommendations.

At the conclusion of the St Vincent meeting, all those attending formally pledged themselves to strong and decisive action in seeking implementation of the recommendations on their return home.

Appendix 2

Useful Addresses

British Diabetic Association (BDA) *Youth and Family Services, 10 Queen Anne Street, London WIM 0BD, UK* Tel: 0171 323 1531; fax: 0171 637 3644

BDA Insurance Motor: Tel: 01903 262 900 Travel: Tel: 0171 512 0890 Life: Tel: 0161 829 5600 Household: Tel: 01903 264464

BDA Directory of Diabetes Specialist Nurses re-Paediatric Diabetes Special Interest Group Tel: 0171 872 0840

Royal College of Nursing *20 Cavendish Square, London W1M 0AB, UK* Tel: 0171 872 0840

British Dietetic Association *7th Floor, Elizabeth House, 22 Suffolk Street, Queensway, Birmingham B1 1LS, UK* Tel: 0121 643 5483

Benefits Agency *An Executive Agency of the Department of Social Security* (see local telephone directory)

Family Fund *Family Fund Director, PO Box 50. York Y01 2ZX, UK* Tel: 01904 621115 (used to be the Rowntree Fund)

Medic Alert *Medic Alert Foundation, 12 Bridge Wharf, 156 Caledonian Road, London N1 9UU, UK* Tel: 0171 833 3034

Diabetes Foundation *177a Tennison Road, London SE25 5NF, UK* Tel: 0181 656 5467

The Juvenile Diabetes Foundation (UK) *25 Gosfield St, London W1P 8EB, UK* Tel: 0171 436 3112

● This Foundation provides free monitors to children < 18 years old. They also provide general literature that needs to be read before giving to patient.

English National Board *170 Tottenham Court Rd, London W1, UK*

● Provides information on Courses for Nurse Specialists.

Royal College of Nursing *20 Cavendish Square, London W1M 0AB, UK*

Royal College of Paediatrics and Child Health *5 St Andrews Place, Regent's Park, London NW1 4LB, UK* Tel: 0171 486 6151

British Activity Holiday Insurance Services *Security House, Frog Lane, Tunbridge Wells, Kent TN1 1YT, UK*

MEDICAL REPRESENTATIVES

Boehringer Mannheim UK,
Bell Lane, Lewes,
East Sussex BN7 1LG, UK
Tel: 01273 480266
Fax: 01273 480266

Monitors — Reflolux S (free)
— Accutrends (free but restricted)
BM Stix/Accutest
Booklets/diaries
Soft-touch blood test pens

Life-Scan (Johnson & Johnson),
PO Box 689, Mandeville House,
62 The Broadway,
Amersham, Bucks HP7 0LD, UK
Tel: 01494 545633
Fax: 01494 729336

Monitors — One-Touch
Leaflets

Medisense Britain Ltd,
PO Box 2159,
Coleshill,
Birmingham B46 1HZ, UK
Tel: 01674 467044
Fax: 01674 467006

Monitors — Exactec and Medisense

Bayer Diagnostics (Ames),
Diagnostics Division,
Bayer House,
Strawberry Hill,
Newbury, Berkshire RG14 1JA, UK
Tel: 01256 29181
Fax: 01256 52910

Monitors — Glucometer IV

Beckton Dickenson UK,
Between Towns Road,
Cowley, Oxford OX4 3LY, UK
Tel: 01865 748844
Fax: 01865 717313

BD Micro-fine Plus Lancets

Lily — 'Diabetes Care',
Kingsclere Road,
Basingstoke, Hants
RG21 2XA, UK
Tel: 01256 315000

BD Pens (free)
Diapens

Novo Nordisk, Pharmaceuticals Ltd,
Novo Nordisk House,
Broadfield Park,
Brighton Road, Pease Pottage,
Crawley, West Sussex RH11 9RT, UK
Tel: 01293 613555

Sherwood Medical Industries Ltd,
County Oak Way,
Crawley, West Sussex
RH11 7YQ, UK
Tel: 01293 534501

Owen Mumford Ltd,
Brook Hill, Woodstock,
Oxford OX20 1TU, UK
Tel: 01993 812021

DIABETES ASSOCIATIONS

American Diabetes Association, Inc: *National Service Center, 1660 Duke St., Alexandria, VA 22314, USA*

Austrian Diabetes Association: *Österreichische Diabetes Gesellschaft, c/o Universitäts Kinderklinik Graz, Avenbrugger platz 30, A-8036 Graz, Austia*

Diabetes Australia: *3rd Floor, 100 Collins St., Melbourne, VIC 3000, Australia*

Juvenile Diabetes Foundation of Australia: *PO Box 1500, Chatswood, NSW 2057, Australia*

Association Belge du Diabète: *Chaussée du Waterloo, 935, B-1180 Brussels, Belgium*

Flemish Diabetes Association: *Vlaamse Diabetes Verenizing, Maaltecenter Block B, Derbystraat 75, St Denijs-Westrem, Belgium*

Danish Diabetes Association: *Diabetesforeningen, Landsforeningen for Sukkereyge, Filosofgangen 24, 5000 Odense C, Denmark*

Association Française des Diabétiques: *14 Rue de Clos, Paris 75020, France*

German Diabetes Union: *Deutsch Diabetes Union, Drosselweg 16, 82 1 52 Krailling, Germany*

Greece: *Hellenic Diabetologic Association, 4 Papadiamandopoulous Street, 11528 Athens, Greece*

Hungarian Diabetes Association: *Magyar Diabetes Társaság, Pihenő út 1, Budapest, H-1529, Hungary*

Italian Society of Diabetology: *Società Italiana di Diabetologia, Via G. Severano 5, 00161 Roma, Italy*

Dutch Diabetes Association: *Diabetes Vereniging Nederland, PO Box 933, 3800 Ax Anersfoont, Netherlands*

Norwegian Diabetes Association: *Norges Diabetesforbund, PO Box 6442, Etterstad, 0605 Oslo, Norway*

Swedish Diabetes Association: *Svenska Diabetes förbunder, PO Box 1545, S 171 29 Solna, Sweden*

Swiss Diabetes Association: *Forstrasse 95, CH-8032 Zurich, Switzerland*

Index

Blood biochemistry, 42
Blood glucose, 22, 24, 25, 27, 42, 47, 173
  control, 63
  meters, 35, 121
  monitoring, 30, 34–5, 44, 127–8, 132
  regulation, 54
  response to exercise, 278–9
  strips, 112
  test, 114
Blood-letting devices, 122
Blood pressure, 100–1, 232, 235
Blood sugar
  control, 190
  records, 94
Blood testing, 44, 72, 110, 113, 121
  review, 102
Breast-feeding, 13
British Diabetic Association (BDA) 38,
  39, 75, 82, 87, 120, 226, 282, 289, 321
  camps 302–3
British Dietetic Association, 139
British Paediatric Association, 87
British Society of Paediatric Endocrinology and Diabetes, 31
Bulimia, 80

Camps, 82, 289–304
  activities, 298–9
  alcohol intake, 301–2
  British Diabetic Association (BDA),
    302–3
  choosing a centre, 292–4
  contingency planning, 299–301
  key elements for success and safety,
    292
  kit list, 307–8
  local development, 289
  medical box contents, 311–12
  medical supplies, 295–6
  participants, 296–7
  planning, 294–5
  pointers to remember, 309–10
  practice points, 303–4
  sample programme, 313
  settling in, 297–8
  see also Holidays
Cannula, 178
Captopril, 231
Carbohydrate, 44–6
  counting, 340
  exchange systems, 36, 142–3

fast-acting, 206
intake, 72, 146, 149, 242, 323
management, 138
sources in diet, 140
unrefined, 146
Cardiovascular autonomic abnormality,
  232
Cardiovascular testing, 231
Care chart, 200
Care model, 87–8
Career guidance, 259–60
Case histories
  exercise, 74
  five- to ten-year-olds, 54–8
  hyperglycaemia, 78–9
  hypoglycaemia, 60
  sport, 74
Cataracts, 232, 234
Catheters, 178
Cerebral oedema, 215–16
  aetiology, 216
  clinical signs, 216
  management, 216, 222–3
Chemical agents, 7
Children's parties, diet, 147–8
Children's stories, 330–55
Chromosome 6, 7
Clinic
  age banding, 89
  and exercise, 283
  geography, 91–2
  PDSN role, 119–20
  practical mechanics, 92–3
  practice, 93–7
  privacy, 91–2
  recording the visit, 94
  role, 87–103
  waiting area, 91
Clinic flow chart, 198
Clinical psychologist ,49, 62–4, 99–100
Coeliac disease, 101, 247
Cognitive function, 319, 320
Colour blindness, 35
Co-morbidity, 93–4
Complications, 38, 156
  acute, 201–23
  factors of significance, 228–9
  long-term, 225–38
  pathogenesis, 228
  prevention of, 227
  teenagers and young adults, 76–80

Index compiled by Geoffrey C. Jones